Feeling blue

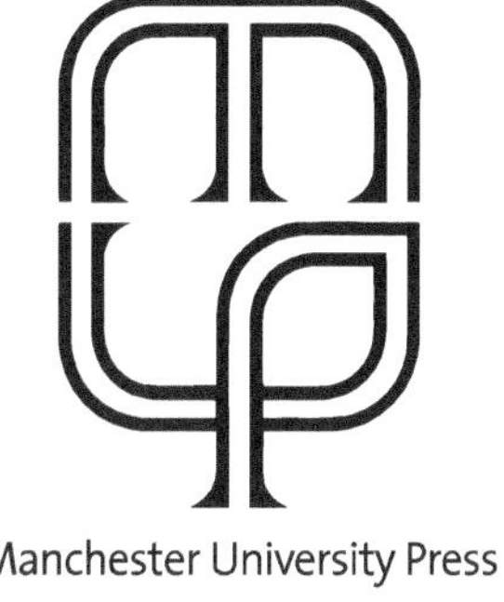
Manchester University Press

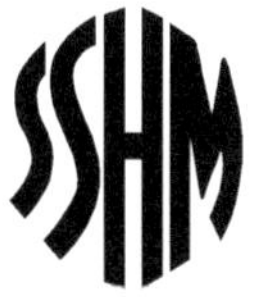

SOCIAL HISTORIES OF MEDICINE

Social Histories of Medicine is concerned with all aspects of health, illness and medicine, from prehistory to the present, in every part of the world. The series covers the circumstances that promote health or illness, the ways in which people experience and explain such conditions, and what, practically, they do about them. Practitioners of all approaches to health and healing come within its scope, as do their ideas, beliefs, and practices, and the social, economic and cultural contexts in which they operate. Methodologically, the series welcomes relevant studies in social, economic, cultural, and intellectual history, as well as approaches derived from other disciplines in the arts, sciences, social sciences and humanities. The series is a collaboration between Manchester University Press and the Society for the Social History of Medicine.

To buy or to find out more about the books currently available in this series, please go to: https://manchesteruniversitypress.co.uk/series/social-histories-of-medicine/

Feeling blue

Colour and the modern British hospital

Victoria Bates

Manchester University Press

With thanks to UKRI Future Leaders Fellowship 'Sensing Spaces of Healthcare: Rethinking the NHS Hospital' [grant number MR/S033793/1 and MR/X022447/1]

Published by Manchester University Press
Oxford Road, Manchester, M13 9PL

www.manchesteruniversitypress.co.uk

British Library Cataloguing-in-Publication Data
A catalogue record for this book is available from the British Library

ISBN 978 1 52616851 1 hardback

First published 2025

EU authorised representative for GPSR:
Easy Access System Europe, Mustamäe tee 50, 10621 Tallinn, Estonia
gpsr.requests@easproject.com

Typeset by New Best-set Typesetters Ltd

This book is an output of the project ‘Sensing Spaces of Healthcare: Rethinking the NHS Hospital’. It is funded by a UKRI Future Leaders Fellowship [MR/S033793/1 and MR/X022447/1].

Most underlying data are available from sources referenced throughout this book. Underlying data from the ‘Sensing Spaces of Healthcare’ research are quoted, and full transcripts are available at the University of Bristol data repository, data.bris, at https://doi.org/10.5523/bris.3b8eg2be3ecw52vt38l7nq9kah (December 2024).

Contents

List of figures

Acknowledgements

The ideas underpinning this book have been in development for many years, through conversations with generous colleagues. One of the earliest papers I gave on hospital colour was at a 'Cultural Histories of the NHS' workshop at the University of Warwick in 2018. I originally intended to develop the workshop paper into a short journal article or book chapter. Thanks to encouragement from people at that workshop, I felt confident to take the leap and write a whole book on the subject. My local colleagues have also been extremely supportive, including giving me feedback on an early draft of the 'white' chapter as part of the University of Bristol and University of Exeter Modern British History group.

Since 2019, I have worked closely with a wonderful small group called the 'Hospital Senses Collective': Marie Allitt, Agnes Arnold-Forster, Harriet Barratt, Rebecka Fleetwood-Smith, and Clare Hickman. On writing retreats, we have not only formed close friendships but have also had rich discussions that have helped me develop my thinking. I am very grateful to this group for the lovely combination of company and conversation. I am also fortunate to have colleagues at the University of Bristol who have provided me with good company, excellent food, and a variety of friendly cat companions on local retreats to carve out some writing time. My parents kindly provided me with never-ending biscuits and their 'view from a window' for a while in 2021 and 2022, which really helped when I was struggling to make time and space for writing. A number of international fellowships also helped with finding space to write, and my hosts on these trips also had really helpful conversations with me about colour, experience, and healthcare design. I am particularly grateful to those who took the time to meet me during fellowships in Montreal, Tampere, and Australia.

The 'Sensing Spaces of Healthcare' project benefits from a brilliant team. Rebecka Fleetwood-Smith led some of the research quoted in the book's conclusion and has been wonderful to work with and learn from. Nicole Andrieu has been invaluable in supporting me from start to finish, keeping my inbox a little bit lighter every day. My ideas have been informed by my brilliant project partners and collaborators at Fresh Arts, GOSH Arts, the National Arts in Hospitals Network, and Architects for Health. For support and advice, I am also grateful to my mentor, Tim Cole, and the project advisory board: Gavin Andrews, Anna Harris, Clare Hickman, Helen Manchester, Mark Paterson, Jonathan Reinarz, Glenn Robert, Charles Spence, and Keir Waddington. A special thanks to Clare and Keir, who also read an early draft of this book, alongside Jennifer Crane, who so kindly originally invited me to the Warwick conference back in 2018, and Jess Farr-Cox, who provided the index.

Many others have helped to bring this book to fruition. I do not have space to list them all, but I am very grateful to every architect, artist, archivist or NHS staff member who has helped me access material. Particular thanks to Angela Whitecross and Charlie Morgan who shared some of the 'Voices of Our NHS' archive and helped me to find references when the British Library Sounds archive was inaccessible. Nick Baldwin from Great Ormond Street Archive helped me to find uncatalogued archival material. Many others have kindly given me their time, for example by participating in an interview, or taking me on a hospital tour. Thanks to editors and reviewers at Manchester University Press for their time, care, and constructive feedback.

Finally, a huge thank you to Sam Goodman and Mr Pickles for being by my side throughout.

Introduction

What is the colour of healthcare? In contemporary England, the answer appears to be surprisingly clear-cut: 87 per cent of people associate the country's National Health Service (NHS) with just two colours: white and blue. The most recognised shade is the so-called 'NHS Blue' or Pantone 300 used in its logo.[1]

Blue seeps into many aspects of hospital life. It is used not only in the NHS 'blue lozenge' logo on hospital signage, but also often in scrubs and nursing wear. On the 'People's History of the NHS' virtual museum, one contributor notes: 'the generic blue curtain found across all hospitals within the UK was the first thing that came to mind when I thought of "the NHS"'.[2] The NHS logo also crosses thresholds between home and hospital, illness and health. It might be found on an information leaflet at the bottom of a drawer.[3] It might be seen on buildings, making a healthcare site more visible from a road. For NHS workers, the colour blue may cross from hospital to home in the form of workplace objects. As Trisha Greenhalgh, professor of primary healthcare, noted in a 2005 piece on lanyards for the *British Medical Journal*: 'How many have you got? I've got a tatty white one with my university ID on it, and a bright blue one with the NHS logo that came with my honorary contract.'[4]

NHS Blue is arguably one of the most successful branding exercises in modern British history.[5] 'It's always been blue', said one respondent when asked about the NHS logo in a focus group about NHS identity.[6] This common perception is remarkable when the colour is examined more closely. The NHS visual identity has not, in fact, always been blue: the current NHS England logo was only introduced in the 1990s. The new coherence and consistency of the NHS – as

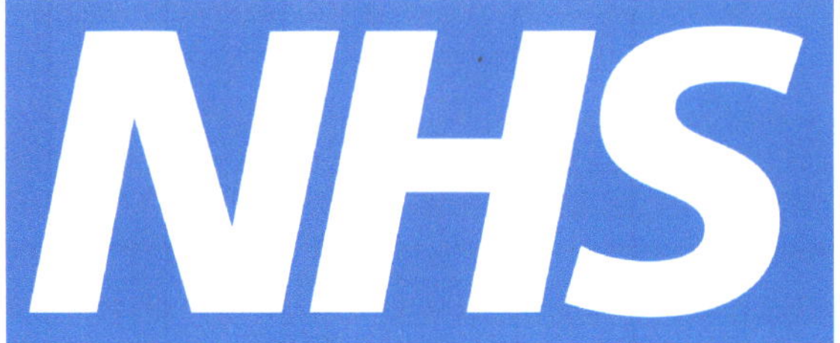

Figure 0.1 NHS Logo. Reproduced with permission of the Department of Health and Social Care.

well as the different logos for NHS England, Wales, and Scotland – makes a political point as much as it seeks to communicate NHS values and to reassure patients. The move towards a single logo for each country was an important, symbolic act that sought to create greater unity – or an impression of greater unity – across what was in practice a still very diverse healthcare system. After the launch of an 'internal market' that made the system more fragmented, and led different arms of the NHS to 'brand' themselves individually, Mathew Thomson notes that, in the 1990s, an estimated 600 different NHS logos were in use.[7]

There might be an argument, at first glance, that the NHS could have chosen any colour for its branding. The meanings ascribed to Pantone 300 have emerged in part *from* its association with the strong emotions attached to the NHS in contemporary Britain (or, for this specific colour, contemporary England). There is also no clear record of how this specific shade of blue was chosen; Sally Sheard ponders '[h]ow were the public and the staff consulted? [...] What's the logic of the colour? (And has the NHS always been "blue"?)'[8] However, the colour blue evidently does have an important and specific place in relation to modern British healthcare. The longer-term connection between blue and staff uniforms has been an important part of imbuing the colour scheme with meaning.[9] Rather than a symbol of corporate branding, this shade of blue has come to represent emotive qualities associated with nursing, such as trust, calmness, and compassion.[10]

The reasons that colour matters lie at the centre of this book. In thinking about the use of colour in twentieth-century British hospitals, with a particular focus on NHS sites in England, it shows how colour was both an important part of hospital design and representative of changes in healthcare politics and philosophies.[11] The blue of NHS branding is just one example of the significance of colour in modern healthcare and its built environments. Colour is a valuable way of understanding meta-narratives of change over time, particularly the layering of new meanings associated with modernity. It is part of the history of everyday experience as well as the history of medicine, design, and architecture. Colour is a visual, cultural, social, spatial, temporal, and affective phenomenon. Despite this importance, or perhaps because of its often 'mundane' or 'everyday' nature, colour is often overlooked as a subject of study.

Colour(ing) in hospital history

Colour is not a neglected area of historical research in general. There have been many conferences on colour studies in relation to art, architecture, materials, and design.[12] The published proceedings of the *International Colour Association* are bulky, and often contain papers on specific buildings and their colour schemes.[13] Much of the leading scholarship in this area has emerged from fields such as art history and archaeology, with their close attention to pigments and materiality.[14] Film scholars have also long argued that viewing colour is a multi-sensory act, and scholars of architecture have often taken a material approach to the colour of buildings.[15] The implications of such work for other aspects of modern British history remain largely unexplored, however, with the notable exception of the history of empire, in which colour has offered new insights into subjects such as power, colonisation, and imperial politics.[16]

The work that does exist on colour in architectural history tends to focus on famous buildings. There are extensive works exploring the relationship between whiteness and Modernist architecture, for example.[17] There is much less work on what might be considered 'mundane' or everyday colour schemes in history. A rare exception is a recent article by Lucy Faire and Denise McHugh in *Urban History*, which emphasised how 'the visual experience of colour was found mainly in the ephemera of everyday life'.[18] They also note that

> [i]n the history of the modern city, physical colour is a neglected topic ... partly due to dependence on written sources. The visual sources we use reveal another view of the city permitting us to see colour as part of the everyday visual sensory experience of the city.[19]

Like Faire and McHugh, this book approaches colour as part of the 'everyday ... sensory experience' of space and place.[20] Much colour – including hospital colour – falls into the category of the everyday because it is prevalent but often unnoticed, by contemporaries and historians alike.

If colour is relatively neglected in modern British history, it is even more overlooked as part of health and hospital histories. Hospital colour schemes – even those integral to architectural histories – have often been skipped over and implicitly treated as purely decorative. When writing about the appearances of hospitals, historians have tended to focus more on the form of buildings than on their decoration.[21] Some recent health histories have dealt more with material culture; for example, the edited collection *Posters, Protests and Prescriptions* engages with such aspects of NHS history.[22] Histories of specific important healthcare objects exist, such as the hospital bed and the birthing pool.[23] However, colour still tends to feature only in passing rather than as a focal point of such research. Occasionally, an historian of health or hospitals will observe the importance of white as a symbol of cleanliness, and a few have written on the emergence of green as a colour of operating theatres and 'modernity', or the cultural influence of NHS Blue, as discussed above.[24] Such work provides insight into the value to historians of thinking with colour, but remains fleeting, and the potential for this subject is largely unexplored. While colour is almost always mentioned as part of any work on built environments, design, and health, colour is rarely placed at the core of these histories. Instead, it is generally discussed as an example, backdrop, 'aside', or accompaniment to the main history of healthcare and its architecture. Colour in these histories is not seen as rich in meanings, representations, or choices.

Colours are important to understanding how experiences of hospitals changed over time, and how the principles of medical care and treatment evolved in dialogue with the built environment.[25] Historians, among others, have long recognised that hospitals must be seen as part of medical work and treatment, rather than just as buildings that 'house' medicine.[26] In this regard, hospital colour schemes and coloured objects in hospitals are just as important as hospital architecture. Surfaces, objects, and people were more dynamic than buildings, and therefore had a particularly important role in the making of healthcare space and place.

Layers of meaning

A history of hospitals, explored through colour, provides a rich opportunity to rethink a range of subjects, from the meaning of modern healthcare to everyday life in hospitals. When the NHS was launched on 5 July 1948, it inherited a huge and diverse infrastructure of 2,688 municipal and voluntary hospitals and 480,000 hospital beds.[27] Colour became an important part of trying to consolidate this diverse infrastructure, and to improve buildings when funds for rebuilding or renovation were limited. The history of colour is a material approach that acknowledges such local and ad hoc redecoration practices, as well as more formal and systematic hospital design. In so doing, it offers a different way of thinking about change over time that complements – but does not entirely align with – narratives of modern British history that centre political or social change.

The book has six chapters, each of which opens with a discussion of colour trends in the built environment, before looking in depth at a specific colour, trend, or association as an example: white and hygiene; green, pastels and emotions; artworks and 'humanisation'; patterns and homeliness; red, vibrant colours, and play; and glass, consumerism, and the connection between hospitals and the outside world. To do justice to the rich subject matter, the chapters draw on a wide-ranging source base, from site visits to archives, interviews, and memoirs. They are broadly organised chronologically to show some of the trends in hospital colour design over the course of the century, and the ways in which the colour palette of hospitals expanded over time. The chapter on white pays the most attention to the early twentieth century because of the importance of modernism to the rise of the 'all-white' hospital. The chapter on green focuses on the post-war period, taking green as a case study for the rise of colour theory and soothing 'natural' and pastel colour palettes. The chapter on artworks shifts to ideas that emerged in the 1960s and 1970s, particularly the goal of '(re)humanising' hospitals and the role of art in pursuing this aim. The subject of patterns follows, with a similar focus on the post-war period, particularly the rise of 'homely' design, textiles, and wallpaper as practical ways to 'humanise' hospitals. The chapter on red attends to the last decades of the twentieth century, as an example of the proliferation of more playful colour schemes in the 1980s and 1990s. The final chapter closes at the end of the century, with the rise of consumerism in healthcare and the role of glass in emulating, reflecting, and connecting to the outside world. This chronological structure is more a matter of emphasis than focus. Each individual chapter takes the twentieth century as a whole, and in so doing complicates the idea of neat shifts or turning points in colour use.

Taking these chapters together, it is possible to identify some trends in colour schemes over the course of the twentieth century. The broad chronological structure of this book traces a shift from shades of white associated with hygiene in the early twentieth century, to pastel shades associated with the soothing of emotions in the post-war period, and finally to more vibrant colours that echoed consumer design at the end of the century. These developments articulated and reinforced shifts in NHS philosophy that mirror those in wider society. This history fits into a narrative of the 'humanisation' of post-war hospitals, followed by their commercialisation in the late twentieth century.[28] Such narratives have appeal because they connect to many other ways of framing modern British history, particularly in terms of chronology. To quote Martin Gorsky on the NHS, '[o]ne explanatory framework sets this arc of change against the sweep of social transformation in Britain, from post-war collectivism to fully-fledged consumer society … The meta-narrative might be described as one of "church to garage" or "communitarianism to marketisation"'.[29] Each stage of this meta narrative has its own colour palette.

Tying in with this meta narrative, the book contributes to histories of so-called 'patient-centredness'. It shows a broad shift in the processes of colour-based design: from design *for* staff and patients, to design *with* them, and finally *by* them, with an increasing emphasis on patients over time. At first glance, this trend appears to align with histories of 'marketisation' and neoliberalism. However, the book also shows how histories of colour complicate this story. It argues that patient-centredness was not just about 'choice' and the 'market', but also about care. It also shows the ways that the rise of patient-centredness materially remade NHS hospitals, sometimes in the short term and sometimes in the longer term, and was about much more than services or consumer rights.

Colour shows how the perceived needs of different people shaped hospitals, and why certain people came to be heard – or overlooked – in design. The growing use of colour to design for disability, dementia, and (later) neurodiversity connects in important ways to histories of ableism, disability, and activism. Successful efforts to reduce the number of long-stay patients are part of the story of a rise in 'stimulating' rather than 'restful' colour interventions for short-stay inpatients or outpatients. Interest in maternity spaces took place in dialogue with feminist advocacy outside of the hospital. Colour can show how and why hospital spaces have been developed to 'include' certain groups of people, but also how this implicitly could mean excluding others, often along lines such as race and class. Overall, particular groups of people gained attention, in relation to colour, at specific points of time. Each group had its own colour palette, and each of these stories is itself an important route into bigger stories in modern British history and the social history of medicine.

The chapter themes – hygienic, emotional, humanistic, homely, playful, commercial – are tied together by the idea of the 'modern' hospital. Some scholars argue that 'modernity' has lost value as an analytical framework because of its ubiquity, but narrowing down to 'modern' hospital colour schemes helps to peel back its layered meanings in a way that makes the concept more stable and less 'elusive'.[30] In general terms, modernity describes both 'major social and material changes ... [and] the growing consciousness of the novelty of these changes'.[31] Over time, the relationship between colour and modernity shifted, but hospitals were consistently using colours thought to be 'modern' – from white in the early twentieth century, to pastels in the post-war period, and brighter shades from the 1970s onwards. This trend raises bigger questions about the meanings of 'modernity', in the late twentieth century, and as a category of analysis.

The history of hospital colour emphasises, though, that these changes were not linear shifts. 'Humanistic' colour palettes, for example, continued to be cognisant of the need for hygiene – or the perception thereof. The book offers an alternative framework for thinking about modernity and change over time: layering. Layering draws on the subject matter of colour, and brings a more nuanced understanding of change as something that builds on, and always exists in relation to, the past. Layering is a gradual and uneven process, in which sometimes the past peeks through or is revealed again; this differs from more abrupt frameworks for change over time such as 'shifts' or 'turning points'. Thinking through layers also helps to understand the multifaceted nature of modernity. As the cover of one 1987 book, *Anatomy of a Hospital*, noted: '[a] modern hospital is a vast and complex institution – an amalgam of humanity, scientific establishment, and hotel'.[32] The concepts of layers and palimpsests, as part of a history of colour, help disentangle this complex modern amalgam. The idea of modernity expanded over time, just as the colour palette of modernity expanded.[33] This story is one of modern Britain, in which multiple modernities have always co-existed.[34] Like paint itself, new meanings of modernity were layered on top of old ones, rather than replacing them.[35]

Putting colour at the front and centre of hospital history in this way allows a rethinking of the chronologies of twentieth-century history. The focus on material trends, and the framework of layering as a way of understanding change over time, helps historians to cut across traditional, politics-based periodisation that have dominated histories of healthcare and contemporary British history.[36] It moves away from the common trend, in British history, to focus on political periodisations such as 'Thatcherism', 'neoliberalism', 'social democracy', and the 'postwar consensus'.[37] Without denying that healthcare was intertwined with politics throughout the twentieth century, and particularly in the post-war period, it is important to consider alternative ways of understanding change over time.[38] Material change, and its meanings in modern Britain, did not always neatly align with political change.

Feeling colour

Hospitals have always been dynamic and diverse environments. To quote Sally Sheard, we must understand 'the NHS as not a monolith but as a composite of hundreds of diverse parts'.[39] Over the course of the twentieth century there was a turn towards larger teaching or general hospitals, which contained an increasingly broad range of activities and people at any given time: birth and death; physical and mental illness; inpatient and outpatient care; acute and chronic issues; research, treatment, recovery, waiting, visiting, eating, working, and much more.[40] Alongside such hospitals, older buildings continued to exist, as did smaller, more specialist institutions that treated particular demographics, communities, or illnesses.[41] Hospitals were also much more than single buildings, and had porous boundaries with homes and with other social or care institutions.[42] The journey to or from hospital could incorporate other healthcare spaces, such as pharmacies, health centres, General Practice (GP) surgeries and ambulances.[43] An expansive and relational approach to histories of colour is therefore necessary, to recognise hospitals as part of a longer healthcare journey and to acknowledge the diversity of people who moved through them. The 'diverse parts' of the NHS – and their diverse people – came with different colour schemes.

Some hospital colours were by design, but others were part of the busy, everyday life of hospitals. Colour entered hospitals in many forms, through objects, inhabitants, and plants, as well as the more obvious paint and other wall or floor surfaces. These 'everyday' colour palettes show how new ideas about 'modernity' were negotiated, brought into being, and sometimes destabilised at a local level. The book's discussion of modernity offers ways to 'read' colour in the past; its discussion of the everyday leans more towards 'feeling' the history of colour as something practised, embodied, and situated. As Joe Moran notes, 'material culture [is] a particularly fertile ground' for investigating everyday life.[44] The mundane is a valuable tool for understanding a range of subjects of crucial importance to historians, ranging from everyday emotional experiences of space and place through to the politics of built environments. It helps us to understand how categories such as 'modernity' sit alongside daily life and experience.

Temporality was particularly important to colour, and people's experiences of it as an everyday phenomenon. The chapters emphasise the importance of repetition and routines, for example in the form of cleaning, maintenance, or other acts of patient care associated with colours. Colour was connected to time in a range of ways, sometimes because of emotions such as boredom, and sometimes because of spatiality, such as long corridors. Colour changed over time even in the absence of human intervention, for example through weather, seasonal change and light patterns. Colour-based design and experience was different for acute, transitory, and chronic patients. Working patterns could shape staff members' experience of light and colour, for example the often overlooked but sensorially powerful experience of working a night shift. Taken together, the chapters show how historical understanding of colour requires consideration of time, as well as space.[45]

'Feeling' colour in history, particularly as part of everyday life, also necessitates recognising the wide variety of ways in which colour was experienced and encountered. Factors shaping experiences of colour could range from shared demographic characteristics to individual people's emotional states. For Tim Edensor 'the experience of colo[u]r belongs to those sensory and affective experiences through which people come to feel connected to familiar place over time' and 'the lived cultural experiences of colo[u]r emphasizes that its effects combine the symbolic and the affective'.[46] To write about colour through the lens of only cultural history, symbols, and meaning-making would miss the crucial way that those cultural histories are interwoven with local and individual affective, emotional, temporal, and sensory histories.

Conclusions

Colour has long been a crucial part of the everyday activity of hospitals. From the uniforms that mark out different staff to the colour schemes that sort hospital waste, colour is essential to hospital life. Wall and floor colours help with wayfinding and spatial organisation, as well as with hygienic practices and attempts to improve the hospital environment. These colour choices have rarely been made unthinkingly. Each colour is often carefully selected for a combination of practical and symbolic reasons.[47] Colour choices have also changed over time, and these changes provide a valuable way into histories of emotions, health, politics, design, architecture, culture, society, modernity, and everyday life.

Colour cuts across many types of history. 'Reading' histories of colour aids an understanding of social, cultural, and political histories. Colour provides a framework for understanding new meanings of modernity, which built up in layers over the course of the twentieth century. As the colour palette of modernity expanded, so did the concept of modernity itself. 'Feeling' histories of colour offers routes into more multi-sensory, more-than-visual histories; to quote Sam Jacob, 'colour is a place as well as a thing'.[48] Colour is a much richer area of study when it is recognised as something unstable, which might change in different light, or get dirty and need cleaning, and which might carry a different meaning on a painted wall than in a blanket. It is also a richer area of study when recognised as something relational, which would have meant different things to the varied populations of hospitals, as well as potentially to the same person at different times.[49]

Colour is also part of the material history of modern Britain. Changing colours of paints, objects, and architecture have made (and regularly remade) built environments over time. In this sense, colour is something that is 'there' as a tangible feature of hospital history. The discussion that follows is to some extent interested in colour as a 'thing' that can be measured through shade, hue, tint, tone, saturation, and in the emergence of standardised colour schemes such as Munsell, Pantone, and BS 2660.[50] However, narratives of colour-based change over time or the rise of standardised colour palettes in healthcare are not the real focus of this analysis. Material change is only part of the history of colour, which is more productively studied in expansive terms as a cultural signifier, spatial and atmospheric quality, embodied encounter, and more. Overall, this book does not just describe what colour was; it asks 'what did colour do?'[51]

Notes

1 There are five different shades of blue within the NHS palette, and different shades of blue are used for the NHS Wales and Scotland logos.

2 People's History of the NHS, 'Blue Curtain', https://peopleshistorynhs.org/museumobjects/blue-curtain/ [accessed: 4 July 2023].

3 For examples of NHS information leaflets found in a home, see *ibid.*
4 Trisha Greenhalgh, 'Lanyards', *BMJ*, 15 December 2005, p. 331.
5 The NHS branding is so strong that other businesses have been criticised for similarities to the logo. For example, see Sarah Marsh, 'WH Smith's "WHS" Rebrand Criticised for Similarity to NHS Logo', https://www.theguardian.com/business/2023/dec/27/wh-smith-whs-rebrand-criticised-for-similarity-to-nhs-logo [accessed: 30 April 2024].
6 Research Works Ltd for NHS England, 'NHS Identity Research: Phase One and Two Combined Research Report June 2016', https://www.england.nhs.uk/nhsidentity/wp-content/uploads/sites/38/2016/08/NHS-Identity-Research-phase-one-and-two.pdf [accessed: 4 July 2023], p. 37.
7 Cal Flyn, 'NHS Blue: The Colour of Universal Healthcare', https://wellcomecollection.org/articles/WyjcSigAACsALDg1 [accessed: 4 July 2023]; People's History of the NHS, 'Branding', https://peopleshistorynhs.org/encyclopaedia/branding/ [accessed: 4 July 2023].
8 Sally Sheard, 'Epilogue: I'm Afraid There's no NHS', in Jennifer Crane and Jane Hand (eds), *Posters, Protests, and Prescriptions: Cultural Histories of the National Health Service in Britain* (Manchester University Press, 2022), p. 324.
9 The colour of NHS nursing uniforms has not been consistent, but blue has long been a feature, despite changes over time. For example, see 'blue is the most familiar nursing colour', in Steve Ford, 'Bristol Trust Replaces Uniforms with Scrubs', https://www.nursingtimes.net/roles/nurse-managers/bristol-trust-replaces-uniforms-with-scrubs-22-08-2013/ [accessed: 4 July 2023].
10 NHS, 'Colours', https://www.england.nhs.uk/nhsidentity/identity-guidelines/colours/ [accessed: 4 July 2023].
11 Some of the hospitals discussed in the book are from Britain (England, Scotland, Wales) and there are a few that include the UK as a whole (Northern Ireland, though its system is called 'Department of Health and Social Care' rather than NHS). The book therefore largely uses the term 'British'. However, it is important to acknowledge that the majority of its examples and its evidence base relates to English hospitals. There were many overlaps in hospital design and architecture trends across Britain and across the UK, but England also has a specific history in this regard. The 1962 Hospital Plan that underpinned much hospital building in the NHS, for example, was only for 'England and Wales'. This book does occasionally dip into the early twenty-first century, but in broad terms it focuses on the twentieth century.
12 'CFP: Colour Matters 2023', https://chromotope.eu/colour-matters-2023/ [accessed: 4 July 2023].

13 International Colour Association, 'Proceedings', https://aic-color.org/publications-proceedings [accessed: 4 July 2023].

14 Natasha Eaton, *Colour, Art and Empire: Visual Culture and the Nomadism of Representation* (I.B. Tauris, 2013); Diana Young, 'The Colours of things', in Chris Tilley, Webb Keane, Susanne Kuechler, Mike Rowlands, and Patricia Spyer (eds), *Handbook of Material Culture* (Sage, 2006), pp. 173–85; Chris Horrocks (ed.), *Cultures of Colour: Visual, Material, Textual* (Berghahn Books, 2012); Carlos Rodríguez-Rellán, Ben Nelson, and Ramón Fábregas-Valcarce (eds), *A Taste for Green: A Global Perspective on Ancient Jade, Turquoise, and Variscite Exchange* (Oxbow Books, 2020).

15 There are many examples that could be given here. To offer one from each field as a sample of extensive scholarship: Sarah Street, *Colour Films in Britain: The Negotiation of Innovation 1900–1955* (Palgrave, 2012); Fiona McLachlan, *Architectural Colour in the Professional Palette* (Routledge, 2012).

16 For example Jordanna Bailkin, 'Indian Yellow: Making and Breaking the Imperial Palette', in Martin Jay and Sumathi Ramaswamy (ed.), *Empires of Vision: A Reader* (Duke University Press, 2014), pp. 91–110; Anne McClintock, *Imperial Leather: Race, Gender, and Sexuality in the Colonial Contest* (Routledge, 1995); Natasha Eaton, 'Excess in the City? Consumption of Imported Prints in Colonial Calcutta, c. 1780–c. 1795', in Martin Jay and Sumathi Ramaswamy (eds), *Empires of Vision: A Reader* (Duke University Press, 2014), pp. 159–88.

17 For example, Brian O'Doherty, *Inside the White Cube: The Ideology of the Gallery Space* (The Lapis Press, 1986); Paul Overy, *Light, Air and Openness: Modern Architecture between the Wars* (Thames & Hudson Ltd, 2007).

18 Lucy Faire and Denise McHugh, 'Twelve Shades of Grey: Encountering Urban Colour in the Street in British Provincial Towns, c. 1945–1970', *Urban History*, 46 (2019), p. 288.

19 Faire and McHugh, 'Twelve Shades of Grey', p. 289; they do note the significant exception of J. Jenkins, 'A System of Joyful Colour and its Disruptions: Architectural Colour in the German Democratic Republic', *Architectural Theory Review*, 19 (2014), pp. 221–42.

20 I predominantly use the word 'space' in this book and occasionally 'space and place'; in line with the work of Doreen Massey discussed in note 49 below, I do not distinguish as neatly between space and place as some geographical scholars. A relational approach to space is inherently meaningful, making it difficult to distinguish between 'objective' space and 'subjective' place. I also use the word 'environment', largely to refer to material environments such as buildings, rooms, and wards rather

than space/place as inhabited. I have written more on this approach to space and place in Victoria Bates, 'Sensing Space and Making Place: The Hospital and Therapeutic Landscapes in Two Cancer Narratives', *Medical Humanities*, 45 (2019), pp. 10–20.

21 A number of architectural and medical historians have worked on modern British hospital design, many of whom are cited throughout this book. The subject matter is therefore relatively well-trodden ground, with some excellent scholarship, but the focus of such work does tend to be on buildings more than on interiors. Examples include Harriet Richardson Blakeman, 'Medicine and Modernity: Fifty Years of NHS Hospital Building in Scotland, 1948–1998' (PhD Dissertation: University of Edinburgh, 2023); Ed DeVane, 'Pilgrim's Progress: The Landscape of the NHS Hospital, 1948–70', *Twentieth Century British History*, 32 (2021), pp. 534–52; Alistair Fair, '"Modernization of Our Hospital System": The National Health Service, the Hospital Plan, and the "Harness" Programme, 1962–77', *Twentieth Century British History*, 29 (2018), pp. 547–75; Jonathan Hughes, 'The "Matchbox on a Muffin": The Design of Hospitals in the Early NHS', *Medical History*, 44 (2000), pp. 21–56; Christina Malathouni, '"In Line with the Modern Conception of Much Mental Illness": Psychiatric Reforms and Architectural Design Contributions in Post-War England', *Architecture MPS*, 24 (2023), pp. 1–21; David Theodore, 'Treating Architectural Research: The Nuffield Trust and the Post-War hospital', *The Journal of Architecture*, 24 (2019), pp. 982–98.

22 Crane and Hand (eds), *Posters, Protests, and Prescriptions*.

23 For a full summary of the historiography of hospital beds, see footnote 10 in Agnes Arnold-Forster and Victoria Bates, 'Care and Crisis: Making Beds in the National Health Service', *Journal of British Studies*, First View (2024), pp. 1–27; Victoria Bates, Jennifer Crane, and Maria Fannin, 'Fluid Modernities: The Birthing Pool in Late Twentieth-Century Britain', *Medical Humanities*, 50 (2024), pp. 312–21.

24 Specific examples of such scholarship are given throughout this book in the relevant chapters.

25 I use 'experience' in this book in line with the work of Rob Boddice and Mark Smith: 'By experience we mean, simply, to capture the lived, meaningful reality of historical actors, whether as subjective or collective reality, and incorporating all the features of past perception in their own terms, be they sensory, emotional, cognitive, supernatural or whatever. We might have used the language of "feeling" to attain a similar position.' Rob Boddice and Mark Smith, *Emotion, Sense, Experience* (Cambridge University Press, 2020), p. 17.

26 There are many examples that could be given to support this point, but perhaps the most obvious is the literature on histories of 'moral treatment' in which the building itself was part of treatment; see Barry Edginton, 'The Design of Moral Architecture at the York Retreat', *Journal of Design History*, 16 (2003), pp. 103–17. On buildings and place as 'treatment' see also Julie Collins, *The Architecture and Landscape of Health: A Historical Perspective on Therapeutic Places 1790–1940* (Routledge, 2020).
27 Geoffrey Rivett, *From Cradle to Grave: Fifty Years of the NHS* (King Edward's Hospital Fund for London, 1998), p. 49.
28 For post-war interest in 'dehumanisation', 'rehumanisation', and the meaning(s) of these terms, see Victoria Bates, '"Humanizing" Healthcare Environments: Architecture, Art and Design in Modern Hospitals', *Design for Health*, 2 (2018), pp. 5–19.
29 Martin Gorsky, 'The British National Health Service 1948–2008: A Review of the Historiography', *Social History of Medicine*, 21 (2008), pp. 440–1. On concerns about the rising threat of neoliberalism to the NHS in the 1980s see also Jennifer Crane, '"Save our NHS": Activism, Information-Based Expertise and the "New Times" of the 1980s', *Contemporary British History*, 33 (2019), pp. 52–74.
30 Miles Ogborn, *Spaces of Modernity: London's Geographies 1680–1780* (Guilford Press, 1998), p. 2; Anne Hugon, 'Maternity and Modernity in the Gold Coast, 1920s–1950s', *Ghana Studies*, 12 (2009/10), pp. 77–95.
31 David Gilbert, David Matless, and Brian Short, 'Historical Geographies of British Modernity', in David Gilbert, David Matless, and Brian Short (eds), *Geographies of British Modernity: Space and Society in the Twentieth Century* (Blackwell Publishing, 2003), p. 2.
32 Julian Ashley, *Anatomy of a Hospital* (Oxford University Press, 1987), dust jacket.
33 This argument echoes those I have made elsewhere, for example in relation to the birthing pool, as an object which similarly managed to 'hold' the apparent tensions of modernity as a medical technology and a symbol of care; see Bates, Crane, and Fannin, 'Fluid Modernities'.
34 Partha Chatterjee, *Our Modernity* (Sephis, 1997); Keir Waddington, 'Problems of Progress: Modernity and Writing the Social History of Medicine', *Social History of Medicine*, 34 (2021), pp. 1053–67.
35 This paragraph is reproduced from Bates, Crane, and Fannin, 'Fluid Modernities'.
36 This quote is an adaptation of the framework of 'cutting across' the century in Emily Robinson, Camilla Schofield, Florence Sutcliffe-Braithwaite, and

Natalie Thomlinson, 'Telling Stories about Post-War Britain: Popular Individualism and the "Crisis" of the 1970s', *Twentieth Century British History*, 28 (2017), pp. 268–304, p. 268.

37 Matthew Hilton, Chris Moores, and Florence Sutcliffe-Braithwaite, 'New Times Revisited: Britain in the 1980s', *Contemporary British History*, 31 (2017), p. 148.

38 Robinson *et al.*, 'Telling Stories about Post-War Britain'.

39 Sheard, 'Epilogue', p. 326; see also Arnold-Forster and Bates, 'Care and Crisis', pp. 1–27.

40 This book speaks to hospital and health histories when they are relevant, but colour is at the forefront of the story. For more detail on the background against which this book is set, it might be useful to consult some survey texts. On health, for example: Helen Jones, *Health and Society in Twentieth-Century Britain* (Routledge, 2014). On the NHS: Geoffrey Rivett, *From Cradle to Grave: Fifty Years of the NHS* (King Edward's Hospital Fund for London, 1998). On architecture: Susan Francis, Rosemary Glanville, Ann Noble, and Peter Scher, *50 Years of Ideas in Health Care Buildings* (Nuffield Trust, 1999); Julie Willis, Philip Goad, and Cameron Logan, *Architecture and the Modern Hospital: Nosokomeion to Hygeia* (Routledge, 2019); Jeanne Kisacky, *Rise of the Modern Hospital: An Architectural History of Health and Healing, 1870–1940* (University of Pittsburgh Press, 2017).

41 In 2018 it was reported that 'Almost 14% of [the NHS estate] pre-dates the NHS and more than 60% is more than 20 years old'; Brian Green, 'Vital Signs: Economics of the NHS', https://www.ribaj.com/intelligence/intelligence-market-analysis-nhs-health-buildings-brian-green [accessed: 30 January 2024].

42 On hospitals as 'permeable', 'fluid', and spaces with 'unfixed boundaries' see, for example, Victoria J. Wood, Sarah E. Curtis, Wil Gesler, Ian H. Spencer, Helen J. Close, James Mason, and Joe G. Reilly, 'Creating "Therapeutic Landscapes" for Mental Health Carers in Inpatient Settings: A Dynamic Perspective on Permeability and Inclusivity', *Social Science & Medicine*, 91 (2013), pp. 122–29; Mia Harrison, Kari Lancaster, and Tim Rhodes, 'The Fluid Hospital: On the Making of Care Environments in COVID-19', *Health & Place*, 83 (2023): 103107.

43 These spaces are not a focus of this book, but are mentioned where they align with hospital trends, emphasising that new colour schemes were part of a journey to hospital and did not start at the hospital door. For example, the whiteness of ambulances, the turn to pastel colour palettes for Boots pharmacy, and the integration of ideas of 'homeliness' and cheerful colour schemes into GP waiting rooms.

44 Joe Moran, 'History, Memory and the Everyday', *Rethinking History*, 8 (2004), p. 51.
45 With thanks to an anonymous reviewer for highlighting and drawing out this aspect of my book, and helping me to articulate it in this way.
46 Tim Edensor, 'What Color is this Place?', *GeoHumanities*, 9 (2023), p. 428.
47 Victoria Bates, 'Cold White of Day: White, Colour, and Materiality in the Twentieth-Century British Hospital', *Twentieth Century British History*, 34 (2023), pp. 1–37.
48 Sam Jacob, 'Colour is a Place as Well as a Thing', in Elena Manferdini and Jasmine Benyamin (eds), *Full Spectrum: Colour in Contemporary Architecture* (RIBA, 2023), pp. 54–65; see also Diana Young, writing on colour in the *Handbook of Material Culture*, 'the idea of colour as involving only the visual is … a limited and culturally bound conception'; Young, 'The Colours of Things', p. 182.
49 The idea of 'relational' thinking about space is often connected to the work of Doreen Massey; though Massey is more focused on human relations, power, and identity, the idea that space is made through relationships can also extend to relationships between people and objects, colours, buildings, and more. The term 'relational' is used broadly, here, to mean that space is constantly being made through interactions with people. The traditional distinction between 'space' as objective and 'place' as subjective is less clear in this relational way of thinking; see Doreen Massey, *For Space* (Sage, 2005). Ideas cited elsewhere in this book such as 'atmospheres' and 'assemblages' are also relational concepts, grounded in the idea that space is always *becoming*. These are connected with slightly different fields of spatial theory, for example: on Gilles Deleuze and Felix Guattari see June Wang, 'Assemblage', *Oxford Biographies*, https://www.oxfordbibliographies.com/display/document/obo-9780190922481/obo-9780190922481-0060.xml [accessed: 4 March 2024]; on atmospheres and the 'relational knotting of forces' see Steven D. Brown, Ava Kanyeredzi, Laura McGrath, Paula Reavey, and Ian Tucker, 'Affect Theory and the Concept of Atmosphere', *Distinktion: Journal of Social Theory*, 20 (2019), pp. 5–24. Each of these theories has differences in meaning and focus, but they are broadly tied together by the idea of space as being in flux, co-produced by the different elements within it, as part of an ongoing relational process. This book is not a spatial theory book and will not focus on these theories in too much depth, but does use concepts drawn from them where appropriate. It explores how histories of colour might be reconsidered when moving from cultural models of colour and meaning, towards a more spatial way of thinking about colour as one actor in a relational process. Its

focus remains largely on humans and human perception, unlike some theorists working in this area, but recognises that colour is also an agent in its own right that can change materially without human intervention. This kind of approach also draws on the ideas of Tim Ingold, who emphasises the importance of recognising materials within materiality; see Tim Ingold, 'Materials against Materiality', *Archaeological Dialogues*, 14 (2007), pp. 1–16.

50 On the history of these standardised colour schemes see Eva-Marie Neumann, 'Architecture, Science and Colour in Britain, 1945–76' (PhD Dissertation: University College London, 1999).

51 Thank you to Shanti Sumartojo for a generous conversation about my book and its focus, which helped me to draw out this distinction.

1

White: modernity and materiality

The earliest colour-based trend in the twentieth-century hospital was the apparent elimination of hues in favour of shades of white, as part of making 'modern', hygienic healthcare buildings.[1] In 1962, the *British Medical Journal* (*BMJ*) summarised the recent history of hospital colour schemes as follows: before 1918, there were 'whitewashed walls above dado height and dark brown below'; in the 1920s, white gloss often replaced the whitewash 'and below dado height some sombre dirt-concealing colour – a dark green or brown'; then, in the early 1930s, 'all-white became a vogue and in the more progressive hospitals white-tiled walls to dado height replaced the sombre colours'.[2] The language of 'progressive' white next to 'sombre' darker colours here is deliberate and significant, highlighting the apparently superior moral and medical qualities of inter-war whiteness.

White is one of the most important colours in the history of hospitals. However, it remains very rare to see whiteness treated as more than a material absence, an erasure, or a background. In 1993, an article in *Hospital Development* magazine described the 'hallmark' of respected architects Powell & Moya as a 'pristine white backcloth for telling colour and natural materials'.[3] However, whiteness was always an important material and symbolic addition to a building, and should not be dismissed as a 'backcloth' for colour or as neutral, pure, silent, plain, or blank.[4] White is neither absent nor blank: it includes 'Lead White, Ivory, Silver, Whitewash, Isabelline, Chalk and Beige'.[5] White should be understood through the analytical lens of colour, even if 'pure' white is not understood as such. Kenya Hara argues, in the opening to the book *100 Whites*, that 'white is not a colo[u]r, but a sensibility or mentality'.[6] If white is taken as the colour equivalent of silence, this must only be done in the spirit of understanding silence as a 'complex acoustical practice' and whiteness as a complex visual–material practice.[7]

A material history of whiteness offers a way to reappraise narratives of the twentieth century, particularly the idea that white was an absence or an instrument of control. Hygiene and germ control were complicated and unstable; white could signify the elimination of germs without eliminating anything, and hygiene was not incompatible with a 'humanistic' hospital. White also maintained its quality as a symbol of hygiene, even after colour replaced it as a marker of modernity. The role of white in hospitals cannot be reduced to a neat narrative, of the sterile white modernist hospital that was replaced by the more patient-centred NHS. White also took on new and shifting meanings in relation to clothing and people, including in the context of an NHS reliant on migrant workers.[8] What was reassuringly hygienic to some was part of an imperial coding of white(ness) to others, which could reinforce racialised labour hierarchies. White was not a static, two-dimensional colour, but rather a dynamic and active part of the making of hospital spaces.

Hygiene: modernism and the early twentieth-century removal of colour

The rise of white in twentieth-century British healthcare built upon late nineteenth-century efforts to make hospitals brighter spaces, filled with sunlight and clean fresh air. Although many commentators would later compare Florence Nightingale's interest in colour with the sterile colour palettes of contemporary hospitals, there was not such a clear-cut separation between the two in practice. Susan Barclay even argues that Nightingale's interest in colour has been over-stated by some historians, when actually she advocated 'pale pink walls' and had a strong preference for 'shiny white surfaces'.[9] In the early twentieth century, there were new associations between whiteness, modernity, and hygiene, which built on and extended these meanings. With the growing influence of germ theory and in the wake of a flu epidemic, hygiene became a driving force for hospital design and for modern architecture more generally.[10] The focus of infection control shifted from the air to water and surfaces; walls were no longer designed to hide dirt, but to *show* dirt – or rather the absence thereof. Germ theory was not a turning point, as many older ideas about disease transmission and healthy architecture continued to co-exist with the hygiene model, but it had a growing influence on architecture over the course of the twentieth century.

Late nineteenth- and early twentieth-century publications on modern or modernised hospitals often commented on the presence of white tiles. This trend can be seen in a range of contexts, including a Birmingham children's hospital in 1890 (with 'modern' cots and walls lined with a combination of square and 'octagonal-shaped white tiles, each marked off by a narrow coloured border'), an operating theatre at the Newcastle Royal Victoria Infirmary in 1906 ('[t]he walls are of white glazed tiles, the floor of marble terrazzo, and the fittings of white porcelain') to an example of a 'Modern Maternity Hospital' in Belfast from 1908 (with its 'smooth white tiles').[11] In 1913, a report in *The Hospital* on the East Suffolk and Ipswich Hospital noted that 'many of the older portions of the hospital have been refloored, and the old matchboarding dadoes have been replaced by white tiles, with a grey-blue glazed moulding at the top'.[12] Such trends were still local, and were examples of more forward-looking hospitals, showing the growing connection between modernity and white, wipe-down surfaces at the turn of the century.

These links between whiteness, modernity and hygiene laid the groundwork in subsequent decades for the rise of white, modernist hospitals in Britain. These hospitals were seen first in inter-war Europe, where, as Margaret Campbell argues, modernist architecture 'philosophically embodied the clean, white world that was so craved for after the carnage and filth of the First World War'.[13] One of the most famous examples of classic modernist healthcare buildings, which inspired British hospital design, was in Finland: Alvar Aalto's Paimio Sanatorium (completed 1933), depicted in Figure 1.1. Another was Zonnestraal in the Netherlands (completed 1928), depicted in Figure 1.2. Both buildings were dominated by the use of white, though in combination with brighter colours such as yellows and blues.[14]

The increasingly extensive use of white in healthcare architecture drew upon wider ideas in European architecture at this time, in

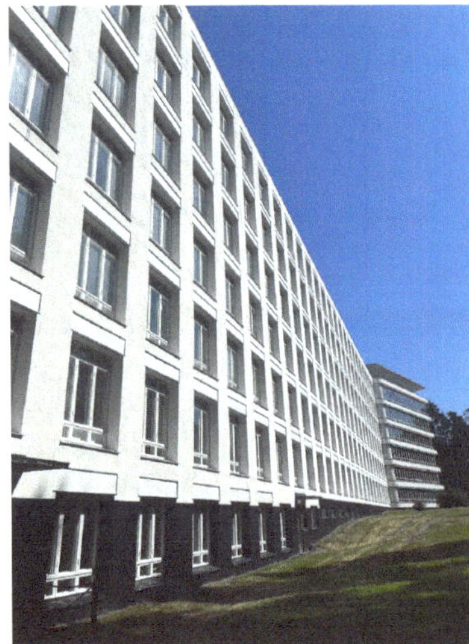
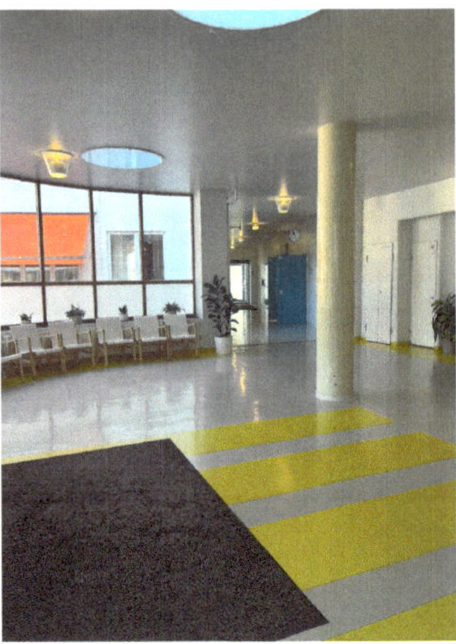

Figure 1.1 Paimio Sanatorium, 2023.

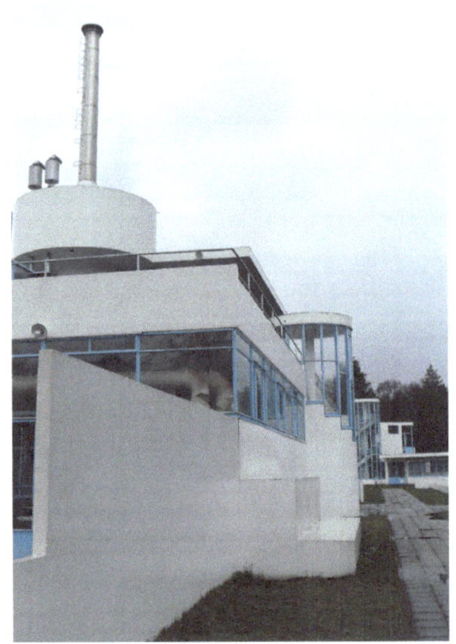

Figure 1.2 Zonnestraal Estate, former sanatorium, 2023.

which the 'white wall' was particularly important under the influence of Swiss-French architect Le Corbusier.[15] Recent scholars writing on 1930s Turkish sanatoria have also shown that whiteness was an important architectural feature, widely noted by patients at the time as key to their experience of treatment.[16] An interest in white, hygiene, and modernity was evident throughout European domestic and public building projects alike. William Rollins, for example, notes that '[w]hite was virtually ubiquitous in Weimar culture, but nowhere did it assume a more prominent role than in the era's landmark project of modern architecture' and that white buildings offer a way to understand 'the self-consciously modern culture of 1920s Germany'.[17] It is rare to find scholarship on the spaces and places of inter-war Europe that does not refer to white walls, even if just in passing, whether in relation to the interiors of 'queer modernity' or the history of surveillance.[18]

The newly 'all-white' hospital offers a valuable case study for historians interested in modernity and the built environment. Wil Gesler *et al.* argue that white clinical spaces were key sites for representing the so-called 'white heat' of modernity, with its emphasis on scientific and technological order.[19] The all-white aesthetic of modernist hospitals – inside and out – was intertwined with the idea of a 'machine for healing'. Stuart W. Leslie notes that this idea was fundamental to modernism: 'just as Le Corbusier considered a house a machine for living […] so he envisioned a hospital as a carefully controlled machine for healing'.[20] This issue of control, and its relationship to whiteness, is crucial for understanding how the all-white hospital has been understood and represented. As Mark Wigley notes, Le Corbusier's extremely influential buildings of the early twentieth century had whiteness at their core: 'the whole moral, ethical, functional and even technical superiority of architecture is seen to hang on the whiteness of its surfaces'.[21] Other scholars of modernist architecture have similarly identified the moral values imbued in white walls. For Lucas Crawford, 'hygiene' itself is part of control and surveillance: 'from the white city to white walls and to white toilets, white operates … as a technology of vision, control, hygiene'.[22] As discussed later in this section, modern/ist whiteness also existed in relation to a powerful legacy of imperialist ideas about race, cleanliness, and social hierarchy. Whiteness, control, and hygiene were inextricably interwoven in these buildings.

These connections between whiteness and hygiene have long historical roots in Europe, in links between white, purity, and cleanliness. Michal Pastoureau's book on white shows that the Romans admired the colour and associated it with purity and beauty in art, and that in Greek and Latin, 'figurative meanings for the adjective "white"' included 'pure, clean, virgin, innocent, empty, intact, bright, luminous, favourable, and so on'.[23] White was associated with money and power, particularly when only the wealthy could afford to keep their clothing white. Whiteness was also associated with purity in the context of the marital ceremony, with cleanliness in restaurants, and with religion in the form of a white dove. As Kassia St Clair argues, even the idea of the existence of a 'pure' white implies some kind of 'transcendent, religious quality'.[24] These meanings have also long been evident in hospitals, even though they were historically more colourful. Whiteness was important in European plague hospitals, in the form of stone, symbols on clothing, and white boats for transporting people and goods.[25] These meanings were not universal. In many other countries, particularly in East Asia, white has long held an association with misfortune, misery, and death.

The all-white hospital trend also came to North America, though a little later than in Europe. As Annmarie Adams notes, in the inter-war period, 'state-of-the-art North American hospitals [...] were far more likely to resemble a Georgian mansion, or [...] a Renaissance palazzo' than the 'slick white villas' of Le Corbusier.[26] Adams looks closely at the examples of hospital architect Edward Fletcher Stevens and his partner Frederick Clare Lee, showing that their version of modern hospital architecture actually drew extensively on historical reference points and looked in many ways distinctly unmodern. Adams shows that this approach to hospital architecture could also be part of communicating new scientific medicine, and the 'white box' was not the only option for hospital architects at this time. The value of all-white design for hygienic and surgical spaces was by no means universally or immediately accepted. By the 1950s, however, Adams notes that the trend for 'undecorated white boxes' was in 'full force' in North American urban general hospitals.[27] The influence of European modernism was broadly global, but scholars have identified modernist architecture – and the ways it entwined with and was shaped by local architects – in different countries at different times. Examples range from female-led modernist architecture in 1930s Palestine, to the influence of British colonialism on modernist African or 'Tropical Architecture' from the late 1940s onwards, to a 1951 Iranian 'modernist white structure – a new hybrid architecture that drew its vocabulary from the main tenets of the Modern movement of Europe and the Zoroastrian fire temples of ancient Iran'.[28]

The early twentieth-century British hospital must be situated in these international architectural and healthcare trends, particularly before the introduction of the NHS in 1948 created a more 'national' hospital history. This history also must not be subsumed within international architectural trends. There is a specific, national story to British hospital design, even in the early twentieth century. Elizabeth Darling and Alistair Fair note that there was 'a specifically English contribution to modernist theory' seen in experimental, landmark projects such as the Pioneer Health Centre, which focused on 'the interplay between environments and people'.[29] These principles would become increasingly important in the years of post-war reconstruction, but it is important not to view the modern British built environment as simply the articulation of European modernism. British modernism was also shaped by local culture, architectural thinking, and – in relation to hospitals – healthcare contexts. In part because British hospitals were a combination of old workhouses and voluntary and municipal buildings, renovation was more likely than large-scale building programmes. Modernist principles made their way into British hospitals often subtly, introduced not as grand architectural initiatives but as local attempts at modernisation. Such localised modernisation efforts would continue to be important throughout the century; the influence of modernist principles went beyond new architecture.

The history of British hospital architecture sits somewhere in the middle of the trends seen in mainland Europe and the later influence of modernist aesthetics in countries such as the US. The premise that white surfaces were the ideal for hospitals seemed to be rapidly accepted. Some hospitals embraced white tiles many years before the 'Modern Movement', and by 1931 one *BMJ Military Health* correspondent stated with confidence that '[t]he meaning of "hospital" has [...] become fixed, and cannot be dissociated from such things as wards, beds, white paint, glazed, tiles, nurses, flowers and charitable lady visitors'.[30] Some hospitals responded to the 'all-white' trend of the inter-war years with a fresh coat of paint or new white tiles. Others integrated these design principles into new architecture, but it would be an overstatement to say that European modernism was instantly integrated into hospital design.

Modernism was dominant by mid-century but – despite some high-profile modernist architectural projects in housing and healthcare – it was still somewhat 'peripheral' in the 1930s, when modernist ideas were appearing in Britain as a 'trickle' rather than a pour.[31] Many British hospitals incorporated modernist principles, rather than building new Modernist architecture with a capital M.[32] That said, some new hospitals did draw explicitly on both the architectural principles and colour palettes of modern architecture in the inter-war years. One example is the 1937 'Modern Movement' style of Kent and Canterbury Hospital, designed by architect Cecil L. Burns (Figure 1.3).[33] The sense of a modern hospital was created through a light exterior and the shapes and recognisable structures of other modern architecture, including curves, light-drenched sunny balconies, and dramatic entrance gates. In 1941 the *Nursing Times* described this hospital as a 'model to copy' for its 'modern style of architecture which combines beauty with efficiency, comfort and ease of performance'.[34] Black-and-white photography enhanced representations of architectural whiteness, and further fuelled efforts to achieve it.[35]

There were a few similar hospitals built in inter-war modernist style. For example, nearby were the spiral ramp of the white-trimmed Kent and Sussex Hospital in Tunbridge Wells (1934), and the curved glass-and-white Lister wing of the Benenden Chest Hospital (1937). Around the same time, routes to the hospital were rebranded, with a turn to white as the dominant colour for ambulances, ensuring that people's first encounter with the hospital left an impression of clean, crisp, white modernity.[36] Light colours require maintenance and these buildings undoubtedly lost some of their impact over time as they weathered, though Wrigley argues that decay of this kind actually draws even more attention to whiteness.[37] By the 1970s, deteriorating white hospital exteriors may have fed wider anxieties of national decline.

White walls combined with other elements to suggest the spatial qualities of efficiency, modernity, and hygiene. Figure 1.4 turns to the inside of the Kent and Canterbury Hospital in 1937, where

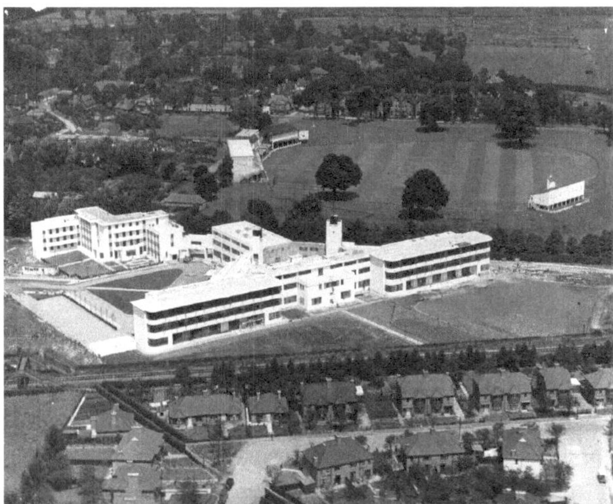

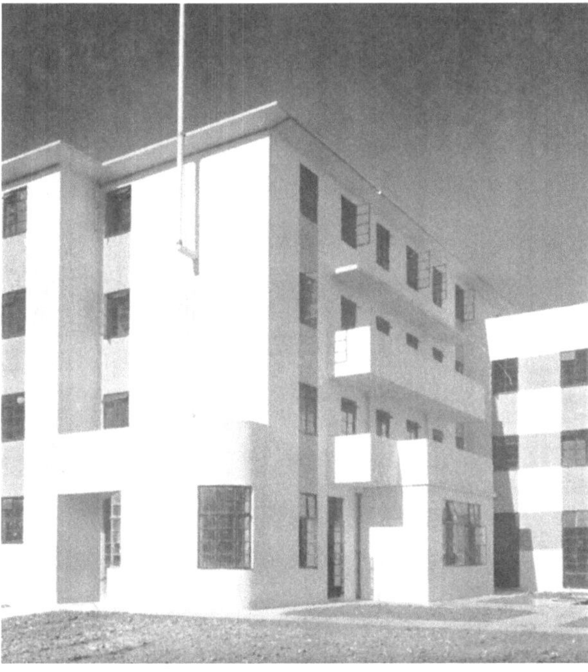

Figure 1.3 Kent and Canterbury Hospital exterior and Nurses Home exterior. New Kent and Canterbury Hospital Archives and souvenir brochure 14 July 1937. © Photograph courtesy of East Kent Hospitals NHS Trust. All rights reserved and permission to use this figure must be obtained from the copyright holder.

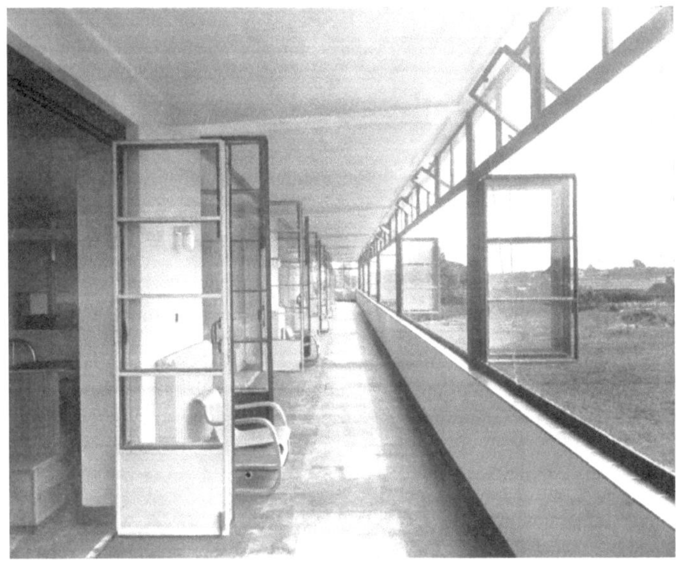

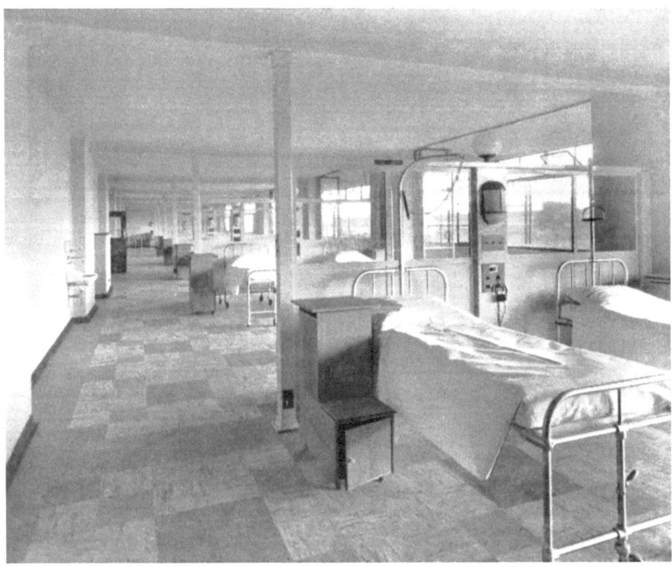

Figure 1.4 Kent and Canterbury Hospital Interior: Ward Solarium and Surgical Ward. New Kent and Canterbury Hospital Archives and souvenir brochure 14 July 1937. © Photograph courtesy of East Kent Hospitals NHS Trust. All rights reserved and permission to use this figure must be obtained from the copyright holder.

white surfaces, walls, and ceilings combined with large windows, fresh air, light, white linen, white doors, white chairs, wipe-down bed frames, and shiny floor tiles. The *Nursing Times* described how the hospital's modern and efficient feel was brought into being through a range of sensory design elements that created 'a sense of space, order and almost silent activity'.[38] The article highlighted rubber flooring, extensive windows, the absence of 'superfluous' design elements, widespread use of anti-glare glass, and carefully directed lighting systems.[39] The use of white was therefore one component in a sensory arrangement that helped to create a feeling of a modern, efficient, light, and spacious hospital.

In practice, colour was rarely absent, even in what might be considered classic modernist buildings. Scholars have started to challenge the idea that modernism was an 'all-white' aesthetic as something of a myth, and this is certainly true of hospital design.[40] Inside the Kent and Canterbury Hospital, white walls were combined with more brightly coloured flooring: a 'lovely blue' in the entrance, with different colours for each department as part of ordering the space.[41] This use of colour is in line with that found in the most famous international examples of modernist hospital design. As already noted, Paimio Sanatorium used white alongside carefully deployed colour and experience-centred design, including white walls with yellow flooring in stairwells, with hints of yellow flooring also visible in Figure 1.1.[42] Such use of colour was a precursor to what have become known as 'wayfinding' measures, in which coloured flooring in different areas of hospitals helps people to navigate the spaces.

It remains true that white dominated in these spaces, and that some patients did find them alienating. However, they were not entirely soulless 'white cubes'.[43] White, light, and brighter colour were often used together carefully. Other famous examples include Lubetkin's Finsbury Health Centre, which opened in 1938 and used light and brightness carefully to create a space that was both modern and 'cheerful'.[44] Some of the key white healthcare buildings of the 1930s might be best thought of as precursors to the patient-centred NHS, rather than in opposition to it.[45] In practice the early NHS did not inherit hundreds of gleaming white 'blank slates' but a disparate collection of buildings that included some predominately (but rarely 'all') white hospitals, alongside a range of older, darker colour palettes, and a number of other colour schemes that hospitals had used to 'modernise' their buildings in more ad hoc ways.

The 'machine for healing' was as much a product of cultural imagination as it was a real dominant architectural form, in modern Britain at least, but it was very powerful. In 1955, *Picture Post* published a story on the 'Modern Kitchen', which noted that the kitchen was 'almost too dazzling, too "hygienic" [in its] whiteness ... so that it looks like part of a hospital'.[46] By this point, the cultural links between whiteness, hygiene, and hospitals were firmly embedded. Implicit, though, in this *Picture Post* article was a critique of 'too "hygienic" whiteness' as too clinical, and as neither homely nor desirable. As Paul Atkinson notes,

> Some people take Le Corbusier's 1923 framing of the house as 'a machine for living in' at face value and consequently see Modernism as inherently dehumanizing. This is frustrating, given that the very roots of Modernism lie in altruistic attempts to improve health and hygiene for all.[47]

The humanistic and hygienic were not incompatible, but the juxtaposition of these ideas in design and architectural rhetoric is an important part of hospital history. The vision of modernism as 'dehumanizing' would become very powerful later in the twentieth century, when the idea of modernist hospitals as all-white and overly sterile would be the basis for a turn towards more 'humanistic' colourful palettes.

Material change: paint

Whiteness is often conceptualised as the removal or absence of colour, but this is misleading. In the early twentieth century many white walls – particularly interiors – were added over old colour schemes. New white paint on existing walls, floors, and ceilings added layers, rather than eliminated the old. Even the 'fresh' paint of new, modernist hospitals must be understood as a material addition rather than an absence. As Mark Wigley emphasises, on modern architecture: 'white is a layer ... this white layer that proclaims that the architecture it covers is naked has a very ambiguous role'.[48] White paint is less comparable to nudity, Wigley argues, and more comparable to clothing: white paint is like wearing white fabric, as a marker of cleanliness, hygiene, and social hierarchies. This conceptualisation of the act of painting, and of white paint in particular, is important for historians. It encourages us to examine the act of painting more closely, as the addition of meaning rather than its removal.

The white walls of many early twentieth-century hospitals were materially varied. Shiny new modern blocks could sit awkwardly alongside older ones that needed 'beautifying', a contrast that could reveal the difference between the 'whiteness' of these buildings.[49] A coat of fresh paint in an old hospital would likely have revealed lumps, bumps, and textures of old walls and previous coats of paint. As Kenya Hara notes in *100 Whites*, walls are never completely flat; this point applies to all walls, but particularly to old ones. Hara argues that 'to see is to observe not only shape but light' in terms of how the light falls on white walls, exposes its textures and blemishes, reflects off its surfaces, and how this might differ day-to-day and hour-to-hour with atmospheric conditions.[50] The reflection of light also varied according to the nature of the paint, the lighting design of rooms, the position and size of windows, and the direction in which people tended to look. As one article in *Architects' Journal* noted in the 1950s, the perceived reflection of surfaces changed when patients' beds were moved from facing windows to being parallel to window.[51] White walls were dynamic, three-dimensional surfaces.

To view white hospital walls as pure, white, controlling spaces is to misunderstand the act of painting as an end-point rather than part of an ongoing process. The meaning of white hospital walls always existed in relation to the colours below, and above, the white paint; a white wall that had been painted over a darker Victorian colour as an act of 'beautification' of old infrastructure, for example, carried different symbolism to a 'fresh' white wall in a new modern hospital. White walls were dynamic and evolving, rather than consistently clean markers of a germ-free space. This is particularly significant in relation to 'all-white' modernist hospitals, which rarely stayed this neat and clean. The challenges of maintenance and cleaning white walls were partly why many hospitals moved to more practical solutions, such as textured or speckled paints mid-century, as discussed further below.

For historians it is useful to conceptualise the act of painting, and the painted wall, as an ongoing process of damage and repair. It is restrictive to focus on neat, clean images of white walls presented in hospital design journals and photographs. White walls were constantly damaged and patched up, and carried visible 'scars'. Paint also changed independently, for example under the influence of sunlight and dirt; as Diana Young notes, such 'a colour change might ... be thought of as the transformation itself not just as symbolic'.[52] These kinds of changes are rarely found in the archive, especially if walls have been cleaned, repaired, or replaced, and the wall itself cannot act as evidence. However, there are occasional references to damage and disrepair buried in hospital records. The causes include plaster failure due to underlying heating, poor plastering that created rough surfaces, knocks and bashes from trolleys, and patches where dado rails were removed.[53] In general, many people would have encountered dirty, faded, or bashed white walls rather than the gleaming white paint found more often in archival images.

The type of white paint that hospitals used was also an important material change over time to hospital walls, whether it was fresh or layered over old paint. David and Beverlie Sloane argue that 'using white paint on walls replaced whitewashing walls [...] but the effect was the same'.[54] I argue, instead, that such material differences should be seen as equally important to the colour. White walls looked and felt different when they were formed by whitewash (a thin coat of plaster) and white gloss paint, which was shiny and showed up the texture of walls. Later, as discussed below, there was a further shift with the use of semi-gloss or textured paints. Although Sloane and Sloane are right in arguing that all of these 'white walls symbolized cleanliness', there were subtle differences in how they symbolised cleanliness and whether they were as clean as they appeared.[55] This distinction became particularly evident when hospitals started to distinguish between the paint finishes required for 'real' hygiene, and those that could create the appearance of hygiene.

White walls that looked clean and white walls that *were* clean were often conflated, and this distinction was sometimes used knowingly in hospital design. King Edward's Hospital Fund for London (hereafter 'The King's Fund'), in the early 1960s, did some experiments on wall surfaces at St Bartholomew's Hospital that illustrated the division between 'real' and 'felt' hygiene.[56] They trialled 59 types of wall surface for the new Central Sterile Services Department (CSSD) at the time. Each name brought into being the paint's materiality and hygienic qualities, reflecting and fulfilling its purpose: 'Dulux hygienic enamel' in vanilla or white, fungicidal gloss, 'Bactol' gloss and tiles.[57] In addition to new colour schemes, many of these were shades of white, though very rarely what might be considered 'pure' white. The report indicated that texture and paint finishes could be used to create a sense of hygiene and cleanliness, rather than necessarily to control dirt. The report's conclusion stated:

> The appearance of dirtiness is not correlated with the actual amount of dirt present. There are some areas where attractive general appearance is the main requirement coupled with ease of maintenance and less frequent cleaning than 'hygiene' areas.[58]

The report continued to recommend light-colour wipe-down surfaces, such as gloss paints, tiles, and plastic sheeting for areas where hygiene was a key consideration. It noted, though, that textured paints and those with slightly darker 'broken or stippled colour' could give the feel of a clean space with a lighter maintenance schedule because they gave 'little evidence of the actual dirt adhering'.[59] A careful balance was negotiated, through colour and texture, between hygienic practices and the portrayal of an area of the hospital as hygienic. Figure 1.5 shows some examples of flecked white paints and textured off-white wall coverings, from this study, that kept the feeling of whiteness without needing regular cleaning.

White paint was used strategically, and in combination with materiality, as part of creating the sense – if not the actual cleanliness – of hygiene for staff and patients. Though this particular study was for the CSSD, which was not a patient-facing department, its principles could apply more widely. The fact that the King's Fund did this research at all is worthy of note. In the early years of the

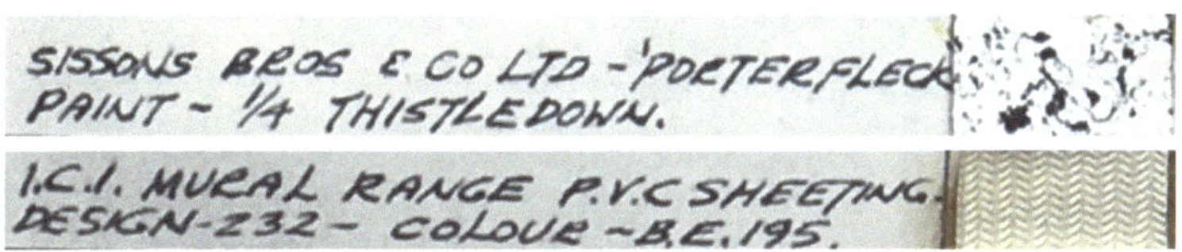

Figure 1.5 Paint and PVC sheeting samples. The King's Fund Wall Surfaces A/KE/I/01/06/002 © Reproduced with permission of the King's Fund.

NHS, research conducted by the charity was crucial to understanding the experiences of those who used and worked in hospitals. The King's Fund was reinvigorated by the NHS and supported the goal of more person-oriented hospitals, treating improving people's comfort and enhancing built environments as key. Their focus ranged from mattresses to noise, and they undertook a range of surveys with staff and patients.[60] Their studies of wall surfaces and paint were part of this wider agenda, not only to improve the hygienic practices of hospitals but to improve people's experiences of hospitals.

This analysis of the King's Fund study suggests that white paint was used to create spaces that reassured staff and patients. In certain contexts hygiene was a person-centred principle or a feeling, as much as it was a measurable quality. Implicitly, in the very existence of this research and the nature of the recommendations made, there was a belief that patients and staff wanted to perceive the hospital as clean and that white walls continued to be an important part of that goal. Later chapters of this book show that white fell out of fashion in the post-war years, as the colour palette of modernity expanded, but this is not to say that it was replaced entirely. White remained important – and appreciated – as a marker of hygiene throughout the century. This is no surprise considering that problems such as hospital-acquired illness and infections were an ongoing risk to staff and patients.[61] There are some limited surveys of patients' experiences of hospitals in the archive, which indicate that the King's Fund was correct that cleanliness was a perpetual concern. Patients who commented on the ward atmosphere in these surveys commonly linked the concepts of lightness, air, and cleanliness: comments included 'light, airy and clean', 'clean and airy', and 'open, bright & light'.[62] Some of this 'lightness' was about windows as much as wall colour, perhaps linking to ideas about the therapeutic potential of ultra-violet light and its power to kill bacteria. Occasionally patients complained that they wanted more vibrant colours as – to quote one respondent – the 'egg-shell white room with the pink window trim was terribly dreary and institutional looking'.[63] These latter comments were generally rare though, and it is unclear from the archive whether they related to the same ward as the other more positive feedback. In general, these surveys indicate that responses to hospital design remained highly personal. There was growing demand for brighter colours and patterns, alongside an enduring, positive connection made by many patients between lightness, 'modern' spaces, and cleanliness. This combination of continuity and change was complementary, rather than in tension.

Some hospital staff resisted the use of textured surfaces in spaces where true hygiene was required. Kresen Kernow archive holds a particularly interesting example from the Cornwall and Isles of Scilly Area Health Authority, relating to a pharmacy extension in 1976.[64] A member of staff pushed back against the ceiling covering specifically on the basis that it was Artex and therefore not 'easily cleaned' or 'washable'. This complaint was in direct opposition to the architect's claim that 'this treatment gives a hard, washable surface well within the requirements of a type B finish', chosen because of its resistance to cracking.[65] Based on practical experience and with the support of the Medicines Inspector, the staff member wrote in firm opposition to this claim that Artex was 'washable'. Significantly, the main area of concern was the Aseptic Suite, in which it was proposed to put a painted ceiling board over the Artex. The use of textured surfaces to create a feeling of hygiene was, then, only possible in certain parts of the hospital and not in those that required true asepsis.

Rooms such as the operating theatre also required genuine asepsis, which could not be satisfied with any strategic use of textured paints or stippled colour. It was actually this requirement that led white to be abandoned in the early twentieth century, in favour of green in the operating theatre. White was – in Jeanne Kisacky's words – 'literally a pain in the eyes for doctors', causing eyestrain in the operating theatre, and green was seen as a more restful colour.[66] These ideas were widely evident in medical literature; Figure 1.6 shows an advert from 1961 for 'green and blue operating materials' to reduce 'the glare of ordinary white materials' in the operating theatre. In relation to seeing blood on clothing or surfaces, it was also increasingly accepted that a red/green colour contrast was clearer than red/white. By mid-century, then, it was known that white was not always the most practical colour in hygiene terms. However, it remained the dominant spatial and social signifier of cleanliness, and many operating theatres remained white throughout the century.

In other parts of the hospital, particularly patient-facing areas that were not '"hygiene" areas', the materiality of paint became

xxiv

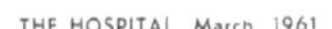

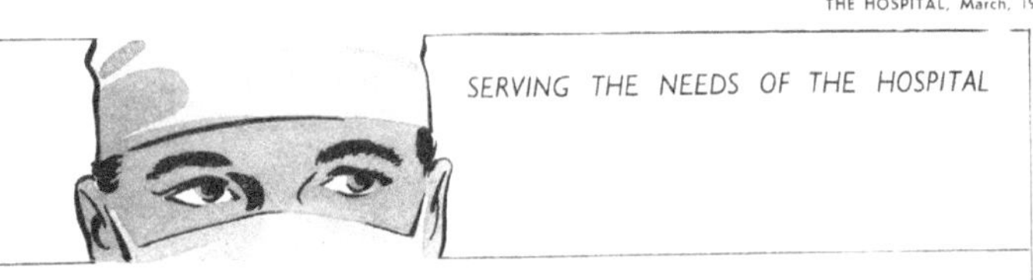

Restful COLOUR FOR THE EYES OF SURGEONS AND NURSES . . .

The glare of ordinary white materials used in the theatre imposes severe strain on the eyes of Surgeons and Nurses. Stethos green and blue operating materials have met with universal approval. They are fast dyed and withstand constant steam sterilisation. J. H. Bounds Ltd. will be pleased to send patterns and prices of Stethos operating gowns, caps, sheets, towels, and all other operating equipment in colours or in white.

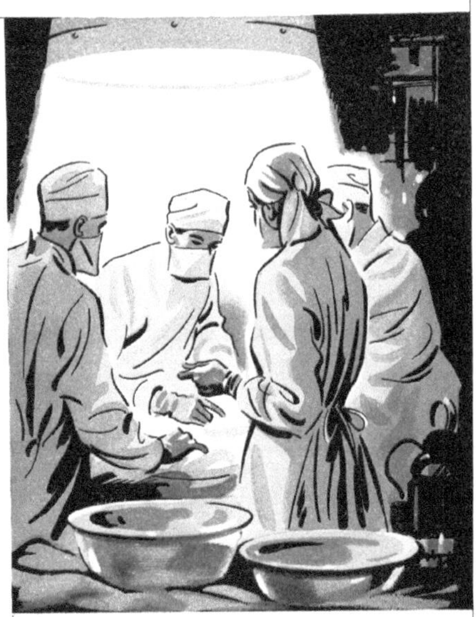

J. H. BOUNDS
LIMITED
STETHOS HOUSE
68 SACKVILLE STREET
MANCHESTER 1
TELEPHONES: CENTRAL 7331-4 · 4 LINES
TELEGRAMS: TENDER MANCHESTER

SPECIALISED CONSULTANCY SERVICE

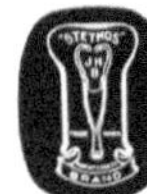

J. H. Bounds Ltd. also offer an efficiently planned textile and Nurses uniform service to Regional Hospital Boards and Management Committees. No problem is too great or small and no region too remote for J. H. Bounds Ltd. to send their consultant specialists.

Figure 1.6 *The Hospital*, March 1961, p. xxiv. Every effort has been made to trace the copyright holders and obtain permission to reproduce this material. Please do get in touch with any enquiries or information about this image or the rights holder. Copy held and scanned by University of Bristol Special Collections. All rights reserved and permission to use this figure must be obtained from the copyright holder.

an important part of the illusion of cleanliness. One 1955 book by the Newcastle Regional Hospital Board, *The Use of Colour in Hospitals*, noted that matt surfaces were difficult to clean and were not advised beyond ceilings. The Board recommended semi-gloss paint, which created a 'restful atmosphere' in wards because 'the slight lustre [...] gives room interiors a more lively and a cleaner appearance than that resulting from entirely matt surfaces'.[67] It is significant, however, that the book also emphasised that semi-gloss surfaces were not the most hygienic. Gloss paint was the most effective for hygiene purposes due to 'the resistance of the hard smooth surface [...] to the collecting of dirt and dust and to the wearing effect of constant washing-down'.[68] However, the 'dazzle' from this surface negatively affected patients, and its reflective sheen highlighted imperfections on wall surfaces. The careful use of paint, even for plain white surfaces, tells an important story. Carefully deployed semi-gloss white paint was not purely an instrument of hygienic control: it was used to create a 'cleaner appearance' for those in the spaces.

Hospital administrators grew increasingly frustrated over time with the distinction between 'real' and 'apparent' cleanliness. This is most evident in discussions over hospital flooring, which carried some of the same properties as the paint discussed to date. In 1966, an article in *The Architectural Review* noted that an Edinburgh hospital extension had terrazzo and vinyl floors that were 'white in colour so as to encourage meticulous maintenance'.[69] However, maintenance and cleanliness should not be taken as synonymous. In the 1980s, *Hospital Development* observed the ongoing conflation in relation to floor cleaning: '[t]he "if it's shiny, it must be clean" syndrome is still very prevalent'.[70] A similar complaint was made in 1985, when it was observed that 'the high cost of keeping up this level of *apparent* cleanliness is not justified in terms of *real* cleanliness because light reflection and true cleanliness are totally and absolutely unrelated'.[71] The difference between 'apparent' and 'real' cleanliness was commonplace, whether in the form of shiny polished floors or textured white walls. The practice of making the hospital 'shiny' was in part for the benefit of patients, who would have been reassured by the illusion of hygiene. By 1985 there was a growing sense that this was no longer true: the *Hospital Development* article also observed that highly polished floors created a 'cold, institutional atmosphere' and could be difficult for elderly patients.[72] The same might have been true for white paint by this time, when the 'all-white' hospital was a thing of the past, and – as Chapter 5 shows – white was being increasingly used to enhance or reflect bright colours.

A careful study of white paint challenges some assumptions about the purpose of white walls and surfaces in hospitals. White walls were probably never as consistently clear, white, and controlling in the early twentieth-century 'machine for healing' as assumed; they were also not incompatible with person-centred design. The careful curation of white paint in hospitals indicates that it was used not entirely for practical purposes, but also to reassure people. Even when 'all-white' walls fell out of fashion, hospitals continued to use white paint carefully, considering factors such as the reflective qualities of gloss paint, to meet the needs of patients for rest and care, rather than to maintain hygiene. The hygienic and humanistic were often intertwined throughout the twentieth century, rather than in opposition.

A clean bill of health: sheets and toilets

White walls became less common in hospitals over the course of the twentieth century, but white objects, fixtures, and fittings remained a feature. They represent continuity amidst change, in two ways. Firstly, these objects were kept as symbols of hygiene, even as there was a shift towards brighter colour as the marker of modernity. Secondly, they show that this association with whiteness was – throughout the twentieth century – materially unstable. White objects represented hygiene because they showed dirt so easily, but this depended on regular and often visible cleaning. In line with Eviatar Zerubavel's influential 1979 study on time in hospitals, these cleaning routines ordered time (and colour in time) through their repeated sequences, durations, locations, and regular rates of recurrence.[73] This section focuses on such cleaning practices in relation to two types of white objects in hospitals, which were materially different: white linen and white toilets.

In 1947, *The Lancet* published an article on Birmingham Home for the Elderly in which it noted that '[w]hite bedspreads, though they look rather bleak, have been deliberately chosen, because the first signs of soiling are easier to detect on white than on coloured materials'.[74] Although this specific article relates to a 'home' for the elderly rather than a hospital, its comments about white linens are equally relevant to hospitals and particularly so-called 'geriatric' wards. The use of the word 'bleak' here might have represented a cultural shift in the meanings and experience of white in healthcare, and an implicit recognition that colourful bedspreads were more desirable by this time. The bedspreads were also 'bleak' for a more practical reason: they showed soiling. In this sense, there was something of a paradox, as the hygienic value of white walls or materials in practical terms (making dirt visible) could undermine the perception of a space as hygienic. White cloth played an important role in the spatial production of hygiene and modernity, but only if it was kept white.

In addition to the problems of soiling on a day-to-day basis, white bedding was discoloured through repeated washing. In a 1966 report by the British Launderers' Research Association on 'Chemical Disinfection of Hospital Woollen Blankets', the problem of 'real' versus perceived hygiene was raised yet again. The process of disinfection through boiling meant that blankets became discoloured, as they needed to be repeatedly boiled in brass machines.[75] Similar concerns can be seen in a trial of mattresses by the King's Fund in the early 1960s, in which extensive tests evaluated how mattress covers responded to the cleaning required in hospitals; some reports focused entirely on discolouration and staining, irrespective of the outcome in sanitation terms.[76] The commitment not only to hygienic practices but to keeping linens *white* is significant here. Even off-white would have served the practical purposes outlined above, indicating that there was a symbolic factor to these concerns as much as a practical one.

White coats provide another symbolically important white linen in the hospital, for which cleaning and germ control is relevant. In experiential terms, encounters with the white coat have always been complex, as it has long operated as both a marker of power and of care. As one Mass Observation respondent noted in 1984, 'to a patient, anyone wearing a white coat is a doctor' even though that was not always the case.[77] As Gesler noted in *Healing Places*, the white coat has also always been highly personal; for some people, for example those with Alzheimer's, the 'white coat may remind one of medical crises' from their past.[78] For others, the white coat represented authority in a way that might have been reassuring.[79] The infamous white coat was phased out in Britain – as it was in many other locations including North America – in the early 2000s, ironically in part because its cotton and/or polyester material was thought to be 'a harbinger of infection'.[80] It is significant that the white coat was kept for so long despite its known impracticality, especially with the decline of on-site NHS laundries. Kenya Hara also emphasises that the whiteness of the white coat is a very specific shade of white: 'not even a vague, unbleached white [...] a fastidious, bright white [...] Perhaps the whiteness forces the wearer to take pains to stay as clean as possible'.[81] This point is an important reminder that different shades of white could serve different functions, and that the brightest shade was designed to hide no speck of dirt.

Though white linens usefully showed dirt quickly, as with white walls it was not always desirable for them to do so. Unlike white paint, however, there was no possible turn to a textured or 'gloss' linen that gave the impression of hygiene without the labour of cleaning. However, these linens were kept throughout the twentieth century; the bright white coat was seemingly kept for symbolic rather than hygienic reasons. As with many of the white surfaces discussed above, then, white linens can be situated in a history of patient-oriented hospitals as much as they can be viewed as mechanisms of power. They also demonstrate that whiteness was never static. The hygienic qualities of white linens and uniforms were brought into being through a range of cleaning practices, rather than being stable or consistent.

Objects of sanitation provide another example of fixtures that stayed white into the late twentieth century, and which required regular cleaning.[82] White baths continued to be used in hospitals throughout the century, including white tiled pools for treatments such as hydrotherapy.[83] Although colourful toilets were becoming more popular in the mid-twentieth century, with coloured bathrooms arguably reaching their zenith in 1970s homes, there is no evidence that hospitals followed this trend.[84] It is only in recent years that there has been a shift to colour contrast and darker toilet seats, as part of inclusive design practices. More commonly, twentieth-century hospitals were dominated by white porcelain toilets and sinks – or even white seats on stainless steel bases.[85] These carried the visual qualities of hygiene, though they were used regularly and only operated as symbols of hygiene if their whiteness was maintained.[86] Surveys conducted by the King's Fund in the late 1960s revealed toilet cleanliness and hygiene to be a recurrent concern, despite the regularity with which cleaners tackled them: 'whilst the baths and toilets were regularly cleaned', one patient complained, 'by virtue of the numbers using them they quickly became soiled'.[87]

Historical sources from the perspective of hospital cleaners are extremely rare, but more recent works show the importance of routine to them. One cleaner, who has worked in NHS hospitals since the 1980s, spoke in a recent interview about the need for constant maintenance of particular objects – including white and wipe-down ones – such as toilets: 'how many times I go round with my toilet? Four times a day, I go around. In the morning, after my break, after my lunch and before I go'.[88] The routine of cleaners and their schedule is also significant here. This work is predominantly done in the daytime, when there is more activity in the hospital and when the light makes dirt more visible. Hygiene is thus a temporal spatial quality, with the clean gleam of white most important in bright light. The meaning of the clean, white toilet is also created through its visual opposition to other, dirty objects. This cleaner notes that equipment is colour-coded: 'the bits for the toilet' are red, while 'high dusting' is blue and the kitchen has a 'green bucket'.[89] This colour-coding is in itself a hygienic practice and ritual of separating and sorting different types of contaminant. It is significant that none of the cleaning products mentioned are white, which thus maintains its status as uncontaminated and pure. Lisa Baraitser notes that 'it is structural to both patriarchy and capitalism that the labour of maintenance remains hidden', and the cleaner indeed has often been an unseen or disempowered figure in the hospital.[90] However, their work is made visible by the maintenance of white objects – such as toilets – at regular intervals.

The use of visible ritual and routine to manage dirt, and mitigate the fear of contamination, is not new.[91] The precise sorting system discussed here is relatively recent, likely introduced as a consistent NHS system as part of the 2007 National Colour Coding Scheme to control harmful bacteria. However, colour sorting in hospitals had a much longer history and was often practised in a more localised way.

There are articles in medical journals from the 1970s and 1980s that do not mention specific colours, but note that there was a colour-based sorting scheme in place in British hospitals for contaminated objects and linens.[92] There is also a long history in pharmacies of using coloured bottles or labels to mark out dangerous substances. Dark colours such as black, red, green, or blue – along with ridged, shaped, or textured bottles – were introduced to avoid accidental poisoning in the nineteenth century.[93] Clear and smooth bottles represent safety and purity. The use of colour in these contexts was not purely practical: the specific colours that were chosen reinforced social, cultural, moral, and spatial hierarchies about the superiority of whiteness or clarity as the marker of purity.

White objects were never abandoned in the modern hospital. Undoubtedly some of this continuity was the consequence of practical and budget concerns, but these objects were also highly meaningful and their whiteness should not be dismissed as simply an 'absence'. White objects remained a key and active part of the material environment of healthcare throughout the twentieth century. They lingered as an important symbol of hygiene in healthcare settings, long after white walls were replaced by brighter colour schemes. This section has also indicated that it is also useful to think more closely about exactly how white operated as a symbol of hygiene and the ways in which it was sometimes undermined. White objects were often soiled or damaged, and required maintenance and cleaning. The meaning and effects of white objects – and the power that they held as symbols of hygiene – were temporal and unstable, depending on whether they were clean. The qualities of whiteness were also created through the act of cleaning itself, and perhaps by the witnessing of this ritual, as part of an ongoing and repeated part of hospital life.

Care and control: populating spaces

White walls, sheets, coats, toilets, and sinks did not simply exist: they needed to be maintained, repaired, washed, cleaned, worn, viewed, and felt. The meanings of whiteness were co-produced with hospital staff, visitors, patients and service users as part of an ongoing process. This section moves on to the different people in hospitals, and how they could shape the meanings and experience of whiteness. It explores factors such as age and race, and the concepts of care and power, to show that whiteness was a relational concept rather than a monolithic one.

The early twentieth-century 'all-white' hospital can be viewed differently when people are put into the picture. Figure 1.7, for example, shows a new clinical block at Great Ormond Street Hospital in 1939. This room not only had wipe-down white walls and tiles, but many other white objects. Symbols of hygiene included white lights, sinks, bedding, tray support, and bed frame, combined with extensive glass and mirrors, and wipe-down tiled floor coverings and shiny fittings. Significantly, there is also a child in the bed; this image differs from many of those available in architectural journals, and from some of the other images discussed, such as the 1937 ward shown in Figure 1.4.

This room presents, at first glance, as a highly sterile space. However, the presence of a person tucked into white sheets in bed, the activity of reading books, and the glimpse of flowers in the corner of the image are important reminders that the ward was inhabited. Colour was brought in through other elements and objects, perhaps chosen by a child or their parents. Missing from the image are other elements that might have contributed to the 'hygienic' quality of this room, from sunlight through the window to the white uniforms of doctors and nurses. Constance Classen reminds us that objects are never just looked at; she notes that by putting 'artefacts' in museum cases, they are 'abstracted from a dynamic context of multisensory uses and meanings and transformed into static objects for the gaze'.[94] Photographs such as Figure 1.7 risk doing the same. This photograph is a staged image of a room that, in practice, would have been dynamic. The child would have been interacting with surrounding objects, for example by using the sink and splashing toothpaste on tiles, or spilling food on the white linen. The white objects and shiny fittings were not necessarily static and clean. Again, a material and relational approach to white objects challenges ideas that whiteness in hospitals always represented order.

Figure 1.7 also raises questions about the different people who used hospitals, and what white objects meant to them. It is difficult to know whether a child would have felt and embodied the ward as a hygienic space, and whether that was positive for a young

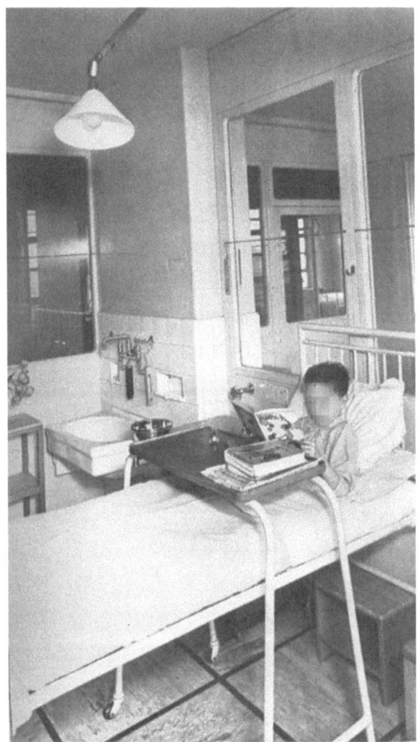

Figure 1.7 Image from Great Ormond Street Hospital 1939 Annual Report © Reproduced with kind permission of Archive Service, Great Ormond Street Hospital for Children NHS Foundation Trust.

person. In general, children's hospitals had long veered towards the brighter end of the colour spectrum in order to provoke distraction and a sense of 'homeliness'. In the late nineteenth century, painted picture tiles offered a colourful and hygienic form of decoration for children's wards in British hospitals.[95] In Figure 1.7, such distraction was offered through other objects and forms of entertainment, while the colourful picture tiles were replaced with plain white. Who, then, were the white and wipe-down objects *for* in children's hospitals, if previous painted tiles had served the same hygienic purpose? As with white walls, ceilings, floors, and corridors, they were intended to create a *feeling* of cleanliness as much as a reality. In this case, the feeling may have been more important for visitors than the children themselves. For anxious parents, the room depicted in Figure 1.7 might have been reassuringly modern and hygienic. It is significant that this image was shared as part of the GOSH Annual Report, as an example of good design practice in the 1930s.

The history of whiteness shifts when it is considered in relation to a specific person, or type of person. The 1930s children's ward requires some speculation and photographic interpretation to demonstrate this point, but other sources make it more explicit. Turning to the more recent history of hospitals, there is great richness in the flourishing of the genre of pathography or published 'illness memoir'. To take just one of many possible examples: encounters with the large, white Computed Tomography (CT) scanner feature regularly in such texts set in the 1990s. In *Patient*, Ben Watt describes the CT scanner as a 'big white doughnut', while in 'Because Cowards Get Cancer Too', John Diamond wrote that '[t]he great thing about the CT scan is that it looks just like prime-time viewers think the medicine of the future ought to look: white, clean, non-invasive'.[96] The initial appearance of the machine and its sleek, white, modern qualities reassured patients in an otherwise difficult and uncomfortable situation. Diamond noted that – despite all the surface-level 'reassuring' qualities of the CT scan's appearance – in practice, encountering the machine also came with a host of unpleasant sensory experiences, anxiety and a feeling of claustrophobia when 'enclosed'.[97] Whiteness was 'reassuring' and futuristic to Diamond, rather than dehumanising and scary; the appearance of the machine was a counter-balance to the stressful sensory experience of the scan. Another person might have viewed this 'white, clean' machine differently, depending on their emotional state, attitude to technology, levels of pain, and more. It is impossible to extrapolate from a single person's impression of whiteness in hospital over time, but such experiences are still noteworthy. Whiteness was a co-produced and relational quality, not simply a colour (or absence of colour) that projected a single, shared meaning into hospitals.

The discussion to this point has provided two very different examples, from the early and later twentieth century, to show that whiteness must be considered in relation to people. Both indicate that what might be stressful and 'sterile' to one person could be experienced as 'care' to another; this has undoubtedly been true across time and place. The viewer of whiteness has always been a co-producer of its meaning(s). People were also part of a wider web of relations in hospitals, and the meanings of whiteness were shaped by human behaviours, acts, rituals, and interactions. The staff delivering trolleys stacked with fresh white linens or white teacups provide one such example.[98] The qualities of care were brought into being through a relationship between white objects, their sensory qualities, and the different people in hospitals. Figure 1.8 depicts a smiling domestic staff member serving tea at Homerton Hospital in 1990, showing a plethora of white plates, cups, bowls, and wipe-down trolley tops. In theory such shiny white surfaces, combined with chrome, should have been signifiers of hygiene but in this context they were symbols of domesticity and care.

Cups, jugs, and plates – such as those on the trolley in Figure 1.8 – did not have meaning on their own. They needed to be part of a ritual to represent care: tea was served at the same time daily, often by the same staff members (or staff in the same uniforms). Tea in white cups was part of a routine involving other sensory stimuli such as sound and smell. As with all white objects, the materiality of the cups was important. Those in Figure 1.8 appear to be ceramic cups and plates, which would make a bright sound when in contact with a teaspoon, and have the comforting feel of non-institutional cups from home. The whiteness of the hospital cups was balanced with the material feeling of homeliness. They differed from the white plastic cups increasingly used for medication or water over the late twentieth century, and from other disposable cups and cutlery that were becoming commonplace in hospitals by the end of the century. These cups were sturdy, firm, and part of the material representation of care.

Figure 1.8 also draws attention to the different people who spent time in hospitals, including not only patients but a range of members of staff beyond the clinical. The 'white coat' discussed above was not the only uniform seen in hospitals, of course. It is difficult to know from the archival image what colour the uniform was at Homerton Hospital, but other records indicate that there were somewhat hierarchical uniform colours at work elsewhere. In Ben Watt's *Patient*, in relation to his time in the recovery ward of a

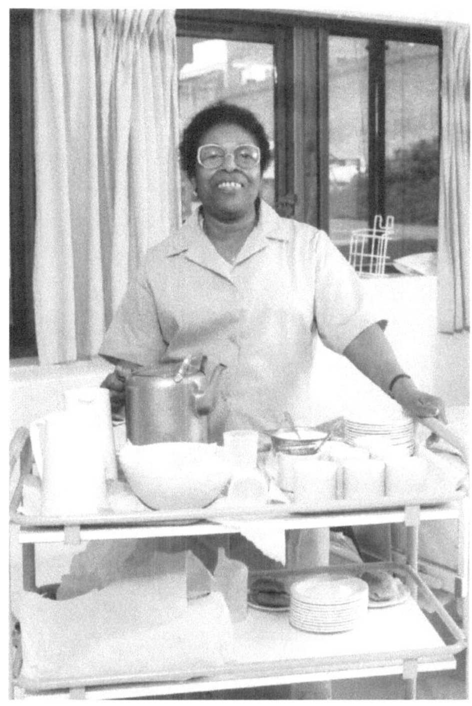

Figure 1.8 Lucia B., domestic at Homerton Hospital. Reproduced with permission of Barts Health NHS Trust archive, 1990. SBHB/MP/4/2/3/12.

London hospital in the 1990s, he notes that, '[a]lmost all the women on the staff were black. They wore bright yellow nylon dresses [...]. Hot, weak tea came round with Marie biscuits at around eleven, and again at four'.[99] Watt emphasises the importance of ritual and of the staff uniform colour, a bright yellow evoking sunlight and cheer. It might be significant that Watt not only notes that Black women were serving tea, but also that they wore 'bright yellow' dresses. The linking of race and yellow clothing here might not be coincidental. Lynda Nead argues that clothing and colour – and their representation in visual culture – have long been key to the construction of race by 'defining both the restrained, neutral look of the white nation and the … excesses of the new black African and Caribbean immigrants'.[100] This point has always been pertinent in the NHS, particularly as the 1948 British Nationality Act brought many (much needed) migrant workers to the health system.[101] Watt's comment about the colourful uniforms of Black staff members must be placed in such a longer history.

The colourful uniforms of domestic staff are in conspicuous opposition to the white coat. While yellow might have been a cheerful colour, white has long been seen as a symbol of superiority. As Philip C. Russell notes, the white coat carried many cultural associations, including 'being morally or spiritually pure or stainless, spotless, innocent; free from malignity or evil intent; beneficent; opposed to something characterized as black (i.e. death); highly prized, precious; fair seeming'.[102] It is no accident that those further towards the perceived 'top' of the hospital hierarchy have been more likely to wear white throughout the twentieth century. In terms of the racial issues raised above, this is a complicated picture. Staffing at all levels of the NHS is racially and ethnically diverse, but there has also always been racial inequality. A recent report by the King's Fund noted that 'as the pay bands increase, the proportion of ethnic minority staff within those bands decreases, from 24.5 per cent at band 5 to 6.5 per cent at very senior manager level'.[103] This means that patients have always been more likely to see white people in white coats. These trends have also long been evident in visual culture; Roberta Bivins, for instance, gives an example of a *Daily Mail* cartoon from 2013 in which 'the racialized nurse figure operates as a stand-in for *all* Mid-Staffordshire nurses, just as its two white male figures – a traditionally white-coated doctor, and a plump and be-suited manager – represent the other hospital professionals'.[104] Bivins shows that there were also representations of Black and Asian doctors in NHS visual culture, but that they were more ambivalent than representations of nurses.

While 'whiteness' is being discussed here primarily in spatial and material terms, rather than in terms of race, the two cannot always be separated. As Kirsty Dootson argues, there are 'intimate connections between the politics of colour-as-hue and the politics of colour-as-race', not least because whiteness is treated as a 'benchmark against which all colours are measured'.[105] Again, this is an important reminder that whiteness – as hue and as race – must be simply treated not as a 'norm', an absence, or a benchmark. Kathleen Connellan notes that 'white has been used architecturally and architectonically to influence or, more specifically, control people especially through white spaces and white places'.[106] In hospitals, Connellan argues, white ensures that there is 'nowhere to hide' and is a feature of large institutions keen on the 'order' of the bodies within them. These meanings apply to white walls and white coats alike. Racial hierarchy is one such type of 'order', power, and control, and the whiteness of hospital spaces, objects, and uniforms was one way of seeking to maintain this order.

Such links between 'whiteness' and 'purity' have long had social implications. Critical race theorists have shown how links between whiteness, cleanliness, physical purity, and moral purity have operated to reinforce racial hierarchies and power systems in a range of contexts.[107] There is also an extensive literature in anthropology and cultural history about the symbolism of 'dirt' and the ways in which control of dirt can be used to manage wider disorder (or disorderly bodies).[108] As Anne McClintock argues, Victorian Britain had shown a 'fascination with clean, white bodies and clean, white clothing'; the legacies of such ideas continued well into the twentieth century.[109] The relationship between whiteness, lightness, brightness, hygiene, purity, and superiority that has long been culturally embedded in Britain cannot be neatly disentangled from the racial implications of whiteness in hospital design.[110] The idea that white walls continued to symbolise hygiene and that white coats continued to mark out superiority, even in the context of the rise of colour as a marker of modernity, was interwoven with the racial and imperial politics of post-war Britain.

This section has highlighted the importance of examining whiteness, and white materialities, in relation to the people who spent time in hospitals. It has explored two very different themes: the ways in which whiteness could operate to produce atmospheres of care, and the role of whiteness in creating social hierarchies. In so doing, it has drawn attention to the fact that whiteness cannot be treated as a 'one size fits all' category with single meanings. This section has explored age and race as two factors that affect the meanings and impacts of whiteness in hospitals, but gender and class would have also been possible and important categories of analysis. Whiteness was a relational category. It was experienced in different ways depending upon the other objects and people in the room, the activities taking place, *and* the social and cultural contexts.

Conclusions

In the 1920s and 1930s, journalist and novelist Joseph Roth travelled Europe and wrote of his 'Wanderings in Europe between the Wars' in a collection later translated as *The Hotel Years*. He wrote, in his reflections on visiting a café, that,

> The colour of the age is white, laboratory white, as white as the room where they invented lewisite, white as a church, white as a bathroom, white as a dissecting room, white as steel and white as chalk, white as hygiene, white as a butcher's apron, white as an operating table, white as death, and white as the age's fear of death! Let's brighten up the ceiling! – Because it is the age's belief that white is cheerful. It wants by brightness to attract cheerful people. And the people are as merry as patients, and the present is as merry as a hospital.[111]

In this extract, Roth draws attention to the prevalence of white in early twentieth-century Europe, the varied connotations of white at the time, and – perhaps most importantly – the notion that whiteness as 'hygiene' or 'operating theatre' or even 'death' was not incompatible with whiteness as 'brightness' or 'cheer'. This latter point is often forgotten by those writing about whiteness in hospitals, as features such as long white corridors are increasingly cited as evidence of bleakness, dehumanisation, and misery. In 1993, junior health minister Tom Sackville commented that 'traditionally, people have thought of hospitals as firstly functional and secondly clinical – complete with very efficient long passages which are often a rather dirty off-white all the way down'.[112] Research on cancer hospitals published in 2013 showed that some patients were vocal about hospital spaces that were thought to be overly white, describing them as 'too clinical, too clean … too cold'.[113] Whiteness was thus situated firmly in opposition to the 'human' in memories of older hospitals.

It is best to understand this trend (pitting functional, clinical white against more humanistic, or stimulating, colours of the late twentieth century) as something of a cultural trope. Whiteness operated in many ways in the twentieth-century hospital at any given time. Depending on the context, white could be: a mechanism to control germs and create asepsis (the pharmacy); a strategy to create the impression of hygiene (textured paint); a symbol of care (the tea cup); a means of promoting rest (the reduced glare of an off-white ceiling); a signifier of power or control (the white coat); or a sign of disrepair or disorder (soiled bed linen). Colour – rather than its absence – came to be the marker of modernity, but whiteness endured as a valuable marker of hygiene and a key part of the everyday life of hospitals.

Notes

1 Much of this chapter is reproduced from Victoria Bates, 'Cold White of Day: White, Colour, and Materiality in the Twentieth-Century British Hospital', *Twentieth Century British History*, 34 (2023), pp. 1–37, though the article has been updated and expanded for the purposes of the book.

2 D. W. A. McCreadie, 'A Hospital Colour Scheme', *BMJ*, 16 June 1962, p. 1687.

3 Peter Scher, 'Northern Exposure', *Hospital Development*, 24 (1993), p. 31.

4 Mark Wigley, *White Walls, Designer Dresses: The Fashioning of Modern Architecture* (MIT Press, 2001), xiv.

5 Kassia St Clair, *The Secret Lives of Colour* (John Murray, 2017).

6 Kenya Hara, *100 Whites* (Lars Müller Publishers, 2019), i.

7 Karsten Lichau, 'Soundproof Silences? Towards a Sound History of Silence', *International Journal for History, Culture and Modernity*, (2019), p. 840.

8 On the role of migrant workers in the NHS see Roberta E. Bivins, *Contagious Communities: Medicine, Migration, and the NHS in Post-War Britain* (Oxford University Press, 2015); and Julian M. Simpson, *Migrant Architects of the NHS: South Asian Doctors and the Reinvention of British General Practice* (Manchester University Press, 2018).

9 Susan Barclay, 'When It's Not the Main Game: Art in Hospitals' (PhD Dissertation: University of Western Sydney, 2015), p. 70. White tiles were also described in a number of late nineteenth-century hospital reports, such as 'The Children's Hospital, Birmingham', *The Hospital*, April 1890, p. 15.

10 Theodora Philcox, 'The Sink in the Hall: How pandemics transform architecture', *Psyche*, https://psyche.co/ideas/the-sink-in-the-hall-how-pandemics-transform-architecture [accessed: 12 August 2021].

11 'The Hospital Workshop', *The Hospital* (April 1890), p. 15; 'The New Infirmary at Newcastle', *BMJ* (July 1906), pp. 91–2; John Campbell, 'Some Modern Maternity Hospitals, with Plans and Illustrations: Belfast Maternity Hospital', *Journal of Obstetrics and Gynaecology* (April 1908), p. 281.

12 Sir Henry Burdett, 'Reports on Hospitals of the United Kingdom', *The Hospital* (December 1913), p. 253.

13 Margaret Campbell, 'What Tuberculosis did for Modernism: The Influence of a Curative Environment on Modernist Design and Architecture', *Medical History*, 49 (2005), p. 487.

14 See Elina Riksman, 'The Colour Scheme', in Nina Heikkonen (ed.), *Paimio Sanatorium Conservation Management Plan 2016* (Alvar Aalto Foundation, 2016), pp. 183–9.

15 Paul Overy, *Light, Air and Openness: Modern Architecture between the Wars* (Thames & Hudson Ltd, 2007). Le Corbusier was also actually very interested in colour, but white was a key feature of his buildings and his name has come to be associated with whiteness; see Maria-Cristina Florian, 'The Myth of Pure White Architecture: How Architects of Modernity Used Color', 3 August 2023, https://www.archdaily.com/1004970/the-myth-of-pure-white-architecture-how-architects-of-modernity-used-color [accessed: 14 May 2024].

16 Cansu Degirmencioglu and Deniz Avci-Hosanli, 'Transient yet Settled: The Rooms for Tuberculosis Patients in Turkish Sanatoria', *Res Mobilis*, 13 (2023), p. 66.

17 William Rollins, 'A Nation in White: Germany's Hygienic Consensus and the Ambiguities of Modernist Architecture', *German Politics & Society*, 19 (2001), pp. 1–2.

18 John Potvin, 'The Writing is on the (Lavatory) Wall: Haptic Presence, Modern Design and the Traces of Community', in Andrew Gorman-Murray and Matt Cook (eds), *Queering the Interior* (Routledge, 2020), pp. 161–71; Peter Jones, 'Building the Empire of the Gaze: The Modern Movement and the Surveillance Society', *Architectural Theory Review*, 4 (1999), pp. 1–14.

19 Wil Gesler, Morag Bell, Sarah Curtis, Phil Hubbard, and Susan Francis, 'Therapy by Design: Evaluating the UK Hospital Building Program', *Health & Place*, 10 (2004), p. 120. On the link between hospitals and modern city design see Jonathan Hughes, 'Hospital-City', *Architectural History*, 40 (1997), p. 268.

20 Stuart W. Leslie, '*Rise of the Modern Hospital: An Architectural History of Health and Healing, 1870–1940* by Jeanne Kisacky (review)', *Bulletin of the History of Medicine*, 92 (2018), p. 392.
21 Mark Wigley, *White Walls, Designer Dresses: The Fashioning of Modern Architecture* (MIT Press, 2001), p. xvi.
22 Lucas Crawford, *Transgender Architectonics: The Shape of Change in Modernist Space* (Ashgate, 2015), p. 143.
23 Michel Pastoureau, *White: The History of a Color*, trans. Jody Gladding (Princeton University Press, 2023 [2022]), pp. 8, 36.
24 St Clair, *The Secret Lives of Colour.*
25 Jane L. Stevens Crawshaw, *Plague Hospitals: Public Health for the City in Early Modern Venice* (Routledge, 2016).
26 Annmarie Adams, 'Modernism and Medicine: The Hospitals of Stevens and Lee, 1916–1932', *The Journal of the Society of Architectural Historians*, 58 (1999), p. 43.
27 Adams, 'Modernism and Medicine', p. 58. For similar comments about the dominance of all-white (or off-white) modernism by the 1960s, see Erika Dyck, 'Spaced-Out in Saskatchewan: Modernism, Anti-Psychiatry, and Deinstitutionalization, 1950–1968', *Bulletin of the History of Medicine*, 84 (2010), pp. 640–66.
28 Talinn Grigor, 'The King's White Walls: Modernism and Bourgeois Architecture', in Bianca Devos and Christoph Werner (eds), *Culture and Cultural Politics under Reza Shah* (Routledge, 2014), pp. 95–118; Sigal Davidi, 'By Women for Women: Modernism, Architecture, and Gender in Building the New Jewish Society in Mandatory Palestine', *arq: Architectural Research Quarterly*, 20 (2016), pp. 217–30; Pyrs Gruffudd, 'Science and the Stuff of Life: Modernist Health Centres in 1930s London', *Journal of Historical Geography*, 27 (2001), pp. 395–416.
29 Elizabeth Darling and Alistair Fair, '"The Core": The Centre as a Concept in Twentieth-Century British Planning and Architecture. Part One: The Emergence of the Idea', *Planning Perspectives*, 38 (2023), pp. 69–98.
30 C. L. Emmerson, 'The Field Ambulance – An Alternative Name?', *BMJ Military Health*, 56 (1931), p. 397.
31 Bruce Peter, 'Review: Re-forming Britain: Narratives of Modernity before Reconstruction', *Modernism/modernity*, 16 (2009), pp. 450–1; Campbell, 'What Tuberculosis did for Modernism', p. 467.
32 Bruce Peter notes that modernism with a capital M tends to focus 'on practitioners and theorists whose modernist credentials are universally accepted'. The capital M usually refers to the more self-aware 'Modern

Movement' than the broader modernist aesthetic, with lowercase m. Peter, 'Re-forming Britain'.

33 RIBA Library, 'Kent and Canterbury Hospital, Canterbury: The Main Entrance', https://www.architecture.com/image-library/ribapix/image-information/poster/kent-and-canterbury-hospital-canterbury-the-main-entrance/posterid/RIBA23618.html [accessed: 25 May 2021].

34 'A Model to Copy', *Nursing Times*, 18 June 1941, pp. 528–9, with thanks to Mark Kerr, Clinical Librarian of East Kent Hospitals University NHS Foundation Trust for sharing this article.

35 See Greg Allen, 'Modernism: Any Color As Long As It's White', https://greg.org/archive/2006/08/16/modernism-any-color-as-long-as-its-white.html [accessed: 30 April 2024]. Thanks to Clare Hickman for drawing my attention to this.

36 'Police, Fire Brigade and Ambulance Services', http://www.igg.org.uk/gansg/00-app1/pfa.htm [accessed: 25 May 2021].

37 Wigley, *White Walls*, p. xvii.

38 'A Model to Copy'.

39 *Ibid.*

40 See Barbara Klinkhammer, 'Creation of the Myth: "White" Modernism', *92nd ACSA Annual Meeting* (2004), pp. 429–34.

41 'A Model to Copy'.

42 Sophie Crocker and David Leatherbarrow, 'The Closed Loop: Ninety Years of Health Care Architecture', *Design for Health*, 2 (2018), p. 24.

43 On the complexities of patients' experiences of sanatoria, see Heini Hakosalo, 'The Walled-in Illness: The Twentieth-Century Finnish Tuberculosis Sanatorium as Lived Space', in Johanna Annola, Hanna Lindberg, and Pirjo Markkola (eds), *Lived Institutions as History of Experience* (Springer Nature, 2023), pp. 213–38.

44 See 'Finsbury Health Centre', *Municipal Dreams*, https://municipaldreams.wordpress.com/2013/04/09/finsbury-health-centre-nothing-is-too-good-for-ordinary-people/ [accessed: 1 February 2022]; and '100 Buildings 100 Years: Finsbury Health Centre', https://c20society.org.uk/100-buildings/1938-finsbury-health-centre-london [accessed: 1 February 2022].

45 On the 'radical' and socialist principles of the Finsbury Health Centre, which might be seen as anticipating the principles of the NHS, see Pyrs Gruffudd, 'Science and the Stuff of Life: Modernist Health Centres in 1930s London', *Journal of Historical Geography*, 27 (2001), pp. 395–416. The other 'landmark' modernist project of this period, the Pioneer Health Centre, broadly differed from NHS healthcare models.

46 'The Modern Kitchen', *Picture Post*, 26 February 1955, np. Thank you to Jennifer Crane for alerting me to this source.
47 Paul Atkinson, 'A Clean, White World', *Design for Health*, 2 (2018), pp. 1–3.
48 Wigley, *White Walls*, xviii.
49 On hospitals as a 'layered landscape' of old and new see also Alice Street, 'Affective Infrastructure: Hospital Landscapes of Hope and Failure', *Space and Culture*, 15 (2012), 44–56. Thank you to Anna Harris for alerting me to this work. On 'beautifying' hospitals see Jeremy Hugh Baron and Lesley Greene, 'Art in Hospitals', *BMJ* (December 1984, p. 1731.
50 Hara, *100 Whites*, pp. 12–13.
51 Richard Llewellyn Davies, 'Furniture and Fittings', *AJ* (July 1954), p. 147; 'Lighting', *AJ* (February 1952), p. 255.
52 Young, 'The Colours of Things', p. 180.
53 London Metropolitan Archives, 'Wall Surfaces (St. Bartholomew's Hospital)', A/KE/I/01/06/001–003.
54 David Charles Sloane and Beverlie Conant Sloane, *Medicine Moves to the Mall* (Johns Hopkins University Press, 2003), p. 108.
55 *Ibid.*
56 London Metropolitan Archive, 'Wall Surfaces'.
57 *Ibid.*
58 *Ibid.*
59 *Ibid.*
60 On the King's Fund's noise surveys, for example, see Victoria Bates, *Making Noise in the Modern Hospital* (Cambridge University Press, 2021).
61 On these wider contexts of concerns about cleanliness, risk, and safety, see Anne Marie Rafferty, Marguerite Dupree, and Fay Bound Alberti (eds), *Germs and Governance: The Past, Present and Future of Hospital Infection, Prevention and Control* (Manchester University Press, 2021).
62 London Metropolitan Archives, A/KE/I/01/059/017–22, 'Completed Patient Questionnaire Forms'.
63 'Completed Patient Questionnaire Forms', A/KE/I/01/059/017.
64 Kresen Kernow, AHA/142, 'Capital Schemes: Pharmacy Extension Royal Cornwall Hospital (Tresilke)'.
65 *Ibid.*
66 Jeanne Kisacky, 'Blood Red, Soothing Green, and Pure White: What Color Is Your Operating Room?', in Marilyn DeLong and Barbara Martinson (eds), *Color and Design* (A & C Black, 2013), pp. 118–24.

67 Newcastle Regional Hospital Board (NRHB), *The Use of Colour in Hospitals* (NRHB, 1955), p. 31.
68 NRHB, *Colour in Hospitals*, p. 32.
69 'Hospital Extension', *The Architectural Review*, 1 August 1966, p. 92.
70 Susan Black, 'Interior Design Trends', *Hospital Development*, 10 (1982), p. 24.
71 'Hospital Floor Maintenance Costs', *Hospital Development*, 13 (1985), p. 33.
72 *Ibid.*
73 Eviatar Zerubavel, *Patterns of Time in Hospital Life: A Sociological Perspective* (University of Chicago Press, 1979), cited in Andrew Georgiou, Johanna I. Westbrook, and Jeffrey Braithwaite, 'Time Matters – A Theoretical and Empirical Examination of the Temporal Landscape of a Hospital Pathology Service and the Impact of e-health', *Social Science & Medicine*, 72 (2011), pp. 1603–10.
74 'Modern Care of Old People', *The Lancet*, July 1947, p. 30.
75 J. C. Dickinson and R. E. Wagg, 'Chemical Disinfection of Hospital Woollen Blankets in Laundering', *Journal of Applied Bacteriology*, 29 (1966), pp. 357–64. It is a reasonable conclusion that the blankets were white based on the reference to 'white fluid' and because in another publication by the same the blankets are described as 'white, all wool, plain weave hospital blankets'; J. C. Dickinson, R. E. Wagg, and Susan Litchfield, 'Residual Bactericidal Action of Wool Blankets Laundered with Formaldehyde: A Hospital Trial', *Journal of Applied Bacteriology*, 33 (1970), pp. 566–73.
76 London Metropolitan Archives, A/KE/I/01/002, 'Plastic Foam Mattresses'.
77 Mass Observation Archive (University of Sussex), Replies to Spring 1984 directive [G224].
78 Wilbert M. Gesler, *Healing Places* (Rowman & Littlefield, 2003), p. 97.
79 'Doctors "Should Wear White Coats"', 13 May 2004, http://news.bbc.co.uk/1/hi/health/3706783.stm [accessed: 1 February 2022].
80 Clare Murphy, 'Death of The Doctor's White Coat', 17 September 2007, http://news.bbc.co.uk/1/hi/health/6998877.stm [accessed: 1 June 2021].
81 Hara, *100 Whites*, p. 100.
82 See Richard Llewellyn Davies, 'Furniture and Fittings', *AJ* (July 1954), pp. 143–7.
83 The Historic England archive has images from the 1980s and 1990s, for example https://historicengland.org.uk/images-books/photos/item/

JLP01/11/54952/06 and https://historicengland.org.uk/images-books/photos/item/JLP01/10/23362 [accessed: 1 February 2024].

84 On the rise of colourful bathrooms in the 1970s see Diana Austen and Gillian Fairchild, 'Just Add Water', *Good Housekeeping*, 103 (1973), pp. 42–7. It is rare for hospital archives or journals to refer specifically to the colour of bathroom fittings, but the fact that there is no reference to colour at all implies that they were considered unremarkable; this points towards the fixtures being classic 'white' rather than fashionable shades. There is also evidence that hospitals that chose colourful palettes often still kept white decorations, such as white tiles, in bathroom areas, and it is likely that this extended to the toilets and sinks; see, for example, 'BUPA Medical Centre: Manchester', *Hospital Development,* 8 (1980), p. 20. Images of wards with sinks (such as Figure 1.7) generally show them to be white. It is possible that some hospitals used stainless steel, as these were increasingly popular in public infrastructure at this time, but white porcelain toilets have long dominated.

85 On the history of toilets, including the materials with which they were made, see Sıdıka Mine Aytaç, 'The Social and Technical Development of Toilet Design' (MA Dissertation: Izmir Institute of Technology, 2004).

86 Satisfaction ratings for NHS toilets have dropped in recent years as they have been perceived as increasingly dirty. On this issue – and many others related to cleaning, soiled sheets, and toilets – on an international level, see Sjaak van der Geest and Shahaduz Zaman, '"Look Under the Sheets!" Fighting with the Senses in Relation to Defecation and Bodily Care in Hospitals and Care Institutions', *Medical Humanities*, 47 (2021), pp. 103–11.

87 London Metropolitan Archives, 'Completed Patient Questionnaire Forms', A/KE/I/01/059/017–22.

88 Teresita P., interviewed by On the Record & ScreenDeep for 'The Texture of Air', https://www.thetextureofair.uk [accessed: 1 June 2021].

89 Teresita P., interview.

90 Lisa Baraitser, 'Touching Time: Maintenance, Endurance, Care', in Stephen Frosh (ed.), Psychosocial Imaginaries. Studies in the Psychosocial (Palgrave Macmillan, 2015), https://doi.org/10.1057/9781137388186_2 See also Anna Harris, 'Sensing and the Shadows: Invisible Work in Medical Education in the Netherlands', *Medical Anthropology*, 42 (2023), pp. 437–50.

91 Beyond hospitals, the role of ritual in managing perceived 'contamination' across many cultural contexts and time periods is also widely acknowledged, for example in anthropology see Mary Douglas, *Purity*

and Danger: An Analysis of Concepts of Pollution and Taboo (Routledge & Kegan Paul, 1966). On the history of sorting and separating soiled items in hospitals, see David Theodore, '"Dirty Dirty Dirt": Automating Segregation in the Friesen Concept Hospital', in Jane L. Stevens Crawshaw, Irena Benyovsky Latin, and Kathleen Vongsathorn (eds), *Tracing Hospital Boundaries: Integration and Segregation in Southeastern Europe and Beyond, 1050–1970* (Brill, 2020), pp. 171–90.

92 For example, 'Isolation System for General Hospitals', *BMJ* (April 1974), 41–4; Lynda J. Taylor, 'Segregation, Collection and Disposal of Hospital Laundry and Waste', *Journal of Hospital Infection: Supplement A*, 11 (1988), pp. 57–63.

93 Peter Bartrip, 'A "Pennurth of Arsenic for Rat Poison": The Arsenic Act, 1851 and the Prevention of Secret Poisoning', *Medical History*, 36 (1992), 53–69; W. A. Campbell, 'Oxalic Acid, Epsom Salt and the Poison Bottle', *Human Toxicology*, 1 (1982), pp. 187–93; Ralph Tapping, 'Poisonous Substance', *The Australian Journal of Pharmacy*, 96 (2015), pp. 4–5.

94 Constance Classen, 'Foundations for an Anthropology of the Senses', *International Social Science Journal*, 49 (1997), p. 403.

95 Barclay, *When It's Not the Main Game*, p. 118; John Greene, *Brightening the Long Days: Hospital Tile Pictures* (Tiles and Architectural Ceramics Society, 1987).

96 John Diamond, 'Because Cowards Get Cancer Too: A Hypochondriac Confronts His Nemesis', *New York Times*, https://archive.nytimes.com/www.nytimes.com/books/first/d/diamond-cancer.html [accessed: 13 August 2021]; Ben Watt, *Patient: The True Story of a Rare Illness* (Viking, 1996), p. 18.

97 Diamond, 'Because Cowards Get Cancer Too'.

98 On trolleys and care see Shanti Sumartojo and Sarah Pink, *Atmospheres and the Experiential World: Theory and Methods* (Routledge, 2019), p. 83.

99 Watt, *Patient*, p. 126. The lower-case 'b' on the word Black is taken from the original.

100 Lynda Nead, '"Red Taffeta Under Tweed": The Color of Post-War Clothes', *Fashion Theory*, 21 (2017), p. 365. The lower-case 'b' on the word Black is taken from the original.

101 See Jennifer Crane, 'The NHS's Forgotten Workforce', *BMJ* (December 2022), p. 379.

102 Philip C. Russell, 'The White Coat Ceremony: Turning Trust into Entitlement', *Teaching and Learning in Medicine*, 14 (2002), 56–9. This article relates primarily to the US 'White Coat Ceremony' but these broader points also apply in the UK.

103 Shilpa Ross *et al.*, 'Workforce Race Inequalities and Inclusion in NHS Providers', https://www.kingsfund.org.uk/sites/default/files/2020-07/workforce-race-inequalities-inclusion-nhs-providers-july2020.pdf [accessed: 13 August 2021], p. 12.
104 Roberta Bivins, 'Picturing Race in the British National Health Service, 1948–1988', *Twentieth Century British History*, 28 (2017), p. 103. On visual culture, photography, and race in the NHS see also Jack Saunders, 'Emotions, Social Practices and the Changing Composition of Class, Race and Gender in the National Health Service, 1970–79: "Lively Discussion Ensued"', *History Workshop Journal*, 88 (2019), pp. 204–28.
105 Kirsty Sinclair Dootson, 'Introduction to the Issue: The Politics of Colour', *Frames Cinema Journal*, 17 (2020), np.
106 Kathleen Connellan, 'The Psychic Life of White: Power and space', *Organization Studies*, 34 (2013), p. 1529.
107 Dana Berthold, 'Tidy Whiteness: A Genealogy of Race, Purity, and Hygiene', *Ethics & the Environment*, 15 (2010), pp. 1–26.
108 Mary Douglas, *Purity and Danger: An Analysis of Concepts of Pollution and Taboo* (Routledge & Kegan Paul, 1966).
109 For example, she shows links between white aprons, Pears soap adverts, hygiene, and race; McClintock, *Imperial Leather*, pp. 31–2, 61–2.
110 Richard Dyer, *White: Essays on Race and Culture* (Routledge, 1997); Kathleen Connellan, 'The Social Politics of White in Design', in Marilyn DeLong and Barbara Martinson (eds), *Color and Design* (Berg, 2012), pp. 65–88.
111 Joseph Roth, *The Hotel Years: Wanderings in Europe between the Wars*, trans. Michael Hofman (Granta, 2015), p. 204.
112 'Sackville Hits Out at "Depressing" Hospital Care Environments', *Hospital Development*, 24 (1993), p. 13.
113 Connie Timmermann, Lisbeth Uhrenfeldt, and Regner Birkelund, 'Cancer Patients and Positive Sensory Impressions in the Hospital Environment – A Qualitative Interview Study', *European Journal of Cancer Care*, 22 (2013), pp. 117–24.

2

Green: from efficiency to emotions

In February 1951, *The Hospital* published an advert by Docker Brothers Ltd for hospital paint. This advert noted that 'there was a time when hospital decoration presented few problems: good, hardwearing and washable paint in safe, sober colours, and that was that'.[1] The advert claimed that there had been a significant change in recent years: 'now the colour specialist asks a host of questions', including what colours are 'cheering to various types of patient' and 'restful for staff'.[2] This advert reflected a growing interest in colour in hospitals by mid-century, and a growing interest in the emotional dimensions of colour. At this time, the architectural symbol of modern efficient hospitals shifted towards high-rise buildings, and white walls fell out of fashion, as they had done in modernism more generally.[3] Pastel shades expanded the colour palette of modernity. This trend connects to wider post-war history, in which Lynda Nead notes that 'colour was the language of the project of modernization' and 'progress' after the Second World War, as symbolised in the Festival of Britain.[4] Martin Moore also notes broad efforts to brighten up post-war British infrastructure, and argues that efforts to brighten General Practice (GP) waiting rooms were connected to the fact that 'brightness [was] seen a way to convince the population of the benefits of post-war social democracy'.[5] Efforts to symbolise modernity through colour were particularly important for the new NHS in its early years, as there was little hospital building at this time; efforts to modernise therefore focused, typically, on enhancing existing infrastructure.

Some commentators were critical that the true potential of 'bright' modernity was not fully embraced at this time, because of a widespread British aversion to apparently garish colours such as those found in the US. In a post-war article on hospital colour schemes, published in the *BMJ* in 1962, one Department of Health Senior Medical Officer – D. W. A. McCreadie – noted that 'pale pastel complementary colours can only be regarded as a sop to modernity and are used by those who are timidly modern'.[6] Only a few sites pursued the 'contrasting' colour schemes that McCreadie viewed as essential to the truly modern hospital. This trend echoes the modern 'brightness' of other urban environments at this time, where colours were also introduced in a relatively 'timid' fashion at first.[7] Many hospitals ended up with a colour palette of pastel shades later also criticised as unadventurous. However, at this moment in time they were an important transition between the light shades of 'hygiene' and the more vibrant colours that hospitals would embrace later in the century.

Pastel shades were increasingly understood in emotional terms in post-war Britain, and fed into a model of a 'modern' NHS that put patient experience at its centre. The chapter first outlines this trend, before turning to green as a case study. Green has been perceived as ubiquitous in hospitals for so long that it features strongly in people's personal, individual memories and in emotions such as nostalgia. It offers a valuable opportunity to delve into the relationship between the theories underpinning hospital design, and how specific colours are felt in embodied and emotional terms. Hospitals had always been emotional spaces: in the mid-twentieth century they were increasingly and more explicitly recognised as such through various shades of pastel and green.

Calm: the primacy of pastels in the 1950s

In 1949, an article on 'Colour Conditioning' in *The Hospital* magazine noted a shift in ideas about colour schemes in the early NHS. The author observed that research in colour conditioning had moved from an emphasis on eyestrain in surgeons to a more expansive notion of the power of colour to provide both physiological rest and 'psychological comfort'.[8] The perceived value of engaging with colour theory for staff had shifted subtly, from improving their work as efficient, modern employees, to improving their psychological state. There was also a growing interest in the ways that psychological 'comfort' and productivity might be interconnected. This kind of theory had already been applied widely in workplaces, for example shaping factory walls and machines in the US, and there was a growing interest at this time in its potential for new hospitals. The author noted that '[w]hile the technique recommends restraint in the use of especially bright distracting and overstimulating hues, colour can be used to create a frame of mind suitable to the state of the patient'.[9] This desire for 'bright' (but not distracting) colours underpinned much of the hospital design that would follow in subsequent decades. The meaning of 'bright' was often left unclear, but seemed to refer to light, clean, fresh, and 'cheerful' shades, more than vibrant or unnatural shades. This form of 'brightness' was commonly found in pastel colours, such as blues and greens. In part, these pastel colours were practical, to compensate for poor lighting or small windows in older buildings, but their use was also grounded in colour theory about the restful and soothing nature of certain colours.[10]

This growing interest in colour and the expansion of colour palettes was supported by a growing body of research. One paint firm produced its own promotional book, *The Function of Colour in Factories, Schools and Hospitals*.[11] Arthur L. Hall also cited research by the 'Colour Consulting Division of the Paints Organisation of our largest Chemicals Group' on a recent example of hospital redecoration: '[s]taff and patients alike appreciate the transformation made by the substitution of pastel tints for the [...] cream [...] with dark green or dark brown to which they have become accustomed'.[12] It is significant that in the early years of the NHS, much of this kind of research was conducted by private organisations, external consultants and paint companies promoting new colour palettes.[13] This might explain, in part, why there are limited records of who chose hospital colour schemes and why. Jean Symons – writing guidance in 1973 on *Improving Existing Hospital Buildings for Long-Stay Residents* – noted that many hospitals were happy to hand colour scheme choices to tiling or paint firms, as 'internal wrangles over colours are best avoided' but that without a design coordinator there was often 'a missing link' that meant designs overall were 'not good enough'.[14] Although pastel shades in hospitals came to be entwined with the principles of the welfare state in the post-war years, particularly once British Standard paints came to be used in public buildings, these early commercial and private influences are important. The commercial roots of some late twentieth-century colour palettes were deeper than they might first appear.

Much was taken from commercial bodies or private colour consultants, though some recommendations were based on government recommendations for other types of building. The Newcastle Regional Hospital Board book on hospital colour explicitly noted that 'much inspiration has been derived and frequent quotations have been included from an excellent Bulletin issued in 1953 by the Ministry of Education and entitled "Colour in School Buildings"'.[15] This tendency to draw upon research relating to other public and private buildings was logical in many ways. Schools had been more rapidly rebuilt after the war, and offered a possible model for new hospitals including – but not limited to – the design of spaces for children. Many rooms in NHS hospitals had to be designed in the expectation that a wide range of people might encounter them. This echoed many other public and private spaces, particularly those of the new welfare state where public infrastructure had to be designed to be increasingly 'universal'. As Lucy Faire and Denish McHugh also note in their work on urban colour 1945–70, a group of architects helped to systematise colour schemes for public buildings around this time, including schools and hospitals, and helped to produce British Standard paints. This kind of standardisation was underpinned by new, more systematic ways of ordering and understanding colour in the twentieth century such as Ostwald that built on other schemes like Munsell.[16] A 'state' colour palette became possible when colour photography and mass production also became culturally important, allowing for replication over time and place not just of 'light blue' or 'light green', for example, but the *exact same* colours.

There was also a growing interest in colour design in workplaces, including factories and offices.[17] As noted above, early research on 'colour conditioning' in hospitals drew on previous work that had been done in international workplaces. There was even a shift towards colour in art galleries around the same time, in a turn away from the 'didactic, focused seriousness' implied by the 'white cube'.[18] This overlap between hospitals and other types of built environment was often made explicit. *The Function of Colour in Factories, Schools and Hospitals* suggested that green could help to counter the impact of factory machinery and employee fatigue.[19] For hospitals, the publication placed similar emphasis on colour schemes that helped the body to rest, and provided more 'cheerful' environments without being overstimulating.[20] The fact that 'factories, schools, and hospitals' were grouped together in this way is in itself very significant, considering the ostensibly very different populations that they housed. All of them were modern environments, though, that needed to provide a careful balance between rest and efficiency, and between the health of body and mind.[21] Hospitals and factories alike were high-technology workplaces, and the distinction between built environments of labour and healthcare was a blurry one in some old workhouses. Some international literature on hospital colour schemes emphasised that there were also many administrative staff in hospitals, and treated their needs as equivalent to those of any office worker. One author in 1960, for example, wrote of administrative hospital personnel that 'the problem of alleviating eye strain is found to be paramount' and that colours such as grey-green or coral offered 'an eye rest for the employee when he looks up from his desk'.[22]

In other ways, those writing on colour in hospitals did have to recognise the particular requirements of these buildings. Specific conditions included the continued importance of hygiene, and the combination of heightened emotions and prolonged periods of boredom that could accompany a hospital visit. *The Function of Colour in Factories, Schools and Hospitals* remarked, in relation to men's outpatient wards, that

> the problem here is the same as in any hospital ward – to create a colour scheme which will be soothing and pleasant when looked at for long stretches of time, and at the same time be, as far as possible, neither monotonous nor depressing.[23]

The publication went on to claim that 'most men dislike all forms of pink' and preferred blue.[24] There was an interesting balancing act undertaken at this time, grouping hospital colour palettes with comparable spaces with the shared goals of making them more 'cheerful' through pastel shades, and recognising the specific emotional dimensions of healthcare settings.

Colour also had a specific meaning in hospitals, because it was so often positioned as a solution to whiteness. Efforts to introduce a new 'light and pastel' colour palette of the NHS emphasised their difference from more institutional colour schemes. Around mid-century, one paint firm wrote that 'broad expanses of glittering white are incredibly inhuman in appearance' in hospitals, and that darker browns or greens offered 'no advantage over the pastel shades in respect of hygiene and maintenance'.[25] Such comments about the 'inhuman' nature of all-white spaces connected with a broader shift towards critiques of the 'institutional'. However, in practice white was still used extensively in combination with pastels. Despite the broad shift away from the all-white hospital at this time, white remained an important feature of hospital design. Many hospitals continued to use white in 'clinical areas' even when wards were made 'brighter' and 'restful' colours were introduced for staff offices.[26] The Newcastle Regional Hospital Board's 1955 book *The Use of Colour in Hospitals* emphasised that white paint should be used, though with care. The book recommended white in specific rooms and spaces; it suggested keeping white ceilings in wards and white walls around windows, for example, but never 'pure white' and with specific finishes to reduce glare (Figure 2.1).

Colours such as 'broken-white, off-white' 'pale cream or ivory' were typically viewed as 'less frigid' than pure white, and could be used in combination with other light and bright pastel colours to modernise hospitals; deeper cream tones, implicitly too dull or old-fashioned, were avoided.[27] Figure 2.1 shows that white was used to enhance, reflect, and complement 'colourful' walls, and the use of 'colours to stimulate interest'. Used with care, white was part of the trend towards an embodied and emotional model of colour, rather than in opposition to it. Therefore, it is best to think of pastels as an expansion of modern colour palettes, rather than the more common narrative of colour replacing 'institutional' schemes.

Against this general backdrop, growing discussion of hospital colour schemes was evident in multiple publications in the early NHS years. Unfortunately only a few publications were printed in colour, so it is difficult to know the exact paints being used. *The Use of Colour in Hospitals* is a rich resource in this regard, because it includes samples of indicative paint colours (Figure 2.2).[28] It is possible that the printed colours in this copy have faded over time, leaving lighter shadows of more vibrant shades, but the colours pictured in Figure 2.2 broadly align with the written descriptions. The book was written with non-experts in mind, as a tool to support

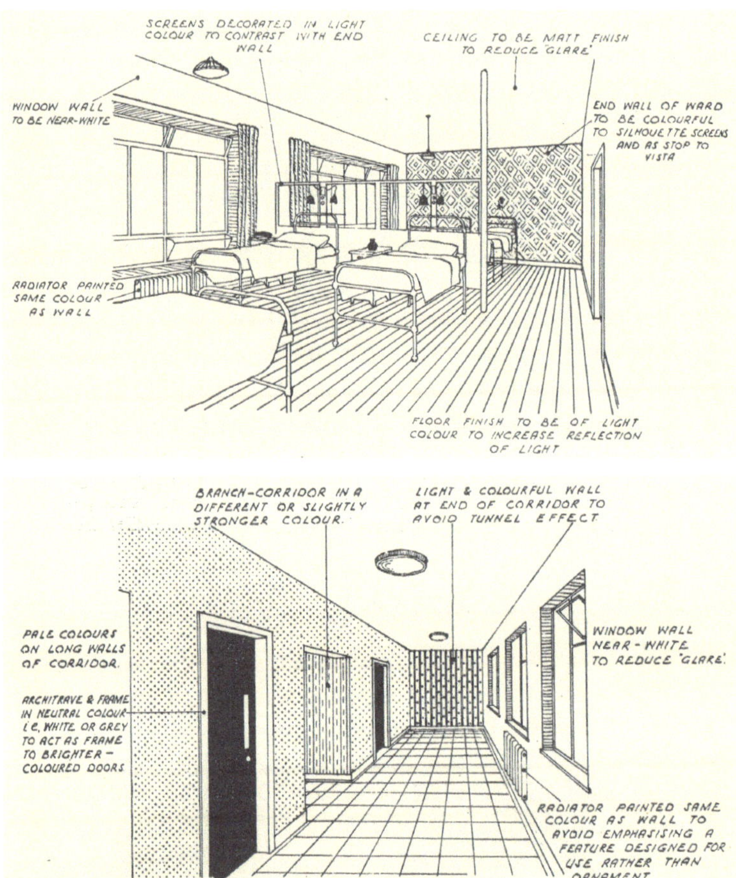

Figure 2.1 Newcastle Regional Hospital Board, *The Use of Colour in Hospitals* (NRHB, 1955), pp. 11 & 24. Every effort has been made to trace the copyright holders and obtain permission to reproduce this material. Please do get in touch with any enquiries or information about this image or the rights holder. Scan provided by the Wellcome Library. All rights reserved and permission to use this figure must be obtained from the copyright holder.

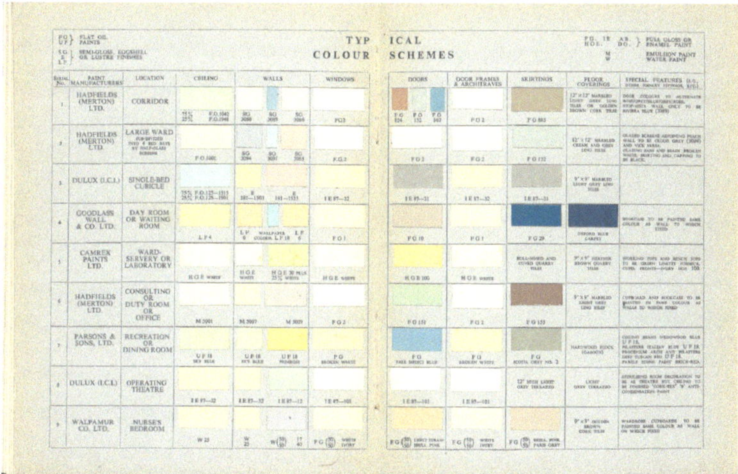

F.O. / U.F. } Flat oil paints
S.G. / E / L.F. } Semi-gloss, eggshell or lustre finishes

TYPICAL COLOUR SCHEMES

F.G. / H.G.E. / A.B. / D.O. } Full gloss or enamel paint
M Emulsion paint
W Water paint

Serial No.	Paint Manufacturers	Location	Ceiling	Walls	Windows	Doors	Door Frames & Architraves	Skirtings	Floor Coverings	Special Features (e.g. other joinery fittings, etc.)
1	Hadfields (Merton) Ltd.	Corridor	75% F.O.1042 25% F.O.1948	SG 3080 SG 3085 SG 3086	FG2	FG 124 FG 152 FG 167	FG 2	FG 883	12" x 12" marbled light grey lino tiles or golden brown cork tiles	Door colours to alternate [illegible] wall only to be Riviera blue (3089)
2	Hadfields (Merton) Ltd.	Large ward sub-divided into 4 bed bays by half-glass screens	F.O.1001	SG 3094 SG 3091 SG 3083	F.G.2	FG 2	FG 2	FG 132	12" x 12" marbled cream and grey lino tiles	Glazed screens adjoining [illegible] wall to be cloud grey (3094) and vice versa. Glazing bars and beads broken white, skirting and capping to be black.
3	Dulux (I.C.I.)	Single-bed cubicle	75% F.O.125–1515 25% F.O.125–1901	E 181–1503 E 181–1533	I.E 87–32	I.E 85–31	I.E 87–32	I.E 87–31	9" x 9" marbled light grey lino tiles	
4	Goodlass Wall & Co. Ltd.	Day room or waiting room	L.F 4	L.F 6 wallpaper colour L.F 18 L.F 6	F.G 1	FG 10	FG 1	FG 29	Oxford blue carpet	Bookcase to be painted same colour as wall to which fixed
5	Camrex Paints Ltd.	Ward-servery or laboratory	H.G.E white	H.G.E white H.G.E 30 plus 25% white	H.G.E white	H.G.E 100	H.G.E white	Bull-nosed and coved quarry tiles	9" x 9" heather brown quarry tiles	Working tops and bench tops to be green linette formica, cupd. fronts—ivory HGE 100
6	Hadfields (Merton) Ltd.	Consulting or duty room or office	M 3001	M 3007 M 3009	F.G 2	FG 151	FG 2	FG 153	9" x 9" marbled light grey lino tiles	Cupboard and bookcase to be painted in same colour as walls to which fixed
7	Parsons & Sons, Ltd.	Recreation or dining room	U.F 18 sky blue	U.F 18 sky blue U.F 18 primrose	F.G broken white	F.G pale medici blue	F.G broken white	F.G Scotia grey no. 2	Hardwood block (Gaboon)	Ceiling beams Wedgwood blue U.F 18. Pilasters Italian blue U.F 18. Proscenium arch and pilasters [illegible] Tuscan red U.F 18. Panels stone paint brick-red.
8	Dulux (I.C.I.)	Operating theatre	I.E 87–32	I.E 87–32 I.E 87–12	I.E 87–101	I.E 85–101	I.E 85–101	12" high light grey terrazzo	Light grey terrazzo	Sterilising room decoration to be as theatre but ceiling to be finished 'Cork-tex' 'B' anti-condensation paint
9	Walpamur Co. Ltd.	Nurse's bedroom	W 25	W 25 W (50/50) 17 40	F.G (50/50) white ivory	F.G (50/50) light straw shell pink	F.G (50/50) white ivory	F.G (50/50) shell pink Paris grey	9" x 9" golden brown cork tiles	Wardrobe cupboards to be painted same colour as wall on which fixed

Figure 2.2 Newcastle Regional Hospital Board, *The Use of Colour in Hospitals* (NRHB, 1955), np. Every effort has been made to trace the copyright holders and obtain permission to reproduce this material. Please do get in touch with any enquiries or information about this image or the rights holder. Image provided by the Wellcome Library. All rights reserved and permission to use this figure must be obtained from the copyright holder.

more thoughtful use of hospital maintenance budgets. It emphasised diversity within hospital colour schemes and an understanding that different people and different medical spaces had specific requirements. Even in the light of this variety, the book fairly consistently advocated light and pastel colours alongside off-white.

Such publications often represented shifts in design philosophies and 'best practice' as much as what was happening on the ground. It is impossible to know how far this specific book informed colour choices, but it seems to have been relatively widely distributed; copies of the book currently exist in libraries including the Wellcome Library and the British Library in London, and the Huntington Library in Pasadena. The colour palette in Figure 2.2 aligns broadly with trends found in architectural journals in the post-war period discussed above, and therefore can be taken as an example of the sorts of pastel shades that were seen as cutting-edge or ideal colour design at this time. A rather critical review of this book in *Architects'*

Journal noted that 'in the text, quite bold recommendations are made and demonstrated in diagrams, but most of the colours selected for the chart are pale pastels'.[29] This review raises an important issue about the meaning of words such as 'bright' at this time, which in practice often meant fairly muted and light colour schemes.

Pastel colours were not thought to be all equivalent, and 'warm' tones such as peach were thought to serve a different purpose to 'cooler' blues and greens. Most advice emphasised that different colours were relevant to different types of space or person. In relation to wards, for example, the 1949 article on 'Colour Conditioning' in *The Hospital* stated that

> Two factors contribute to the decoration of the wards, the psychological aspect and the orientation of the building and rooms. Warm tones tend to be stimulating and are suggested for maternity wards and others where rapid convalescence is desired. For those wards where long stay or chronic patients are installed, cool colours are claimed to achieve a passive and restful effect ... Rooms with a north exposure can be painted in warm tones to compensate for the relatively bluish outdoor light.[30]

Despite the apparent specific needs of different patients, and the distinction made between 'warm' and 'cool' colours, most hospitals shifted slowly towards similar colour palettes at this time, which included a balance of light blue, green, pink or peach, and cream. As another article in *The Hospital* noted in September 1951, '[l]ight and pastel colour schemes are becoming more widely accepted as the colours for decoration schemes in hospitals and the old dark and dirt concealing "institutional" colour schemes are slowly being replaced as the backlog of work to be done since the national health service came into operation is gradually being overtaken'.[31] Pastel colours offered an alternative both to dark 'institutional' colour schemes and, as discussed above, to all-white 'inhuman' ones.

There is plenty of evidence of local initiatives to brighten up hospitals in the 1950s, when the focus was on redecoration and renovation rather than building. Architect Arthur L. Hall gave the example of an old day room from an 1860s hospital that was redecorated on a limited budget 'from the small but charming range of Standard Colours for wall decoration selected by the B[ritish].S[tandard].1. for subsidized housing and made by most paint firms'.[32] Similar examples can be found in records held by The National Archives of hospital inspections, such as a report from 1952 on assistant nurse training at Thornbury hospital, which noted that the old hospital (which had blocks built as long ago as 1900) had been redecorated with a lighter paint.[33] The same language was evident in a visitors' book for a nurses' home at Hinckley Hospital in 1955 in which a member of the Hospital Management Committee noted: 'we thought the iron bed steads … could do with a coat of light paint'.[34] Harriet Richardson Blakeman makes similar observations for Scotland at the same time where, she notes, '[i]nteriors of new buildings in the 1950s contrasted with the drabness associated with Victorian and Edwardian hospitals. They were brighter, painted in lighter colours, particularly in entrance spaces and on the wards'.[35] None of these examples offer detail on what colours were considered 'charming' or 'light', nor do they describe who chose the paint schemes, but they remain useful in broad cultural terms. They show how important redecoration was in early NHS modernisation processes. Based on the general pastel trends outlined above, it is also reasonable to assume that in the 1950s, references to 'light' colours implicitly meant pastel shades.

The introduction of pastels was slow in some places, and white remained popular. In another article for *The Hospital* magazine, on 'Colour in the Hospital' in June 1951, Hall noted criticisms of 'whitewashed' walls without brighter colour for long-term inpatients who were sometimes bed-ridden for years.[36] He emphasised that progress remained slow for both practical and cultural reasons. 'There has been no sudden flowering of colour schemes in [hospitals]', Hall noted, but there was slow progress by 'infiltration'.[37] In 1959 an article in *Architects' Journal* noted that even when architects from the Nuffield Trust designed a hospital building, at Musgrave Park in Belfast, they used

> off-white walls and trim dark grey skirting, light grey linoleum tiles … The only relief to this is the incidentals of curtains and furniture. The colour scheme can be considered as architecturally a forthright and clear statement of the structure. On the other hand, one cannot help feeling that the opportunity has been missed to produce some degree of variety by colour, less a clinical and more domestic atmosphere in keeping with the planning.[38]

Considering that the Nuffield Trust were leading voices in hospital architecture and design at this time, including a 1955 publication that declared 'there is scope for experiment in a far bolder use of colour' in hospitals, there was a disjuncture here between principles and practice.[39] Interestingly, *Architects' Journal* gives an example of a Scottish Casualty Block at Dunfermline in 1959, in which they noted 'colours generally tend to be in the cream and pastel range, being a committee responsibility and outside the architect's sphere of influence'.[40] This might indicate that Scotland embraced pastels more rapidly than England, but it also indicates a difference between professional architects and local decision-makers at this time. Architects may have stayed wedded to the white box of modernity for longer than others. There was great variation at this time in practice in terms of whether interior design schemes fell into architects' remits, and this may partly explain the unevenness of colour schemes.

A range of professionals, from architecture to healthcare, advocated in writing for even bolder use of colour over subsequent years. As early as 1954, when pastels were still taking off as a trend in many places, an article in *Architects' Journal* complained that 'it is time to get away from the timid, pastel colour schemes which still persist in most hospitals'.[41] In 1969, geriatrician John Agate wrote of the need for more colour in hospital, particularly for long-stay patients such as those in geriatric hospitals, and gave examples of a recent successful project using 'vivid, challenging colour schemes'.[42] He also recognised how unusual the project was even over a decade after Hall's pleas for change: elsewhere 'pastel distemper or emulsion colours have crept in here and there, only to fade almost as soon as applied, but few wards and corridors have so far contained any bright splashes of colour'.[43] However, there was a clear growth of support for making hospitals more 'cheerful environments' – to cite Agate again – and for shedding the 'drab colour schemes' and stigma of the old workhouse buildings within which many hospitals, particularly those housing long-stay patients, were situated.[44] Overall, the 'pastel turn' was uneven but clearly visible throughout British hospitals by the post-war years.

Fifty shades of green: mint, misty, sage, and spinach

Pastel colours often repackaged traditional colour palettes. Though typically painted directly over white, colours such as blue and green had much longer histories in hospitals. The early twentieth-century 'all-white' hospital had itself replaced older colour palettes that often included dark green. New hues and shades of green offered new layers in this ever-changing palimpsest. Colours such as blue and green were not new in late twentieth-century hospitals, but were lightened, brightened, and modernised. This section takes green as an example of a colour that was regularly refreshed, redeveloped, and revisited in hospitals. It outlines shifting ideas about the function of colour, with late nineteenth- and early twentieth-century greens often used to hide dirt or reduce eye strain in hospital staff, and later greens being used to emotional ends.

Histories of green tend to focus on the story of the operating theatre, which is worth outlining briefly here because of its importance in the scholarship.[45] Much is often made of the work of Harry M. Sherman, who in the 1914 *California State Journal of Medicine* advised that green should be used in operating theatres: 'The particular shade of green to be selected was that which was complementary to h[a]emoglobin, and it was found to be the green of the spinach leaf'.[46] This article was followed by another commonly cited 1924 piece by Palugi Flagg who recommended the use of a bluish green.[47] However, these works did not trigger a wave of green operating theatres, and the fact that they are repeatedly cited is probably significant in itself. In 1943 in *The American Journal of Surgery*, Richey L. Waugh and Ester M. Welch reported that they had changed the colour of operating room linens from white to green to reduce eye strain, drawing on their knowledge of the successful use of green in other contexts to do so. At this point, though, they noted that 'the literature on the subject is scanty' and had to refer to literature from over three decades prior to find reference points.[48] Such practices were seemingly still fairly localised and ad hoc at this point. The same is likely to have been true in the British context, where there was an awareness of the idea that green was a more 'restful' colour to reduce eyestrain in surgeons, but there was no systematic redecoration campaign.[49] There is some evidence that washable greens such as 'foam green hard gloss paint' were part of operating theatres by mid-century, and Pilkington tiles offered a blue-green option for surgery, but many operating theatres remained white even under the NHS.[50]

The history of green outside the operating theatre is equally important, but more often neglected in scholarship. Dark green was the backdrop of many Victorian hospitals, and in the 1920s it was common to find colours such as dark green remaining below dado height. Significantly, considering how important they would come to be as a marker of 'old-fashioned' hospitals, some NHS patients strongly remembered these colours: one Mass Observation response in 1997 said that 'I am of an age to remember pre-NHS hospital waiting rooms ... always either a green or a brown painted dado'.[51] This trend was similar to that seen in the US at the same time, where – as one commentator from the American Institute of Architects' Committee on Architecture for Health later observed – 'many of the university hospitals' corridors and rooms were also green; three shades of green with a dark green wainscot, a darker green dado, and a lighter green above'.[52] New shades of green were introduced to brighten and modernise hospitals, apparently in opposition to the darker Victorian shades. Some older hospitals and workhouses even refreshed their colour palettes in green and cream in the 1920s, rather than opting for the white of modernist buildings.[53]

In broad terms, green was thought to be an important colour for rest and relaxation for much of the twentieth century. Though colour theory and interest in hospital colour schemes grew around mid-century, some hospitals had opted for fresher greens in the 1930s when other sites were going all-white. Brian Abel-Smith's work on the history of British hospitals gives an example of green and cream being introduced in the 1930s as a colour scheme that was restful and – quoting *Hospital* – a 'delight to the eye'.[54] A Canadian Red Cross Hospital based in England in 1940 apparently had 'pale green walls ... and darker green dado, which is considered soothing and therapeutic'.[55] Commentators in the 1930s and 1940s were already using emotional language, such as 'delight[ful]' and 'soothing', to describe green in interior decoration. Abel-Smith positions this colour-based trend as part of a broader trend to make hospitals more appealing to patients, including smaller rooms and improved waking hours. This indicates that NHS patient-centredness had its roots decades earlier, and supports the argument that colour design was a key part of this agenda.

The ad hoc use of colours such as green and cream in early twentieth-century hospitals echoes trends in other workplaces.

Abel-Smith's emphasis on rest also is as important as his comment about 'delight', as in the 1930s green-and-cream colour schemes were chosen as much (if not more) for their perceived value of rest for the body, including for workers, as for the soul. Vicky Long's work on factories shows many parallels with hospitals, in terms of renovations starting often with localised efforts at ad hoc improvement, although the turn to colour seems to have taken place earlier in factories. She quotes a report from 1920 that noted how companies had made 'attempts to carry out effective colour schemes', including those later seen in hospitals such as 'pleasant shades of green'; Long also notes that by 1930 colour schemes such as green and primrose were described as 'in line with prevalent psychological theories'.[56] Even with the rise of white as the colour of modernity in the 1930s, there was evidently a growing interest in the value of other colours for body and mind. As in hospitals, such interest picked up in the post-war years, when *The Lancet* noted that the 'report for 1945 by the Chief Inspector of Factories ... draws attention to the awakening of interest in colour schemes, which many firms are introducing during renovations; light colours are usually chosen and pastel shades of light green, buff, and blue are especially popular'.[57] In 1951, *The Hospital* reported on 'new developments at Clatterbridge General Hospital' and noted that in a new extension to the maternity department 'the colour scheme was that in use elsewhere in the hospital, namely light green and cream'.[58]

By the early post-war period, any shade of green perceived as dull, dark, outdated, or old-fashioned was rejected. In 1950, for example, the Liskeard Hospitals' House Committee visited one local hospital and noted that 'we would suggest that ... the walls should be painted a more pleasing tint than the present green. We would suggest, perhaps, a warm cream'.[59] Mass Observation records also show that people considered hospitals decorated with dark greens to be old-fashioned; in response to the 1997 Spring Directive on the NHS, for example, one respondent noted that 'I didn't use the NHS much in the '70s ... One accident ([A]chilles tendon) landed me in hospital; the medical treatment was outstanding – but Florence Nightingale would have recognised the Ward – 60 beds, and dark green walls'.[60] The reason for such a rejection of green walls might be because of the particular shade of green, and its specific associations with older buildings such as renovated workhouses. In this example, the colour combined with the architecture of the old Nightingale ward to create a sense of an old-fashioned hospital building.

Green endured but evolved, with the introduction of new hues, hints, tones, and shades. Light and pastel greens gained emotional power because they were always compared to older shades of the colour, or other older wall colours. Layers of green paint were also physically, and materially, in dialogue with what came before; the layering of meaning did not take place only in texts. Walls have always been – in Sarah Bennett's words – 'memory archives', which continue to be reshaped and 'wounded' by the daily activities of the hospital.[61] Figure 2.3 shows a layer of cream underneath a later layer of hospital green – seemingly peeling paper – at an abandoned

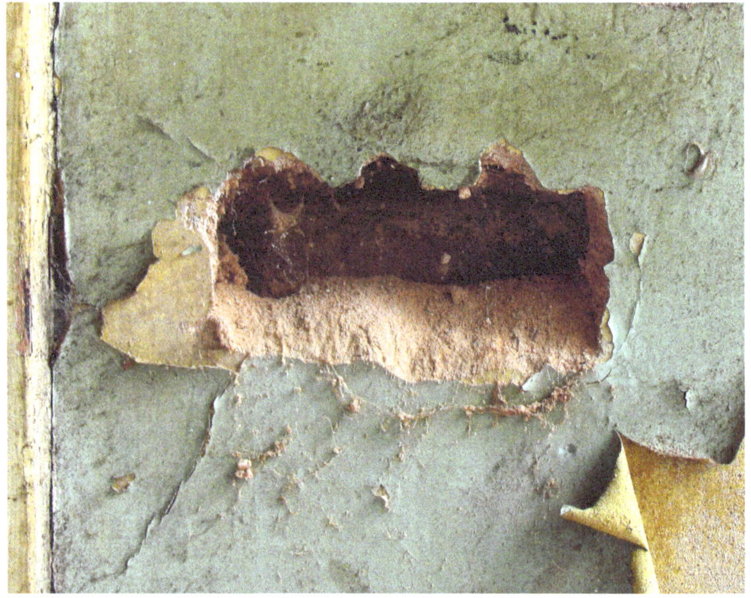

Figure 2.3 'Wall-wound (found) DCH-4' (2010). Bolt hole at the old Exe Vale Hospital, formerly known as the Devon Mental Hospital and Devon County Lunatic Asylum. 1845. Rights Reserved Sarah Bennett 2021. Reproduced with permission.

hospital for mental health patients, revealed by the passage of time and the removal of an old bolt.

Any freshly painted green wall continually evolves in feel and appearance, sometimes revealing older layers where it is bashed and bruised. By taking paint and the wall itself as an archive, or a form of palimpsest, it is possible to understand how paint and its meaning evolved over time. As Serena Dyer notes, writing on twelve layers of wallpaper held at the Museum of Domestic Design and Architecture: 'the wallpaper sandwich acts as a material time-capsule'.[62] Additionally, the existence of multiple layers of paint (or wallpaper) at any given time was a part of making its meaning; the layers did not just mark the frozen years of a 'time capsule', but continued to exist in relation to each other at any given point in time because the paint underneath was often exposed through wear and tear. New layers of green always existed in relation to what came before, both conceptually and materially.

A specific shade of blue-green started to grow in prominence in the early post-war years, in a shift towards a more 'modern' version of the colour. This drew on trends in North American hospitals, where there emerged a particular shade of 'misty green'. David Pantalony writes that colour theorist Faber Birren actually developed this 'misty green' in mid-century, based on another colour scheme that he developed for the US navy.[63] In itself this connection is significant, as the colour was drawn from a very different context that also sought to evoke modernity and efficiency. It is possible that references to 'mist green' paint in British archival records refer to a similar colour.[64] Figure 2.4 shows two objects first made by The British Oxygen Co. Ltd in the 1950s, to provide anaesthetic and analgesia. This company's repeated choice of similar shades of light blue-green, close to the 'misty green' that Pantalony identifies, might be significant in relation to brand identity. Other products had smaller touches of green, including a portable respirator for polio patients in the early 1950s. The specific blue-green also came to represent hygiene, a meaning that was found in other uses of the colour, from surgical scrubs through to the 'sterilisation pouch' from the 1980s (Figure 2.5). There was a growing use of blue-green for medical equipment in the NHS, but white and chrome remained dominant as signifiers of hygiene and modernity in medical equipment.

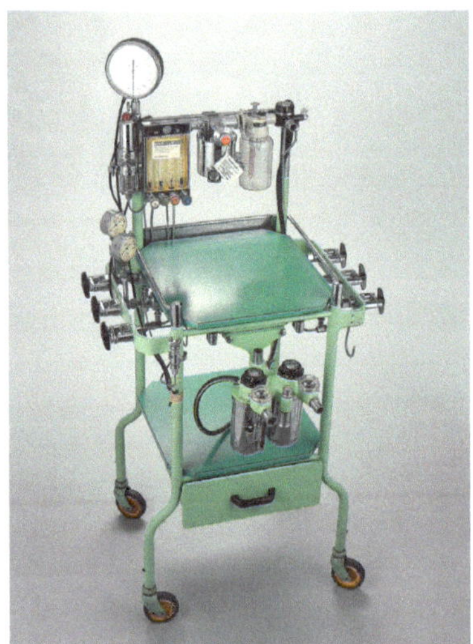

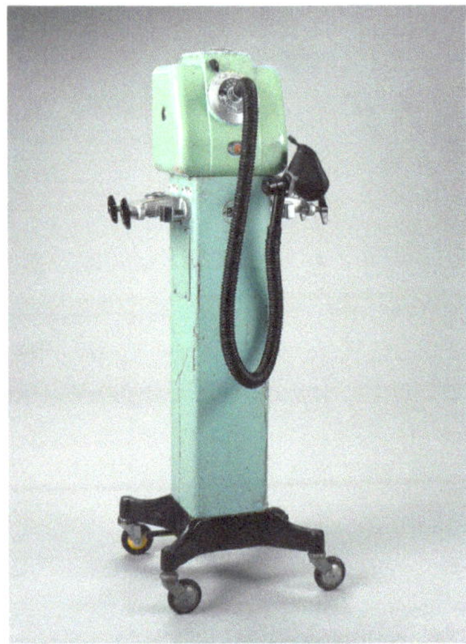

Figure 2.4 Trolley with drawer for Boyle's-type anaesthetic machine. Object number 1986-1067/7; Lucy Baldwin analgesia apparatus, used in midwifery. Object number 1984-1743.

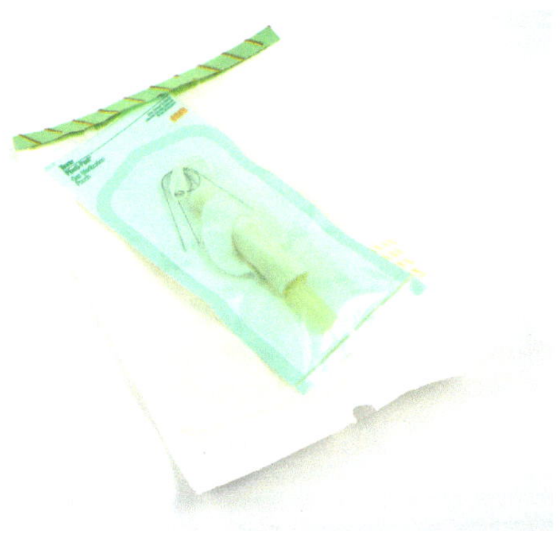

Figure 2.5 Gas sterilisation pouch in packaging for the Jarvik Artificial Heart System, donated by The Papworth Hospital, c.1980. Object number 1999-834 Pt10.

The 'misty green' shade also seems to have found its way into the British healthcare system in what might be considered non-medicalised objects. Instead of being only a symbol of high-technology and modernity, it was also used for bedside cabinets, bins, and railings. The Bristol Maid brand, for example, was founded in 1953 to manufacture NHS office equipment and filing cabinets, and soon expanded its range; it now has a catalogue of over 400 pages. Bristol Maid has made the 'misty green' shade core to its product range, including furniture and fittings. In such objects, 'misty green' represented both hygienic and humanistic principles.[65]

It is also important to remember that colour entered hospitals in a range of ways, and that green was prevalent outside hospital design. Patients might have seen blue-green in non-medical contexts; for example the Science Museum holds a hospital clergy stole in this colour.[66] They also encountered green as part of everyday rituals in hospital, which were not 'designed in' as part of medical equipment. Patients noticed whether their peas were bright 'chemical' green or pale 'processed' green, and whether pot plants were vibrant green or 'dusty'.[67] Each of these carried very different symbolic meanings and helped to create different embodied and multi-sensory encounters, affecting everything from emotions to taste. Such greens are more difficult to historicise than those found in interior design, object design, and architecture, but are important to bear in mind when considering colour and meaning in healthcare. Colours such as pastel green or 'misty green' have clear cultural and emotional histories that can be traced, but people encountered a much wider range of greens that also – subtly or implicitly – shaped their experiences. Any effort to write a neat history of green is destabilised and complicated when considering green objects more broadly such as plants, food, and non-medical clothing. Hospitals were awash with greens, but it was only walls and objects that expressed institutional values.

The history of green in hospitals takes many shades, and many forms. This section has outlined how older greens were regularly refreshed and replaced by more modern versions of the colour, as part of formulating and expressing the values of the early NHS. Modern 'misty green', in particular, brought together concepts such as hygiene and humanisation. Green played an important role in formulating concepts such as the 'modern', through conceptual and material dialogue with the past. Green could only be 'bright' or 'optimistic' in opposition to something 'dull' and 'depressing', and it could only be 'modern' when positioned against something 'old-fashioned'.

These trends continue to this day. In a recent interview with creative health consultant Jane Willis, for example, I asked her to reflect on change over time in her work and she responded:

> I think one of the biggest changes is that people now appreciate the importance of the environment and really when I started working at Barts in London there seemed to be no sense that it mattered and all the paint was cream and peppermint green and the waiting rooms were kind of plastic chairs. So, one of the first things I did there was trying to persuade the estates department that maybe we could have a colour scheme that went beyond cream and green and looking at

Figure 2.6 Hospital wall in Accident & Emergency, Bristol Royal Infirmary, 2022 © Image: Victoria Bates.

> how to make that manageable and sustainable for them in terms of maintenance.[68]

At the same time, many contemporary NHS Trusts continue to opt for green and cream in their hospitals. This colour combination has thus always been simultaneously traditional and modern, and it would be a mistake to take at face value the repeated references to it as 'old-fashioned' (Figure 2.6). References to green and cream as 'old fashioned' were part of the ongoing process of constructing, reconstructing, redefining, and repainting modernity.

Green-tinted glasses? Emotion and memory

This section takes a closer look at the emotional language of hospital green, and individual emotional encounters with green spaces and objects. It shows that, in practice, green was something of a catch-all emotional container that served any purpose. Rather than carrying an innate emotional quality, green was an emotional colour that operated in a wide range of ways. The same shades of green that were 'modern' and bright for one generation were 'depressing' and 'sombre' for the next. Green was a colour onto which anxieties about the modern hospital were repeatedly projected, particularly by external commentators for whom 'hospital green' was a short-hand for 'outdated' or 'old-fashioned'. This section also shifts beyond the lens of society and culture, to consider individual encounters with colourful surfaces and objects. To quote Sasha Handley and John Morgan, emotions in history are best understood not as purely cultural or mental, but as 'embodied and as constituted by a network of interactions between bodies, environments and materials'.[69] Many people who spent time in hospitals went 'off script' in terms of their responses to greens, for example finding old-fashioned greens to be reassuring or nostalgic rather than 'depressing', or situating the colours in individual life stories.

A common feature of mid-century colour research was its emphasis on the psychological and emotional aspects of colour. Ideas about colour and healing had long roots, though the new colour psychology was conceptually distinct. Chromotherapy has been traced back centuries, across the world, and shared some concepts with colour theory in its understanding of colours such as blue or green as 'cool' and orange or red as 'stimulating'. By the twentieth century, there was a new emphasis on the body–mind relationship, and on emotions or psychology, rather than the 'healing energy' of coloured light waves.[70] American architect William Ludlow, for example, noted the specific emotional value of different shades of green in hospitals in the early twentieth century, and advocated the 'soft greens, pale blues' that were 'positive colours' associated with nature.[71]

In Britain, the First World War fuelled interest in such questions, as the emotional power of colour was seen as particularly important in relation to the mental health of soldiers. In 1917 *The Lancet* reported on the work of Kemp Prosser, who 'holds the opinion that the colour of the surroundings has an enormous effect on the recovery of the sick, especially those who are depressed for one reason or another or are suffering from shell shock', and had decorated a ward in line with these theories.[72] He used blue on the ceiling to resemble the sky and remove the 'idea of being shut in', and chose 'greenish yellow' for the walls to represent the colour of spring foliage to make the space more 'cheerful'.[73] The walls were yellow with a green undertone, while the floor had more green and evoked grass. The idea that the careful application of colour to hospital design could improve physical and psychological health was relatively unusual at the time, and Prosser's 'colour wards' were widely reported upon.[74] Despite the cultural association between Modernism and whiteness, many key Modernist architects were also interested in colour theory; Le Corbusier, for example, published a book in 1931 called *Polycromie Architecturale* (*Polychrome Architecture*) that – in part – addressed the role of colour in evoking emotions.[75]

The colour psychology and colour theory of the late twentieth century, then, did not emerge from nowhere. One of the most influential post-war American colour theorists, Faber Birren, had been writing on the subject since the 1920s. However, it shifted from being an unusual or fringe interest into something much more mainstream.[76] Le Corbusier expanded his book in 1959 to include 20 further colours, which were more 'powerful and dynamic'.[77] In 1961, Birren bemoaned the plethora of English 'colour cultists ... devoted to chromotherapy, colour-breathing, the human aura' as 'romantic and superstitious' and advocated the more scientific approach of the psychological scientists to understand the relationship between colour, emotions, and health.[78]

It is unsurprising that hospitals came to be an important focus of colour psychology. They were emotional spaces. They could house people with mental health conditions, alongside others with physical ailments – or awaiting results for themselves or others – who could be feeling anything from high anxiety to boredom. They were also workspaces, in which thoughtful colour use was thought to promote productivity or efficiency and reduce stress. At first, emotional management was seen as part of the work of the 'healing machine'. Birren classed hospital colour use as 'functional', differing from buildings that were more decorative such as hotels and restaurants. This approach connects with a trend noted by Thierry Pillon in relation to colour in post-war French workplaces, of a growing interest in the 'functional' aspects of colour in terms of something that was useful and that played a clear, defined role in a given built environment.[79] The turn towards pale blues and greens was, for Birren and those influenced by him, part of the 'function' of hospitals as therapeutic environments that supported rest and recuperation. In 1961, Birren wrote: '[i]f the decoration of a home should properly gratify the aesthetic fancies of the owner, the hospital should serve the ends of medicine, look upon colour as a psycho-therapeutic agent rather than a mere frill [...] beauty should be a by-product of utility'.[80] This is similar to comments made by some of his contemporaries in Britain, who emphasised the utility of colour; in 1949, for example, an article in *The Hospital* described 'colour conditioning' not only as a technique to prevent eye strain, but also as a potentially valuable way 'to create a frame of mind suitable to the state of the patient'.[81] The author drew on research in the US and Australia, which was part of growing international research into the 'functional' aspects of colour and its power potentially 'to create moods more conducive to favourable reaction under treatment'.[82]

The goal, in this 'functional' framework, was to improve emotions in the pursuit of better treatment and recovery rather than for their own sake. This was part of the shift towards 'humanistic' hospital design, but it differed from some of the later models of the 'humanistic' hospital, which would come to use art, colour, nature, and more as an apparent counter-balance to high-technology medicine.

For Birren, colour was *part* of medicine, and he viewed his model of 'humanistic' colour palettes as more 'scientific' than those who pursued pure 'beauty' or decoration as routes to the same end.[83] This is not to say that he thought colour was in itself a form of treatment, in the chromotherapy model. In his article for *The Hospital* magazine in 1951, architect Arthur L. Hall noted that Birren had said in 1946 that colour does not 'cure' but that it could shape human moods, which could in itself be 'therapeutic'.[84]

As Figure 2.7 shows, in practice 'functional' and 'decorative' colour palettes were not dramatically different; hotels were also sites of rest, and colour palettes had to be perceived as pleasant 'decoration' to serve their therapeutic functions. Apart from a couple of notable exceptions – such as 'flamingo' pink – both colour palettes were relatively muted and only subtly different, with pastel colours appearing in both the 'functional' and 'decorative' categories.

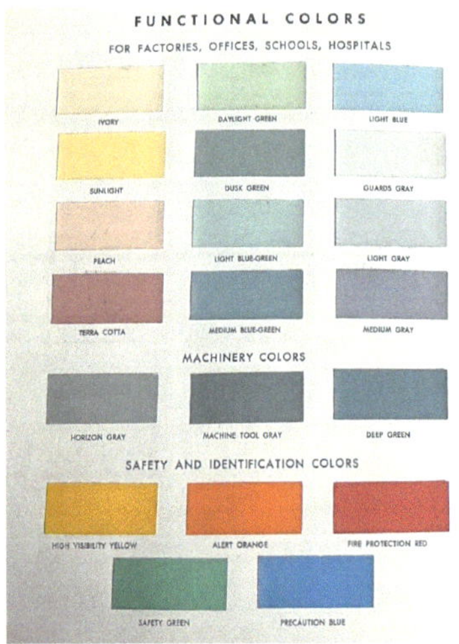

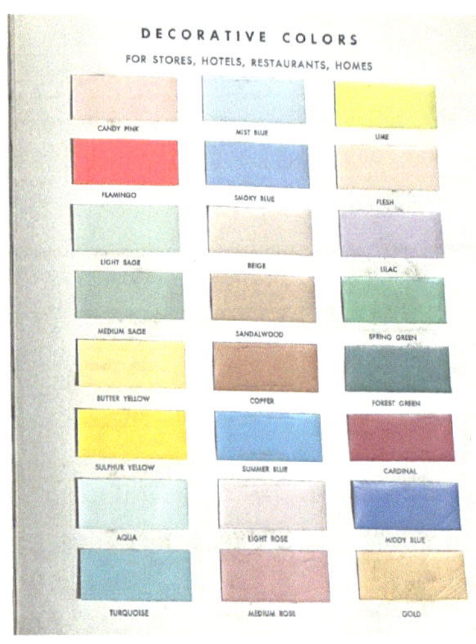

Figure 2.7 Faber Birren, *New Horizons in Col*or (Reinhold Publishing Corporation, 1955), np. Every effort has been made to trace the copyright holders and obtain permission to reproduce this material. Please do get in touch with any enquiries or information about this image or the rights holder. Image taken by Victoria Bates from a personal copy.

The names of the colours are also worthy of some attention. As Michel Pastoureau notes, such labelling was important: 'Words possess infinite chromatic powers. Any adjective associated with any colour term bestows upon it a particular nuance'.[85] Birren gave some of his 'functional' shades of green names that evoked nature, such as 'daylight green' and 'dusk green', which might be considered decorative rather than utilitarian. The main distinction appears to be a leaning towards so-called 'cooler' colours for functional spaces, a wider colour palette for decorative spaces, and the most vibrant shades used for safety purposes.

Birren's work was not universally accepted. A critical review of one of his books in 1970 in *Architects' Journal* declared that

> The author is simply not qualified to discuss history, philosophy, aesthetics or anything else apart from the limited sphere where apparently he is expert. His colour code for safety, devised in 1942 for the US Navy, has become a national [i.e. US] standard. This book is not likely to become a standard anywhere.[86]

However, there is extensive evidence that such colour theories had direct impacts on colour schemes in British hospitals, even if those choosing the colours were not engaging in depth with the psychological theories underpinning them. The 'Arts for Health' archive collection of work in Manchester hospitals, held at the Wellcome Library, includes international literature about colour and colour psychology throughout the late twentieth century (1960s–1990s) and substantiates the direct influence of Birren on NHS hospital design.[87] In the 1960s Pilkington's Tiles Ltd even directly engaged Birren as their colour consultant for a publication on ceramic tiles for hospitals.[88] In a study on colour commissioned by NHS Estates Research and Development, published in 2006, Dalke *et al.* note the long-term legacy of these ideas in NHS hospitals:

> Much conventional application of colour has been built on the earlier advice of colour design consultants such as Faber Birren who prescribed certain colour schemes [...] these have become dated, yet they have established conventions which are still in use today. The overuse of blue or green, for example, in medical interiors has been widely observed especially in older institutional buildings.[89]

Other developments in international colour psychology and colour theory had slightly less influence on hospitals over the course of the late twentieth century. The famous colour 'Baker Miller pink' for example, tested in US prisons and psychiatric institutions as an anti-violence shade in the late 1970s and early 1980s, has been used only very selectively in British contexts, including NHS hospitals.[90]

The separation of hospitals from more 'decorative' spaces of shops, hotels, and homes is important in understanding what the perceived function of colour was in early post-war healthcare design. This separation was challenged as hospitals looked increasingly to hotels and homes in the 1960s and 1970s as models for 'humanisation'.[91] By the mid-1970s, official DHSS guidance on hospital colour schemes shifted away from the idea that all colour in hospitals was 'functional'.[92] It started to distinguish instead between 'hard' clinical areas, requiring neutral palettes, and the 'soft' areas of hospitals, where more decoration might be beneficial as part of 'a pleasant reassuring atmosphere'; the latter apparently included relatives' waiting areas, day rooms, dining rooms, entrances, and children's rooms.[93] Both frameworks attended to the emotional aspects of colour and its therapeutic potential but there was a subtle discursive difference between colour as 'functional', which was grounded in scientific research about its psychological and physiological effects on patient health, and colour as something more atmospheric, which could have emotional benefits for everyone in the hospital. The rhetoric around colour, emotions, and the hospital shifted in tone over time, from the management of emotions as part of the function of the hospital to improving emotional experience as a valuable goal in its own right. 'Function' would later reappear in the form of evidence-based design, but it was not core to the 'humanisation' agenda.

This background is important for understanding what was meant by often generic statements about 'cheerful' colours in healthcare settings. Literature on subjects ranging from GP waiting rooms to hospital wards emphasised the value of 'cheerful' and 'bright' colour schemes, but often without explaining what that meant.[94] As noted above, 'bright' at this time often actually meant light and pastel, rather than the vibrant shades that would come later in the century, and 'cheerful' was seemingly rooted in broad ideas about the psychological merits of different colour palettes. In colour theory, including colour theory for hospitals, blues and greens were commonly conceived of as optimistic or cheerful. These emotional qualities are perhaps surprising for 'cool' colours, though the concepts of 'warm' and 'cool' are malleable. Michel Pastoureau notes that blue had traditionally been considered a 'warm' colour that began to 'cool' in the seventeenth century, and only gained its 'true status as a cool colour' in the nineteenth century because of its growing association with water.[95] In general, 'cooling' and 'restful' qualities were not deemed incompatible with 'cheer' if designed with care, for example with warm undertones, or in combination with other colours to avoid making a space feel 'cold'.

Describing such colour-based and emotion-centred design as 'with care' is deliberate, to recognise that material environments and design decisions could be part of care practices. This approach links to the work of Christina Buse, Daryl Martin, and Sarah Nettleton, on 'materialities of care', who note that materials and architecture can 'sometimes "stand in" for caring relations, and may shape, enable, or constrain practices of caring … materialities are not merely a backdrop for care interactions, but play an active role in constituting relations of care'.[96] Though care is itself a complex and disputed concept, it is widely agreed that care is an ongoing practice rather than a single act. In line with the principles underpinning this book, Buse, Martin, and Nettleton also argue that 'a focus on mundane or taken for granted materials can unfix understandings of care'.[97] Here, it is colour that is 'taken for granted' and which is an often overlooked component of the assemblages of people, objects, spaces, and practices that constitute the ongoing process of 'care'.

In some ways, the goal of creating 'cheerful' environments was nothing new. Clare Hickman, for example, shows that emotional states such as 'cheerful' and 'tranquil' often underpinned the design of asylum gardens in the nineteenth century.[98] White was thought of by some as a cheerful colour.[99] 'Cheerfulness' and 'calm' can be seen as similar to 'modernity', in terms of being consistent design goals but with new colour palettes over time. What *was* new, in this model of mid-century modern 'cheer', was the role of colour psychology and colour theory. Colour theorists often combined ideas about the physical and psychological impacts of different colours through the concepts of 'warm' and 'cool' colours. An article in *The Hospital* in 1949, for example, observed that 'the emotional qualities of colour, it is said, can be utilised to stimulate or stabilise and create sensations of warmth or coolness as many be required'.[100] There was long-standing debate among theorists of emotion about whether physiological symptoms were the articulation of mental emotions or *vice versa*, but for many contemporary writers on colour and emotion the two were not clearly separated.[101] The idea of green as a colour that was cooling, soothing, and restful, for example, embraced rest for the eyes and soul alike.

For other post-war thinkers, a 'warm' colour was a social or cultural signifier of meaning, rather than an innate value. In 1968 Jean Baudrillard noted, for example, that

> in a sense we are no longer dealing with colours *per se* but with more abstract values [...] it is not so much a question of blue and green as of one of *hot and cold* [...] colours lose their unique value, and become relative to each other and to the whole. This is what is meant by describing them as 'functional'.[102]

This comment draws direct comparisons with Birren's 'functional' colours and the value of understanding colours in relative terms (for example 'functional' versus 'decorative', 'cool' versus 'warm'). For Baudrillard, though, the 'function' was purely symbolic. Colour and materials could create 'functional' warmth through the 'abstract synchrony of a perpetual "warm-and-cold" which in reality continually defers any real "warm" feeling. This is a purely signified warmth'.[103] There were thus a range of different ways of thinking about colour, emotion, and the importance of 'warm' and 'cool' shades at this time, and it was an emerging area of interest to researchers from colour theorists to psychologists and sociologists. Each field had different conceptual frameworks for thinking about colour, though they shared an interest in concepts such as 'warmth' and 'coolness'.

Returning to green as a case study of emotions and colour, the idea of green as a colour of cheer, hope, and optimism had wider cultural origins.[104] For example, David Howes and Constance Classen note that purple, white, and green, stood for 'dignity, purity and hope' respectively in the suffrage movement.[105] White and green, as colours of purity and hope, held similar meanings in the twentieth-century hospital. The optimistic quality of green was also linked to its association with nature.[106] It is no coincidence that so many shades of green paint had 'natural' names. However, not all greens were thought to be equally cheerful. Old shades of green were widely deemed 'depressing' and 'sombre' as a point of comparison with the 'optimism' of new, fresh, bright pastel colour palettes – usually including pastel greens – of the early NHS.[107] In 1969, John Agate was still bemoaning the presence of 'the old style cream-and-green painted wards'.[108] The *BMJ* later described the dark greens of the 1920s as 'sombre' colours, pre-dating more 'progressive' white walls.[109] In *The Lancet* in 1956, a psychiatrist wrote about a mental health ward that was 'drab and depressing' in part because it 'had not been painted since 1925, and the prevailing colour scheme was olive-green and black'.[110] When the ward was 'entirely redecorated in modern pastel shades' in September 1955, they noted improvements in verbal and social engagement from patients.[111] Later commentators made similar comments about replacing the old-fashioned colour schemes of the mid-century, often with a focus on green and cream. Green was constantly both 'optimistic' and modern, and 'depressing' and old-fashioned at any given time.

For every article that spoke of green as cheerful, calming or modern, there was one that dismissed green as depressing or outdated. In 1955, Viscountess Ridley – a member of the Newcastle Hospital Board – complained that '[t]he chocolate and mustard of the old Public Assistance Institution or Orphanage has been replaced in our generation by a sickly green and cream, which to my mind is even more depressing, for it reflects a dullness and lack of imagination'.[112] She was referring particularly to the trend towards these colour schemes in old charitable institutions, creating a colour-based division between the apparent gleaming white modernity of new hospitals such as those in Kent discussed in Chapter 1, and the green-and-cream 'dullness' of old workhouses and other such institutions. This trend was repeated throughout the twentieth century. In *Hospital Development* in 1987, one author noted that the NHS hospital was characterised by 'green paint, clinical smells, Victorian institutionalism at its most daunting'.[113] Susan Barclay similarly notes that, by the 1980s, green paint was a symbol of depressing institutionalisation, citing 'pop artist Richard Hamilton's art installation titled *Treatment Room* (1983–84), which was 'a visual metaphor for the 1980s ward, with a bare bed surrounded by green and magnolia painted walls and no evidence of human comfort'.[114] At the same time, certain greens – such as the 'misty green' discussed above – were still deemed 'modern' and optimistic. Green also had specific emotional connotations in particular geographical locations: in some port cities, for example, green was considered unlucky as part of local fishing history and superstition.[115] Green was therefore not neatly the colour of optimism and hope, as might be assumed from reading colour theory.

As Rob Boddice notes in *The History of Emotions*, '[a]rchitectural intent tends not to map onto how people feel once the building is, for want of a better word, alive'.[116] Staff, architects, designers, and patients could differ in their responses to green. Interior designers, architects, and even some popular artists continued to deride green as a depressing colour of dehumanised institutions. For many, it took on similar symbolism to white, in terms of being clinical. However, patients did not always agree. By the 1980s, new understandings of 'patient-centredness' meant that genuine consultation was increasingly prioritised (designing with, rather than designing for). *Hospital Development* reported in 1983 that in a Ramsgate geriatric hospital 'the patients were asked to choose the colours and decided upon dark green, light green and beige'.[117] In 1982, the same journal quoted the principal assistant interior designer to the North East Thames Regional Health Authority, saying that the most popular colour was '[d]ear old green – much maligned by many hospital staff!'[118] In 1987, a 'Patient Perception Group' at South Tees Health Authority did extensive research into patients' experience and chose décor 'to soothe and reassure: a pale green predominates with splashes of bright yellow', alongside other careful sensory design, including sound and lighting. This was published in the very same issue, however, that lumped 'green paint' in with 'clinical smells' and 'Victorian institutionalism'.[119] The institutional association of green(s), or a nostalgia for colours associated with hospitals, may even have been the basis of their appeal for some. History was part of the reason that green was reassuring to some people, and depressing to others.

Nostalgia is both a personal and cultural emotion, and individual life stories have often altered the meaning of hospital green dramatically.[120] In people's stories of hospitals, green objects are cited fairly regularly in association with memories. Remembering work at Wythenshawe Hospital in the 1960s, for example, one nurse focused on the uniform's different shades of green and white: '[i]t changed year by year so as to give easy recognition of the nurse's seniority' with dark green denoting the most senior.[121] Another remembered that 'private patients [...] were not given much attention really [...]

but they did get a tray with green crockery rather than white'.[122] One nurse recalled that 'we had our own bedrooms. They were green', while another remembered sneaking back into their accommodation through 'the green door opposite the laundry'.[123] In theory, the mention of 'green' is not significant in all of these memories; the story of sneaking in through a laundry door, for example, does not rely on any description of the door. However, the colour was clearly significant to their memories and to the nurses' feelings about the past.

For others, green objects stand out as reminders of traumatic or difficult experiences. In one recent oral history interview, the interviewee noted that 'I do remember [being] in hospital at three, because I had to go in to have my tonsils out, so I do remember that. I remember the green cot that I was in, the metal, the smell of it. And I didn't like being back there at all'.[124] In a recent survey of people's sensory memories of the hospital, one respondent replied: 'Possibly linked to trauma of visiting someone after a serious accident – walking in to a long, dark ward (green?) with metal framed beds (cream) in long rows either side'.[125] One interviewee for the 'Sounds of our NHS' project made similar comments when remembering visiting her father in hospital in the 1960s as a child: 'Catching two buses to get to North Staffs. I can still remember the green walls and the black floors … and having to wait outside because children weren't allowed in the wards, so I used to have to sit in the corridor'.[126] The colour green is a shorthand in some of these accounts for embodied nostalgia or difficult memories, and is particularly powerful when combined with other sensory memories. The colour was genuinely a significant part of people's experiences and interaction with the hospital, but these stories are also powerful because of the emotional symbolism of hospital green.

The examples given to this point are people's memories, in which hospital green is the focus. Such emotional memories can also be reversed, with life experiences outside the hospital informing people's experiences of hospital green. As Sarah Hosking and Liz Haggard note, reflecting on NASA's findings about the individual nature of emotional relationships to colour, '[i]n other words, if as a child you were scratched by a ginger cat or had an unpleasant aunt who wore a violet dress, you will remain conditioned to dislike these colours. This does not augur well for the universality of

Dr Cleo Hanaway-Oakley
@CleoHanaway
Replying to @hospital_senses and @WellcomeLibrary
My husband proposed at Claridges so it has very strong (positive) associations!
Bristol Maid
12:23 PM · Nov 2, 2021 · Twitter for iPhone

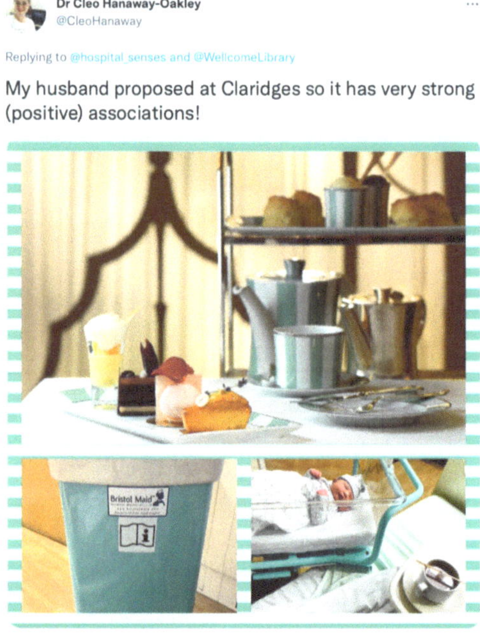

Figure 2.8 Cleo Hanaway-Oakley tweet, 2 November 2021. With thanks to Cleo Hanaway-Oakley for permission to share this image. Images © Cleo Hanaway-Oakley. All rights reserved and permission to use this figure must be obtained from the copyright holder.

colour reaction'.[127] Though Hosking and Haggard's examples are somewhat tongue-in-cheek, they are making an important point that is borne out by historical and contemporary evidence. A colleague from the University of Bristol recently told me, via social media: 'I was obsessed with the mint green in my room on the maternity recovery ward. It reminded me of the tea sets at Claridges!' where her husband had proposed.[128] Figure 2.8 shows images of these greens together, with a focus on non-medical objects and the shared sensory elements such as cups of tea. The materiality of the objects, their function, the shade of green, the context of childbirth, and individual memories or feelings all combined to give meaning to this colour.

Individual life stories, and the social, cultural, and demographic relationships between colour and emotion – which have their own histories – have shaped encounters with hospital colours over time. Taking green as a case study shows how the colour carried some significant cultural emotional associations throughout the late twentieth century, and into the present day. It seems no coincidence that the 2024 play *Nye*, about Bevan and the founding of the NHS, used various shades of green (alongside another key symbol of the NHS, the hospital bed) heavily in its set design as part of evoking nostalgia in the audience.[129] Green was also, though, always relational and co-produced with other actors in hospitals. To quote Birgitte Schepelern Johansen on the materiality of emotions, emotions can also be found 'beyond the individual: in spaces, atmospheres, objects … dispersed, across and in between'.[130] Colour itself can be seen as an actor in emotional networks, shaping what is broadly conceived as the 'atmospheres' or 'affective atmospheres' of hospitals.[131]

Conclusions

In post-war Britain the colours of modernity expanded, and the hospital new palettes, such as pastels, helped to freshen and modernise hospitals. In 1965, architect Dorothy W. Strachan noted that – partly for reasons of economy – 'for more than a century' British hospitals 'did get by, inside and out, on virtually three colours – brown, cream and green gloss'.[132] With the expansion of colour palettes in post-war Britain, brighter and lighter shades – though by no means vivid at this stage – replaced those three colours and white as the markers of a modern, hygienic hospital. Hospital green brightened and lightened over time, with the goal of making hospitals more pleasant for patients, visitors, and staff alike. Green was thought to serve a multitude of purposes, from Faber Birren's 'functional' therapeutic goals through to the creation of a reassuring, modern healthcare space. It was part of expanding the remit of the modern hospital and the NHS itself, to acknowledge and address the emotions of workers, patients, and visitors.

The use of green in hospitals reveals the growing importance of an emotion-led way of thinking about hospital colour. New layers of green existed in dialogue with 'old-fashioned' green. However, this was not a one-off event but a cycle that was repeated over the late twentieth century as new 'modern' or 'brighter' greens replaced older ones. In each of these cycles, green maintained its importance as a colour not only of modernity but also of emotion: each new green was apparently the best suited for the psychological and therapeutic needs of staff and patients, and represented progress from 'depressing' or 'dull' old shades. Through close attention to subtle shifts in the colour green, and the ways in which it was discussed over time, it becomes possible to see how concepts such as 'modern' and 'old-fashioned' were brought into being through emotional and colour-based rhetoric. The colour combination of green and cream continues to hold great power in healthcare settings today, as a shorthand for outdated or old-fashioned colour schemes.

Criticisms of colour schemes as 'old-fashioned' were inextricably bound up with emotive language such as 'depressing'. Post-war British hospital design was greatly influenced by new work in colour theory, and colour schemes were increasingly designed not only with staff efficiency but also patient experience in mind. Each criticism of 'depressing' old, dark colour schemes and their replacement with 'modern' fresh colours – even if just, in practice, slightly different shades of green and cream – helped to express some of these patient-centred principles. Its strong association with the hospital means that green has also, over time, taken on significance for individuals as a relational emotional experience, whether in the form of nostalgia or traumatic memories. The emotional dimensions of green were produced through intersections of cultural, individual, and material factors. Though a similar claim could be made for any other colour, 'hospital green' is particularly resistant to a neat cultural history approach to meaning. As Michel Pastoureau notes: 'Green seems to be an ambivalent, if not an ambiguous, colo[u]r'.[133] It was a crucial part of the making of the affective atmospheres of hospitals, albeit never in a consistent way. Green was always an emotional colour and became more explicitly so in the NHS.

Notes

1 'Bringing Colour to Life in the Hospital World', *The Hospital*, February 1951, p. ix.

2 'Bringing Colour to Life'.
3 Jonathan Hughes, '"The "Matchbox on a Muffin": The Design of Hospitals in the early NHS', *Medical History*, 44 (2000), pp. 21–56.
4 Lynda Nead, *The Tiger in the Smoke: Art and Culture in Post-War Britain* (Yale University Press, 2017), pp. 134–5. On modernity and colour beyond Britain, see also Nicholas Gaskill, *Chromographia: American Literature and the Modernization of Color* (University of Minnesota Press, 2018).
5 Martin D. Moore, '"Bright-While-You-Wait"? Waiting Rooms and the National Health Service, c. 1948–58', in Jennifer Crane and Jane Hand (eds), *Posters, Protests, and Prescriptions: Cultural Histories of the National Health Service in Britain* (Manchester University Press, 2022), p. 214.
6 D. W. A. McCreadie, 'A Hospital Colour Scheme', *BMJ*, 16 June 1962, p. 1689.
7 For more detail see Chapter 5, which discusses 'brightness' in more depth.
8 'Colour Conditioning for Hospitals', *The Hospital,* January 1949, p. 45.
9 'Colour Conditioning for Hospitals'.
10 On pastels as a way to brighten up dark buildings in the US see 'Cycles and Cures', *Hospital Development*, 15 (1987), p. 45.
11 Jenson and Nicholson, *The Function of Colour in Factories, Schools and Hospitals* (Jenson and Nicholson, c. 1940s/1950s). The exact date of this publication is unclear. Vicky Long cites it as the 1940s, though the text I saw is undated. The British Library lists it as the 1960s, though the company merged with another in 1960 and had a different name so this seems incorrect. The book references Cuprinol, which they apparently distributed from 1945 onwards, so this book is seemingly from some point between 1945 and the late 1950s. On the history of the company, which informed this date estimate, see https://www.gracesguide.co.uk/Jenson_and_Nicholson [accessed: 10 June 2025].
12 Arthur L. Hall, 'Colour in the Hospital', *The Hospital*, June 1951.
13 On use of private consultants on colour schemes by regional architects in the early 1960s see The National Archives, MH158/187, 1961–66, 'Employment of Interior Designers on the Staff of Regional Hospital Boards Architects'.
14 Jean Symons, *CEH Design Guide 1: Improving Existing Hospital Buildings for Long-Stay Residents* (CEH: London, 1973), p. 9.
15 Nuffield Provincial Hospitals Trust, *Studies in the Functions and Design of Hospitals*, preface.

16 Hall, 'Colour in the Hospital', p. 384.
17 Nuffield Trust, *Studies in the Functions and Design of Hospitals*, p. 111; 'Colour in Factories', *Architects' Journal* (*AJ*), 5 July 1961, p. 17; see also the Dockers' Paint advert 'Putting Colour to Work?', *AJ*, 24 June 1954, p. xxxii, which refers to the importance of colour for 'soothing, guiding and classifying' in office buildings, hospitals, schools and factories.
18 Melanie Bühler, 'Why the White Cube is No Longer White', http://www.metropolism.com/nl/features/39062_colour_critique_reflections_17 [accessed: 16 August 2021].
19 Jenson and Nicholson, *The Function of Colour*, pp. 14–47.
20 *Ibid.*, pp. 75–6.
21 As Jackson and Moore note '[d]uring the twentieth century it became customary to mobilise concepts of balance and imbalance to capture the multiple dimensions of human, non-human and planetary health"; Mark Jackson and Martin D. Moore, 'Introduction: Balancing the Self in the Twentieth Century', in Mark Jackson and Martin D. Moore (eds), *Balancing the Self* (Manchester University Press, 2020), pp. 1–30, 4.
22 Francis J. Blaise, 'The Color Prism in Today's Hospital', *Hospital Management*, 89 (1960), p. 38. This article was published in the US journal *Hospital Management* but clearly had an influence in the UK, as it made its way onto the 'Colour in Hospitals: Sources of Reference' list of The British Health Care Arts Centre.
23 Jenson and Nicholson, *The Function of Colour*, pp. 79–80.
24 *Ibid.*
25 *Ibid.*, p. 74.
26 'Hospital in Dunbartonshire', *Architects' Journal*, 3 November 1955, p. 603.
27 Newcastle Regional Hospital Board (NRHB), *The Use of Colour in Hospitals* (NRHB, 1955), pp. 14 and 40; Nuffield Provincial Hospitals Trust, *Studies in the Functions and Design of Hospitals* (Oxford University Press, 1955), p. 111.
28 NRHB, *Colour in Hospitals.*
29 'Miscellaneous: Colour in Hospitals', *Architects' Journal*, 3 November 1955, p. 609.
30 'Colour Conditioning for Hospitals', *The Hospital*, January 1949, p. 46.
31 'Notes on Equipment Supplies and Services', *The Hospital*, September 1951, p. 671.
32 Hall, 'Colour in the Hospital', p. 384.
33 The National Archives, DT 33/1326, 8 February 1952, Report on Inspection of Hospital for Assistant Nurse Training: Thornbury Hospital.

34 Record Office for Leicestershire, Leicester and Rutland, DE9471/29, 1955, Hinckley Hospital Visitors Book.
35 Harriet Richardson Blakeman, 'Medicine and modernity: fifty years of NHS hospital building in Scotland, 1948–1998' (PhD Dissertation: University of Edinburgh, 2023), p. 127.
36 Hall, 'Colour in the Hospital', p. 379.
37 Hall, 'Colour in the Hospital', p. 384.
38 'Hospital Extension', *Architects' Journal*, April 1959, p. 563.
39 Nuffield Provincial Hospitals Trust, *Studies in the Functions and Design of Hospitals* (Oxford University Press, 1955), p. 114.
40 'Building Illustrated: Hospital Extension', *Architects' Journal*, 10 September 1959, p. 177.
41 'Technical Section', *Architects' Journal*, July 1954, p. 147.
42 Wellcome Library, ART/AFH/A/9/9, Colour/Environmental Effect: Articles and Papers, 1960s–1990s. John Agate, 'Colour Can Transform Our Older Hospitals', *Health*, 6 (1969), p. 13.
43 *Ibid.*
44 *Ibid.*
45 For example, Jeanne Kisacky, 'Blood Red, Soothing Green, and Pure White: What Color Is Your Operating Room?', in Marilyn DeLong and Barbara Martinson (eds), *Color and Design* (A & C Black, 2013), pp. 118–24; David Pantalony, 'The Colour of Medicine', *CMAJ*, 181 (2009), pp. 402–3; Julie Willis, Philip Goad, and Cameron Logan, *Architecture and the Modern Hospital: Nosokomeion to Hygeia* (Routledge, 2019), p. 83.
46 Harry M. Sherman, 'The Green Operating Room at St. Luke's Hospital', *California State Journal of Medicine*, 12 (1914), p. 181.
47 Palugi J. Flagg, 'A Scientific Basis for the Use of Color in the Operating Room', *Modern Hospital*, 22 (1924), pp. 555–9.
48 Richey L. Waugh and Esther M. Welch, 'The Use of Color in the Operating Room', *The American Journal of Surgery*, 60 (1943), pp. 309–11.
49 See, for example, Historic England, 'The Interior of an Operating Theatre at West Dorset County Hospital', 8 April 1987, https://historicengland.org.uk/images-books/photos/item/JLP01/10/26678 [accessed: 9 February 2024].
50 A. Ashworth, 'Conversion Project at King's Mill Hospital', *The Hospital*, November 1951, p. 775; Dorset History Centre, D-PPY/A/4/3/8/1, Pilkington's, *Hospital Tiling* (nd).
51 Mass Observation Archive (University of Sussex), Replies to Spring 1997 directive [R1418].
52 'Cycles and Cures'.

53 For example B. S. Platt, T. P. Eddy, and P. L. Pellett, *Food in Hospitals: A Study of Feeding Arrangements and the Nutritional Value of Meals in Hospitals* (Oxford University Press, 1963) described 'an old poor-law hospital with additions in 1927 and later … Green and buff paint', p. 123.
54 Brian Abel-Smith, *The Hospitals, 1800–1948: A Study in Social Administration in England and Wales* (Heinemann, 1964), p. 403.
55 'Canadian Red Cross Hospital', *BMJ* (June 1940), p. 1031.
56 Vicky Long, *The Rise and Fall of the Healthy Factory: The Politics of Industrial Health in Britain, 1914–60* (Palgrave Macmillan, 2010), pp. 65–6.
57 'Health in the Factories', *The Lancet*, 25 January 1947, p. 151.
58 William J. B. Groves, 'New Developments at Clatterbridge General Hospital', *The Hospital*, February 1951, p. 91.
59 Kresen Kernow, AHA/372, 'Minutes, Liskeard Hospitals' house committee', 1948–54.
60 Mass Observation Archive (University of Sussex), Replies to Spring 1997 directive [N1592].
61 Sarah Bennett, 'Re-forming the Institution: The Wall as Memory Archive', *Journal of Media Practice*, 11 (2010), pp. 199–214.
62 Serena Dyer, 'Masculinities, Wallpaper, and Crafting Domestic Space within the University, 1795–1914', *Nineteenth-Century Gender Studies*, 14 (2018), np.
63 Pantalony, 'The Colour of Medicine'.
64 London Metropolitan Archives, A/KE/I/01/06//002, 'Wall Surfaces (St. Bartholomew's Hospital)'.
65 Most recently, see their 'Next Generation Bedside Cabinet' designed with Kinneir Dufort in 2010. This piece of furniture is used for personal objects and not medical purposes, but is explicitly designed – and named – to be hygienic.
66 Science Museum Group, 'Clergy Stole, England, 1991', https://collection.sciencemuseumgroup.org.uk/objects/co8012326/clergy-stole-england-1991-clergy-stole [accessed: 9 February 2024].
67 Platt *et al.*, *Food in Hospitals* described how '[p]rocessed peas were extremely pale when served to the patients, but the same peas were a bright and chemical green when served to the staff, to the surprise of the hospital secretary, who exclaimed: "Good God, have they been dyed?"', p. 170. There are many examples of contemporary comments on the health or presence of green plants in hospitals, though this quote about dusty pot plants is taken from Susan Barclay, *When It's Not the Main Game: Art in Hospitals* (PhD Dissertation: University of Western Sydney, 2015), p. 210.

68 Jane Willis interviewed by Victoria Bates, 21 February 2023. Victoria Bates, 'Sensing Spaces of Healthcare' interviews, published December 2024, https://doi.org/10.5523/bris.3b8eg2be3ecw52vt38l7nq9kah
69 Sasha Handley and John Emrys Morgan, 'Environment, Emotion and Early Modernity', *Environment and History*, 28 (2022), p. 356.
70 Samina T. Yousuf Azeemi and Mohsin Raza, 'A Critical Analysis of Chromotherapy and its Scientific Evolution', *Evidence-Based Complementary and Alternative Medicine*, 2 (2005), p. 482.
71 Cited in Pantalony, 'The Colour of Medicine', pp. 402–3.
72 'A Colour Ward', *Lancet* (October 1917), p. 542. See also E. N. Snowden, 'Report on the Kemp Prossor Colour Scheme', *The Lancet*, March 1919, pp. 522–3.
73 'A Colour Ward'.
74 On the international impact of his work see Jim Berryman, 'The Colour Treatment: A Convergence of Art and Medicine at the Red Cross Russell Lea Nerve Home', *Health and History*, 18 (2016), pp. 5–21.
75 Eduardo Souza, 'Le Corbusier's Color Theory: Embracing Polychromy in Architecture', 18 July 2023, https://www.archdaily.com/1003880/le-corbusiers-color-theory-embracing-polychromy-in-architecture [accessed: 14 May 2023].
76 'Colour Conditioning for Hospitals', *The Hospital*, January 1949, pp. 45–6; see also Katharina Cichosch, 'Thinking in Colors? On the Revolutionary Ideas of Josef Albers', 15 July 2016, https://www.schirn.de/en/magazine/context/josef_albers_interaction_of_color_peter_halley_color_theory/ [accessed: 9 February 2024].
77 'Architectural Polychromy', https://www.lescouleurs.ch/en/the-colours/colour-system/ [accessed 14 May 2024].
78 Faber Birren, 'The Rational Approach to Colour in Hospitals', *The Hospital*, September 1961, p. 565.
79 Thierry Pillon, 'The Colours of Atmosphere: The Example of Offices in the 1950s and 1960s', *Communications*, 102 (2018), pp. 199–209.
80 Birren, 'The Rational Approach to Colour in Hospitals'.
81 'Colour Conditioning for Hospitals', p. 45.
82 *Ibid.*
83 Birren, 'The Rational Approach to Colour in Hospitals'.
84 Hall, 'Colour in the Hospital'.
85 Michel Pastoureau, *The Colours of Our Memories*, trans. Janet Lloyd (Polity, 2022 [2010]), p. 136.
86 David Pearce, 'Reviews: Designs of "Colour"', *Architects' Review* (16 September 1970), p. 681.
87 Wellcome Library, ART/AFH/A/9/9.

88 Dorset History Centre, D-PPY/A/4/3/8/1, Pilkington's, *Hospital Tiling* (1964).
89 Dalke *et al.* 'Colour and Lighting in Hospital Design', *Optics & Laser Technology*, 38 (2006), pp. 353–4.
90 Alexander G. Schauss, 'The Physiological Effect of Color on the Suppression of Human Aggression: Research on Baker-Miller Pink', *International Journal of Biosocial Research*, 7 (1985), pp. 55–64.
91 Chapter 3 explores 'humanisation' in more depth, and it continues to be a theme in Chapter 4.
92 The National Archives, MH166/1136, Harness Interiors produced by the interior designers from the Regional Health Authorities and the Department of Health & Social Security, part of the papers of the 'Technical Design Group', 1973–75.
93 The National Archives, Harness Interiors.
94 Moore, '"Bright-While-You-Wait"?'
95 Michel Pastoureau, *Blue: The History of a Color*, trans. Markus I. Cruse (Princeton University Press, 2001 [2000]), p. 181.
96 Christina Buse, Daryl Martin, and Sarah Nettleton, 'Conceptualising "Materialities of Care": Making Visible Mundane Material Culture in Health and Social Care Contexts', *Sociology of Health & Illness*, 40 (2018), p. 245.
97 Buse, Martin, and Nettleton, 'Conceptualising "Materialities of Care"', p. 245.
98 Clare Hickman, 'Cheerfulness and Tranquillity: Gardens in the Victorian Asylum', *The Lancet Psychiatry*, 1 (2014), pp. 506–7.
99 See Chapter 1.
100 'Colour Conditioning for Hospitals', p. 45.
101 For a high-profile early example of this ongoing debate, see Walter B. Cannon, 'The James-Lange theory of Emotions: A Critical Examination and an Alternative Theory', *American Journal of Psychology*, 39 (1927), pp. 106–24.
102 Jean Baudrillard, *The System of Objects*, trans. James Benedict (Verso, 1996 [1968]), p. 35.
103 *Ibid.*, p. 37.
104 See Michel Pastoureau, *Green: The History of a Color*, trans. Jody Gladding (Princeton University Press, 2014 [2013]).
105 David Howes and Constance Classen, *Ways of Sensing: Understanding the Senses in Society* (Routledge, 2014), p. 77.
106 On nature in hospitals see also Chapters 3 and 6.
107 Agate, 'Colour can Transform'.
108 Wellcome Library, ART/AFH/A/9/9, Agate, 'Colour in Hospital', p. 15.

109 D. W. A. McCreadie, 'A Hospital Colour Scheme', *BMJ*, June 1962, p. 1687.
110 A. R. May, 'Changes of Social Environment: Their Effect on Mentally Deteriorated Patients', *The Lancet*, April 1956, pp. 500–2.
111 May, 'Changes of Social Environment'.
112 NRHB, *The Use of Colour in Hospitals*, p. iv. This was even quoted in the news: 'Green and Cream Out of Date', *Manchester Guardian*, 6 October 1955, p. 10.
113 Jane Green, 'Profit by Design – An Inside View', *Hospital Development*, 16 (1988), p. 26.
114 Barclay, *When It's Not the Main Game*, p. 210.
115 I was told, anecdotally, that hospitals in Hull avoid green though I have not been able to verify this in text. However, the link between green, boats, and bad luck is widely reported as a 'superstition'. For example, see 'Boating Superstitions and Good Omens to Abide By', https://www.boatinternational.com/yachts/editorial-features/yachting-boat-sailor-superstitions-sea [accessed 25 September 2024].
116 Rob Boddice, *The History of Emotions* (Manchester University Press, 2018), p. 170.
117 'Viewpoint', *Hospital Development*, 11 (1983), p. 6.
118 Susan Black, 'Interior Design Trends', *Hospital Development*, 10 (1982), p. 24.
119 Bill Murray, 'Changing the Face of Patient Care', *Hospital Development*, 16 (1988), p. 25.
120 On nostalgia, see Agnes Arnold-Forster, *Nostalgia: A History of a Dangerous Emotion* (Pan Macmillan, 2024).
121 Manchester University NHS Foundation Trust Library, 'Memories of Nursing at Wythenshawe Hospital 1966–2008'.
122 Roger Sim and Helen Kitchen, *More than a Place of Healing: An Anthology of Memories, Memorabilia and Anecdotes of Withington Hospital* (Hospital Arts, 1999), p. 54. Thanks to Manchester University NHS Foundation Trust Library for access to this publication.
123 Sim and Kitchen, *More than a Place of Healing*, p. 84.
124 British Library Sounds, C1559/14, Richard Rieser Interviewed by John Hargreaves, Oral Histories of Disabled People's Experience of Education © The Alliance for Inclusive Education.
125 'Sensing Spaces of Healthcare: NHS Sensory Memory Bank', Memory 15, https://hospitalsenses.blogs.bristol.ac.uk [accessed: 9 February 2024]. Research conducted by the author.
126 British Library Sounds, C1887/216, Vivian Lowe interviewed by Stephen Rydzkowski, October 2018, Voices of Our National Health Service © University of Manchester.

127 Sarah Hosking and Liz Haggard, *Healing the Hospital Environment: Design, Management and Maintenance of Healthcare Premises* (E. & F. N. Spon, 1999), p. 120.
128 Cleo Hanaway-Oakley, https://twitter.com/CleoHanaway, Tweet from 2 November 2021, quoted with permission.
129 'Nye at the National Theatre – Reviews Round-Up', https://www.westendtheatre.com/225398/news/reviews/nye-at-the-national-theatre-reviews-round-up/ [accessed: 30 April 2024]. Thanks to Clare Hickman for drawing my attention to this set design.
130 Birgitte Schepelern Johansen, 'Locating Hatred: On the Materiality of Emotions', *Emotion, Space and Society*, 16 (2015), pp. 48–55. Thanks to members of The Centre of Excellence in History of Experiences (HEX) in Finland for introducing me to this work as part of a visiting scholarship in June 2023. On emotions, space, place, and architecture see also Sara Honarmand Ebrahimi (ed.), 'Exploring Architecture and Emotions through Space and Place', *Emotions: History, Culture, Society*, 6 (2022), pp. 65–177.
131 There is extensive work on atmospheres and affective atmospheres; some scholars use the terminology explicitly, though historians tend to write more in terms of emotions, space, and place. The work of Sara Honarmand Ebrahimi, for example, speaks in important ways to emotions, space, place, and hospital buildings in history, with a focus on colonial contexts. Ed DeVane also writes on 'emotional communities', 'emotional ecologies', and engages explicitly with the concept of affective atmospheres in relation to early NHS healthcare planning in his PhD thesis; Edward Patrick DeVane, 'Building the NHS: Planning, Publics and Britain's New State Healthcare Facilities, 1945–74' (PhD Dissertation: University of Warwick, 2022). Agnes Arnold-Forster also writes on 'emotional landscape' as a spatial as well as emotional concept. See, for example, 'The Emotional Landscape of the Hospital Residence in Post-War Britain', in Agnes Arnold-Forster and Alison Moulds (eds), *Feelings and Work in Modern History: Emotional Labour and Emotions about Labour* (Bloomsbury, 2022), pp. 58–75. The actual concept of 'atmospheres' is used more explicitly in relation to current-day healthcare settings and theoretical frameworks. See Deborah Lupton, 'How Does Health Feel? Towards Research on the Affective Atmospheres of Digital Health', *Digital Health*, 3 (2017), pp. 1–11; Daryl Martin, Christina Buse, Nik Brown, Sarah Nettleton, Alan Lewis, and Lynne Chapman, 'Assembling Atmospheres, Encountering Care: Risk, Affect, and Safety in the Cystic Fibrosis Clinic', *Wellbeing, Space and Society*, 3 (2022), pp. 1–9; Daryl Martin, Sarah Nettleton, and Christina Buse, 'Affecting Care: Maggie's Centres

and the Orchestration of Architectural Atmospheres', *Social Science & Medicine*, 240 (2019), pp. 1–8; Shanti Sumartojo *et al.*, 'Atmospheres of Care in a Psychiatric Inpatient Unit', *Design for Health*, 4 (2020), pp. 24–42; Shanti Sumartojo and Sarah Pink, *Atmospheres and the Experiential World: Theory and Methods* (Routledge, 2019), pp. 81–6.

132 Dorothy W. Strachan, 'Colour in Hospitals', *Nursing Times*, 7 May 1965, np.

133 Pastoureau, *Green*, p. 7.

3

Arts: humanising healthcare

From 1960 onwards, there were two important trends in hospital architecture and design.[1] Firstly, the 1962 Hospital Plan for England and Wales marked the first significant investment in NHS infrastructure. The Hospital Plan led to the building of new, larger District General Hospitals. At the same time, internationally, there was growing interest in patient experience. Julie Willis, Philip Goad, and Cameron Logan argue that this had consequences for hospital design: '[a]s popular taste began to move away from functional modernism and anti-institutional feeling grew, particularly from the late 1960s, the designers of hospitals sought to distance the hospital from its overly institutional feel'.[2] These two trends were entwined and at times in tension. The NHS was constructing large institutions, many of which were high-rise structures that built on the post-war preference for functionalist 'matchbox on a muffin' design, or 'brutalist megahospitals' of around 600–800 beds, just when there was a cultural turn away from such large and overly 'institutional' buildings.[3] These parallel trends can be explained, in part, by a time-lag of around ten years from design commission to building for many hospitals; new, large District General Hospitals in the 1970s did not represent contemporary trends in architectural thought.[4] Indeed, many quickly became seen not only as 'white elephant' projects but as large, dehumanised institutions. Paint schemes and decoration within such institutions could adapt more rapidly to the changing winds of contemporary thought, and therefore were often key to 'humanising' the institutional feel of old and new hospitals alike.

Many contemporary commentators emphasised the need to 'humanise' hospital buildings, and the concept of 'humanisation' became increasingly embedded with the rise of patient-centred care as an NHS principle. Despite the prevalence of this design goal, the concept of 'humanising' a space has rarely been defined or interrogated in depth. This chapter first outlines the history of 'humanisation' as a concept and then focuses on art as a case study, with close attention to representations of nature in hospital art and the uses of art for wayfinding. It shows that artwork reflected wider shifts in healthcare philosophies; the hospital echoes many trends in public art and culture, in which 'co-production' and more participatory (rather than philanthropic and paternalistic) models took hold over the course of the late twentieth century. Over time, hospital arts – and their colour palettes, which shifted from soothing to bright, like other elements of interior design – helped to bring some of the values of the 'modern' NHS into being.

Humanisation: the rise of an idea from the 1960s

In the early 1980s, an article in the *BMJ* made the following passing comment: 'of course we must humanise hospitals'.[5] Its casual use of 'of course' is highly revealing, implying that this comment was made in a context of general acceptance that hospital care needed reform. A few years later, the design journal *Hospital Development* observed that

> in hospital design matters ... [a] strong trend is towards 'humanisation' – a principle first voiced by a few concerned people in the late 1960s. It was badly neglected then but is now in full bloom, as can be seen in both the external and internal aspects of many of the latest projects in the UK.[6]

This section outlines some of these intellectual 'voices' in the 1960s and 1970s, and the forms in which these ideas entered medical literature and design practice by the 1980s. Each of these forms could be the subject of an in-depth analysis but there is also value in considering them together in relation to a bigger conceptual framework: the 'human'. One important finding from taking this bird's eye view, is that the idea of humanistic design was both highly influential and underexamined.

Calls to (re)humanise British hospitals had indeed increased over the post-war period, and were part of wider international trends.

In 1958, the French Ministry of Health had produced a circular on 'humanisation des hôpitaux', which articulated the need for humanistic hospital care under a system of universal healthcare.[7] Nor were these concerns a product only of welfare states. In 1981, architect James Falick wrote an article for *Hospitals* journal under the heading 'Humanistic Design Sells your Hospital', arguing for the value of paying attention to hospital aesthetics as well as function in the more consumer-driven US.[8] By the end of the century, projects seeking to humanise hospitals were evident across the globe, from Japan to Brazil.[9] Some of these initiatives focused on daily life in hospitals or on specific contexts of apparent 'dehumanisation', most commonly maternity care. Many others advocated the humanisation of hospitals in broad terms, which included reference to hospital architecture, layout, and interior design.

References to 'humanising' hospitals have been made in a range of social and political contexts across the world, a fact that raises questions about the meaning of the term. Humanistic design undoubtedly had very different implications when its end goal was to support universal hospital care in France in the 1950s, as opposed to 'selling' an American hospital in the 1980s, but few commentators ever drew out such differences. The term was widely used across different decades, countries, healthcare systems and types of patient in the late twentieth century, but often uncritically. This section seeks to unpick some of the different ways in which the term was used in this period, in order to understand better its rhetorical power and continued influence over hospital design. The NHS drew on design theory both from Europe and the US and this section also makes comparisons with these geographical contexts, where relevant, to highlight similarities and differences in the meanings of humanistic design.

The multiple meanings and ideological underpinnings of 'humanistic design' are worthy of detailed attention, and are important to understanding the forms that 'humanisation' took in hospitals. 'Humanisation' was a broad-ranging concept that should first be understood in its own right, before turning to the specific subject of hospital art. Part of the value of understanding this language is, of course, that it will enable a better understanding of trends in 'humanistic' healthcare design in practice. However, it is important also to remember that the growing influence of an *idea* and *practice* are not synonymous. Indeed, for practical and economic reasons, there were limits on the extent to which 'humanistic' design principles could be implemented in practice. 'Humanisation' should not be read through the lens of a progress narrative. That said, these practical limits also should not prohibit recognition of the ideological significance or power of 'humanisation' as a concept.

Different forms of 'humanisation' were bound together by a shared goal of person-centred, rather than science- or technology-centred, medicine. The 'human' aspects of design have increasingly sought to address the needs of staff and visitors, but patients have been the primary focus of concerns about 'dehumanisation' and its effects.[10] The 'human' operated as an umbrella term in opposition to constructions of 'dehumanised' medical care, with its apparent loss of patient agency, individualism, and holism. With the continued prevalence of the language of humanisation in healthcare design today, the political and social contexts in which these ideas were initially produced must be acknowledged. Historicising the language of 'humanistic' medicine is a significant task, due to its overlaps – and sometimes interchangeable use – with terms such as 'humanitarian', 'humanism', and 'humanity'.[11] While linguistic definitions are not the focus here, it is worth noting that the very language of humanistic medicine carried with it a much longer history of ideas about good medical care and the relationships between healthcare practitioners, patients, and communities. Its root alone, 'human', carries with it the weight of big questions about 'what makes us human?' that connect to themes such as human rights, identities, emotions, creativity, sensibility, and culture.[12] The word 'human' was used broadly to imply a shared humanity, but the term also has a complex politics and history linked to imperialism and colonialism: some groups of people were seen as 'more' human than others, and other groups were actively dehumanised.[13]

The concepts of humanisation and dehumanisation in hospital design often rested, albeit almost always implicitly, upon culturally specific assumptions about what the human was and – in particular – what it was *not*. The 'human' stood increasingly in opposition to the 'technological'. Humanisation was increasingly seen as the marker of civilisation in the late twentieth century, a shift from previous Western imperialist and colonial ideas about 'machines as the measure of men'.[14] That said, neither humanistic design nor the principles underpinning it were entirely new in the late twentieth century, and people in imperial Britain never entirely rejected the 'human' in favour of scientific progress. Ideas about the importance of holistic models of healthcare, of the value of spaces for reflection when unwell, of cheerful spaces and distraction for the ill, and of the healing powers of nature can be traced back for centuries.[15] *The Lancet* commented in 1866 on the 'humanising influence' of 'neatness and beauty of arrangement in the wards' of one typhus hospital.[16] A number of the features later identified as 'humanistic' ideals were also evident in famous examples of Victorian design, such as Florence Nightingale's emphasis on visual stimulation, nature, and colour in wards. They were also found in some outstanding early twentieth-century modernist hospitals, despite the tendency later to align modernism with 'dehumanisation', such as Alvar Aalto's famous Paimio Sanatorium in Finland and Berthold Lubetkin's Finsbury Health Centre in London.

These longer histories are key to understanding why the 'humanistic' value of certain design features – such as arts, gardens, and homeliness – were rarely questioned in British hospital design. However, 'humanisation' also represented something new. These design features took on a specific meaning in relation to the language of 'dehumanisation' and a perceived need to (re)humanise hospitals, which indicated a new sense of loss. Humanistic design was constructed in opposition to particular features of modern medicine, particularly technologies and practices that diminished the patient's voice or individuality.[17] It was also constructed in opposition to health planning processes that focused on impersonal 'technical knowledge of clinical functions and medical procedures', to quote one recent publication on mid-century Australian hospital design, which has been subject to similar critiques.[18] Concerns about the loss of the individual may have reflected some of the wider – albeit highly complex and much debated – tensions surrounding modernity itself and its impact on the individual. Modernity, capitalism, industrialism, and globalisation simultaneously encouraged and threatened individualism.[19] This model of the 'human' is culturally specific, with its focus on the individual and self-expression.

The language of humanisation seemed to grow in a wide range of contexts at a similar time, often as part of wider critiques of Western healthcare and big institutions. These trends related in part to social shifts that promoted social equality and sought to provide voices for the marginalised (including patients) in the 1960s and 1970s. Some work in this area was done by philosopher and priest Ivan Illich, for example, who is well known for critiquing the medicalisation of society and medical iatrogenesis in *Medical Nemesis*; Illich travelled widely and his ideas gained significant attention in Europe and the US.[20] Perhaps less well known is that Illich published similar ideas in an edited collection entitled *Humanizing Hospital Care*, showing how interwoven these wider critiques of medicine were with the hospital humanisation agenda.[21] Although this collection focused on human relationships in hospitals, rather than design, these two issues have never really been separable. Many such broad, international contemporary critiques of modern medicine came from outside the profession. In the 1960s and 1970s, concerns circulated in print about the growing power of medical knowledge, the rise of technology and the consequent shift of patient from subject to object, and the move towards large impersonal large institutions. Many of these works focused on psychiatric institutions, but others made broader critiques of medical knowledge about the body and of clinical spaces.[22] As a high-technology space, the built environment of the hospital came physically to represent many of these wider critiques.

Mechanisation and technology were particularly prominent themes of literature on medical 'dehumanisation', and on wider social dehumanisation. Concerns about the negative impact of modern technologies on human relationships and health had a longer history, famously articulated through Victorian disease categories such as 'railway spine' and neurasthenia.[23] Fears about the loss of the 'human' aspects of medicine with the rise of technologies grew after the many ethical abuses of science and technology witnessed in the Second World War. In the context of NHS hospitals, the health benefits of technology were rarely in doubt, but such high-technology spaces were still widely seen as 'dehumanising'. There was a fear that holism was being lost as the (increasingly voiceless) patient's body was fragmented in modern medicine, with the hospital seen as a 'machine for healing'.[24] An editorial in the *American Journal of Public Health* in 1978 neatly summarised the prevailing intellectual mood: 'for the past century, the more rapid the advance has been in technology, the less emphasis there has been on the caring and human aspects of medical practice'.[25] These kinds of comments relied on the construction of binaries, between care/humanity and cure/technology. Such ideas were undoubtedly problematic in many ways, and some contemporaries recognised them as such. In a sociology-driven article for the journal *Medical Care*, Howard *et al.* argued that 'technologies of the health-care industry can be humanizing or dehumanizing depending on how and for whom they are applied', but noted that they still had a negative reputation.[26] 'In light of its humanizing potential', they asked 'why is technology so often considered a crucial source of dehumanization?'[27] In seeking to challenge this idea, they acknowledged its power and prevalence.

Humanisation was also emerging as an agenda in wider medical practice, including education, and in other architectural contexts such as workplace design.[28] One Canadian commentator noted the link between hospital and wider design trends, writing that

> internationally renowned architect Eberhard Zeidler [saw an] increasingly complex hospital technology and scientific approach threatening to turn [the] vulnerable human into a faceless case. It is not mere coincidence that, in the wider world, the word in office design today is 'humanize'.[29]

Zeidler also worked in healthcare, designing the McMaster University Health Sciences Centre. Concerns about the human aspects of design and health were thus part of wider culture – including international circulation of these ideas – and were not limited to the medical sphere.

There was also a wider shift in ideas about experience and architecture at this time, towards a more human-centred way of thinking about space and design.[30] Historians have shown that experience has long been important to architectural thought, particularly in the modern world. Sigrid de Jong, for example, shows that, from the eighteenth century onwards, there was a 'move in perspective' towards thinking about the viewer's experience and a 'growing prominence of the experience of buildings in architectural thought'.[31] H. Horatio Joyce and Edward Gillin also argue that 'in the nineteenth century more than ever before, architecture was built to be experienced'.[32] What they mean by this is that 'architecture was seen, smelt, felt, heard in, interpreted […] evoked emotions and conjured up memories' but was also expected 'to embody specific cultural values', including those associated with a modern, industrialising society.[33] It would, then, be erroneous to claim that architects suddenly became interested in 'experience' in the post-war years. Rather, there was a subtle shift in the nature of the concept over time. Earlier ideas about experience still tended to privilege the architect as the designer of a form of embodied encounter, but in the post-war years the idea of putting 'experience' at the centre of architecture increasingly meant listening to users' voices (not just their imagined, embodied or visual encounter with a space).

This trend was part of a theoretically more democratic turn, particularly in public architecture, considering *users* rather than just aesthetics or values. More collaborative approaches to British architecture had been growing for some time, but there was a post-war trend towards more human-centred architecture and design, including what it meant to 'humanise' modern buildings.[34] Sociologists were increasingly influential in building the post-war welfare state, particularly in relation to housing, and there was a growth of user and occupant surveys across a wide range of contexts.[35] Schools were also increasingly designed with the user in mind, particularly in more 'progressive education authorities', some of which hired architects to design buildings that an imaginative teacher 'could use effectively' in the post-war years; the process incorporated everything from layouts to working with paint companies on colour schemes.[36] Post-occupancy studies and interest in revisiting buildings were also features of 'humanistic' post-war architecture. The hospital was no exception to such trends. As David Armstrong notes, a 'series of reports and publications during the 1950s and early 1960s proposed measures to humanise the hospital'.[37] Armstrong argues that there was no specific political or economic agenda to these studies, but that they resulted in 'a wide-ranging technical critique of the hospital'.[38] Many of these proposed measures related to daily routines, but many others related specifically to hospital aesthetics. The King's Fund gathered feedback from patients and staff, including on new buildings and on some elements of sensory design in maternity units such as the use of background music.[39]

The emphasis on 'human' elements of design could be viewed as a new form of anti-modernism from the 1970s onwards. It is, though, more productively understood as a new form of modernity rather than anti-modernity. In a PhD thesis on architect James Stirling, for example, Michael W. Farr considers this question in some depth in relation to the turn towards more 'humanistic' colour and architecture.

'Stirling's use of colour combined with identifiable motifs of technology and modernity', Farr argues, is 'a shift from a techno- to an anthropocentric approach to a building's finished appearance'.[40] This included '[r]elying on plants, trees, and the impact of weathering' to show 'the effects of the passing of time on his structures; the ultimate criterion by which human existence and experience is measured'.[41] However, Farr emphasises that

> Stirling's elevation to primacy of the human experience of architecture was not a rejection of either technology or modernity, but rather a re-assessment of man's relationship to them and, by implication, the modern world. Stirling's combinations of bright paintwork and coloured materials are here interpreted as an attempt to address mass-production's tendency to subjugate the individual.[42]

Similar arguments can be made about humanisation, and its colour palettes, in the hospital context. It was a reaction to and against a specific form or idea of modernity, but it was not intended to be 'regressive'.

A wide range of practical, political, and economic factors limited the ability to implement humanistic design. Important questions also remain about what humanistic design meant to patients, staff, and visitors. The human in the hospital has never been homogeneous; as noted in the chapter on white, some people feel soothed by high-technology spaces. It is therefore important not to assume that human-centred design has always reflected the diverse wishes of patients, visitors, and staff. However, there are also plenty of examples of hospitals introducing new architecture, colour schemes, artwork, gardens, and more, under the heading of making them more 'human'. Many of these schemes did include extensive consultation processes, and were increasingly participatory in nature.

Biophilia: nature in hospital arts

Histories of hospital art echo broader narratives in the history of hospital architecture and design. There is a common tendency for narratives to emphasise a long, deep tradition of hospital arts that was destroyed by medicalisation and modernism, before being revived with the post-war '(re)humanisation' of hospitals. Writing on the history of art in hospitals, Hugh Baron emphasised that, from the 1920s to the 1960s, 'patients had to suffer environments in which colour and decoration were taboo'.[43] It is significant that many of these narratives were written by people who helped to integrate arts into hospitals in the late twentieth century, rather than by historians. They are not entirely inaccurate, but tend to ignore the role that colour played in modernism, and to over-emphasise the impact and coherence of post-war arts and health movements.

Hospital art was not new in the 1960s, nor was it a simple revival of what came before modernism. Previous hospital artworks had tended to focus on spiritual or religious themes in the medieval years, through to more philanthropic messages in the Victorian period.[44] Some of the large, famous artworks in historical hospitals were only 'for' staff, rather than patients.[45] What artwork was thought to do is a more productive question than 'how many artworks were on the walls?' This section does not seek to offer a simple progress narrative of the 'humanisation' of hospitals in the post-war years, but rather to consider the question of why – and in what form – art was thought to be a key solution to the perceived 'dehumanisation' of hospitals at this time.

There was a rise of professionalised or organised hospital arts in the post-war years.[46] This interest was intertwined with the growing profile of public arts in Britain at the same time. Historic England note that the 'post-war institutional promotion of sculpture and other art forms' was 'characterised as bringing art to the people' as part of regeneration and reconstruction, and driven by educational authorities and local councils.[47] Hospitals cannot be understood outside this relationship to wider post-war reconstruction. Indeed, some artists commissioned for hospitals were hired specifically because of their work on other high-profile public arts schemes.[48] Hospitals were increasingly conceptualised as 'public' spaces through which a local population would flow, and which could act as a type of gallery for this purpose. The principle of democratising access to art – and including a range of people in choosing that art – was also an important part of movements to introduce artwork to hospitals. Some hospitals also came to benefit from the government 'Percent for Art' scheme of the late 1980s onwards, which encouraged public architecture to commit funds to artwork. These principles explain why hospital artworks adhered to the principles of 'public art' in terms of typically being there primarily to be ‘enjoyed’; they overlapped with the types of artwork found in galleries, but did not tend to include the more provocative or challenging works. Hospital arts were thus entwined with the principles of the welfare state, though they were less neatly connected to state principles than some other forms of public art, because they were driven at first by charities and individuals rather than institutions.

The charity Paintings in Hospitals was founded in 1959 and gradually built up a collection of thousands of paintings that it loaned out to hospitals.[49] The Paintings in Hospitals Communications and Development Manager Thomas Walshaw recently wrote that such interventions were based on holistic models of health such as that written up by the World Health Organization in 1948 (‘Health is a state of complete physical, mental and social wellbeing and not merely the absence of disease or infirmity’).[50] Art offered an alternative to what Walshaw describes as the ‘austere environment’ of a ‘purely medical approach to care’, arguing that ‘[a]rt and medicine together allow us to stop simply treating patients and instead to care for whole human beings’.[51] This kind of argument was key to the link between hospital arts and the growing ‘humanisation’ agenda. Many early loans were requested by people who wanted to brighten up their wards, for example, rather than by professional interior designers or arts coordinators, and offered them a form of ownership over the spaces in which they worked.[52] Paintings in Hospitals worked on the principle that everyone should have access to ‘real’ art, rather than just prints or reproductions, and that people did not need to be experts in art to access it. It was more important that the work was ‘authentic’ than ‘current’, though in the early years it was often both. This interest in authenticity was its own form of modernity.

Other organisations soon followed, many of which thought more expansively about what ‘hospital arts’ were. Hugh Baron and Peter Senior set up local hospital arts projects in Manchester and London in the 1970s, and then separate national organisations (Arts for Health and British Health Care Arts) in the 1980s. British Health Care Arts was based in Dundee, with Malcolm Miles as director and Baron as Chair, funded by the Gulbenkian Foundation. These organisations had important relationships with others seeking to improve hospital environments in the post-war years, including the King’s

Fund, Nuffield Provincial Hospital Trust, the Medical Architecture Research Unit (MARU), The King's Fund, Chase Charity, Health Boards, and Regional Health Authorities.[53] They also were part of, and influential within, international arts and health networks. Susan Barclay, writing about one distinctive large artwork in an Australian hospital, notes that the one designer had actually 'recently returned to Australia from London where he had been influenced by the emerging arts-in-health movement established in Manchester' during the 1970s.[54] Government funding in the late 1990s also gave the field a significant boost. By the end of the century NHS art coordinators or consultants promoted the idea that hospitals should be vibrant, not just soothing. Occupational therapists have also played important – and often overlooked – roles in decorative and artistic colour schemes, particularly when considering specific sensory needs and/or neurodiversity.[55] British hospitals have been an important part of the history of healthcare arts, both through local practices and national organisations.

It is important not to make this story seem too tidy. Though hospital arts-related roles were increasingly common in the NHS over the course of the late twentieth century, they were often unsystematic part-time or freelance roles at first, or staff might be hired temporarily for new capital projects. It is only in recent years that it has been common to find such jobs core-funded in hospitals, and this is still an uneven practice.[56] In interviews with some of the important early hospital arts coordinators and advocates, I asked whether they felt that they were unusual or part of a community. They typically could list just a handful of 'big names' in healthcare arts and noted hospital arts networks that were short-lived.[57] Progress in some regards, such as professionalisation, has also been counter-balanced to some extent by challenges in the NHS. Retired art coordinator Anne Greer recently reflected: 'I think hospitals have changed a lot. The pressure on staff is so great now that I can't imagine having the leisure to get department heads, cleaners together at a meeting and look at colours. And I feel very sad about that aspect. In some ways I feel that I worked during a kind of golden era.'[58] That is not to diminish the importance of those people or networks, but rather to emphasise that many hospital art practices remained local and unsystematic. Different NHS hospitals have always had specific local priorities, and hospital arts are no exception; in interviews about the history of this profession, the emphasis has often been on the importance of individuals or local organisations in advocating for and supporting the arts. Despite this somewhat unsystematic and uneven development of hospital arts, there was something of a sea change in late twentieth-century hospitals, as the 'humanisation' agenda started to become visible.

Whether acquired, borrowed, or commissioned, hospital artwork was typically selected to suit the specific needs of healthcare settings and to provide beauty, balance, distraction, and even a form of care. This differs from art designed, for example, to challenge or disrupt. One of the most common trends in 'humanistic' artworks was 'natural' colours and imagery. Pictures of landscapes, flowers, and trees made up a large proportion of the Paintings in Hospitals collection from the start. One of their earliest acquisitions in 1961 was Julian Trevelyan's *Penne-du-Tarn*, an impressionistic representation of the French countryside.[59] Alongside such pieces, they collected more abstract art by high-profile artists such as Bridget Riley and Gillian Ayres (an artist described as 'impatient with landscape').[60] But even in more abstract pieces, natural shapes, colours, and other signifiers of nature were common. Such trends reflected the organisation's belief, stated more recently on their website, that

> Art that features the landscape is not only one of the most popular artistic forms, it is understood to be one of the most therapeutic too. Pictures of soaring mountains, green valleys, flowing rivers, open skies, and beautiful clouds not only reconnect us with the natural world but lower our levels of anxiety, reduce stress, and stimulate positive mental health.[61]

'The natural world' was actually a very specific vision of 'nature' in such artworks: 'flowing', 'soaring', and 'beautiful'.[62] Typical collections represented English or European landscapes. Many of these artworks were chosen because of familiarity, as well as the perceived democratising value of having gallery-style artworks in hospitals. Landscapes were recognisable as part of a long tradition in 'Western' high art, and represented what the Romantics had considered the 'sublime' value of immersion in – or awe at – 'nature'.[63] These choices and cultural reference points spoke to a specific group of people, and may have alienated or excluded others. Decisions about landscapes in some ways echoed those made about waiting room music, in which 'Western' and classical music were dominant in the post-war years.[64] Such aesthetic choices implicitly carried value judgments about what type of landscape ('green' or 'blue', European) were morally and spiritually uplifting.

Imagery with violent or dark themes (such as stormy weather) was also avoided. Unlike other nature-based interventions in hospital, such as horticultural therapy, many early versions of biophilic art took the wildness and agency out of engagement with nature.[65] This is not to say that they took the senses out of nature. As Constance Classen notes, in line with ideas about synaesthesia, even a traditionally beautiful garden scene in a Monet painting could be 'vibrant' and 'almost aromatic'.[66] Many hospitals also introduced sculptures that used natural materials, sat within water features or gardens, or emulated the natural world, and which encouraged touch or multi-sensory engagement.[67] Engaging with 'beauty' was not, then, a purely passive experience, but a specific type of sensory encounter.

In line with some of the trends in general hospital design, artworks became more ambitious and brighter over time, shifting from paintings of landscapes to large-scale murals or installations. Pioneering examples of such artworks were found in continental Europe, and show how the colours of nature could actually be grey or brown; artists often went beyond the more predictable ideas of 'green' and 'blue' in such pieces. Rigshospitalet in Copenhagen, for example, had geometric figurative wall reliefs chiselled into concrete in the 1960s by artist Svend Saabye (1913–2004). To quote the hospital's arts guide, 'try to touch the patterns of the reliefs, which are inspired by the beach, stones and beach bottom, fish and birds'.[68] The artwork was thus integrated, multi-sensory, and 'inspired by' nature without being a literal representation of the sea. Figure 3.1 shows some images of this wall.

Such ambitious, integrated art schemes were still unusual in 1970s Britain but there was certainly growing demand, and an awareness of some of the international examples and contexts in which more experimental artwork was taking place. As noted, there were several national networks and an increasing professionalisation of 'arts for health' at this time. There was also increasing support for public art interventions, of which hospitals were seen to be a good example, by organisations such as the Arts Council. In 1982, Colchester

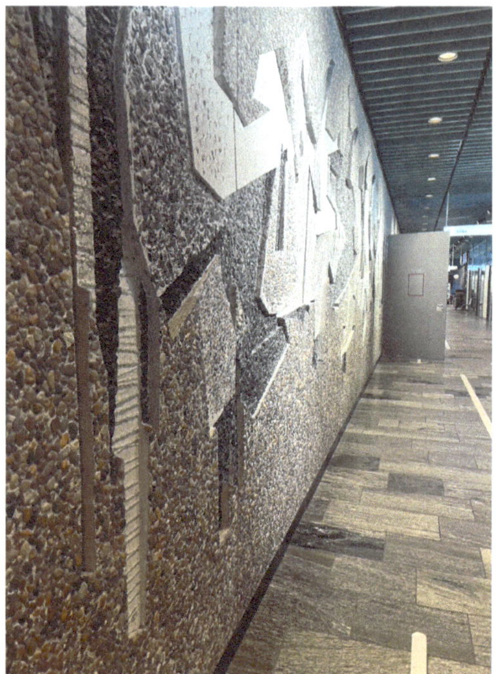

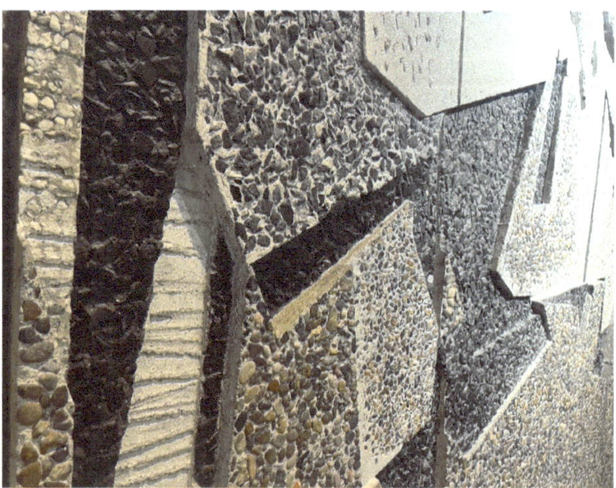

Figure 3.1 Figurative wall reliefs, 1964–68, Svend Saabye (1913–2004) at Rigshospitalet, Copenhagen. © The artist. Image: Victoria Bates. Awaiting permission.

District General Hospital had an arts scheme because of 'an intense local appeal' and 'Art[s] Council catalysts, like Art for Public Places' encouraged private sponsorship. As one write-up of the project noted, this arts scheme incorporated everything from murals to garden sculptures, and most importantly 'shows how art can be used as a vehicle for the "appropriation" of a public building by its community of users'.[69] This example further shows the importance of local initiatives, and the way that hospital arts could be part of community-building and ownership, rather than just an end 'product'.

By the 1980s hospital artworks were often explicitly 'humanistic' in intent, and were part of a 'total environment' strategy. There was a general interest in nature in architecture at this time, and a cultural turn towards the belief that 'there's some sort of deep, spiritual … link between us and plants' as part of counter-culture in the 1970s.[70] In the 1980s, the idea of 'biophilia' took off, defined by biologist Edward O. Wilson as 'the innate tendency to focus on life and lifelike processes', including landscapes.[71] This context fuelled the use of natural imagery in hospital arts. In 1984, for example, the *BMJ* published an article on 'Art in Hospitals' that included a picture of the brightly colour 'Tree Frieze' at Southampton General Hospital, commissioned by its 'humanising committee' the previous year (Figure 3.2).[72] This mural is interesting in part because it reframes colours such as red and orange as natural, rather than as unnatural or garish. Its use of a rainbow of colours echoed shifts in modern art, in which 'the Newtonian spectrum began to be deployed in its full range' in the twentieth century.[73]

Natural imagery continued to be the most common theme of hospital artworks, in colours beyond blue and green. As seen in the Southampton 'Tree Frieze', artists were inspired by a range of natural colours, including autumnal shades of red and orange. An impetus to the biophilic trend came from Roger Ulrich's famous 1984 study from the US showing more rapid healing in patients with a view of hospital gardens.[74] While there are many critiques of the limits of this study, it certainly provided a boost for those seeking to justify investment in views of nature. Guy Eades, in relation to St Mary's Hospital, which opened in 1990–91 on the Isle of Wight, noted that Ulrich's work was a direct influence on the decision to choose 'nature' as the theme for the hospital arts programme.[75] Where windows were absent or the views from them limited, art

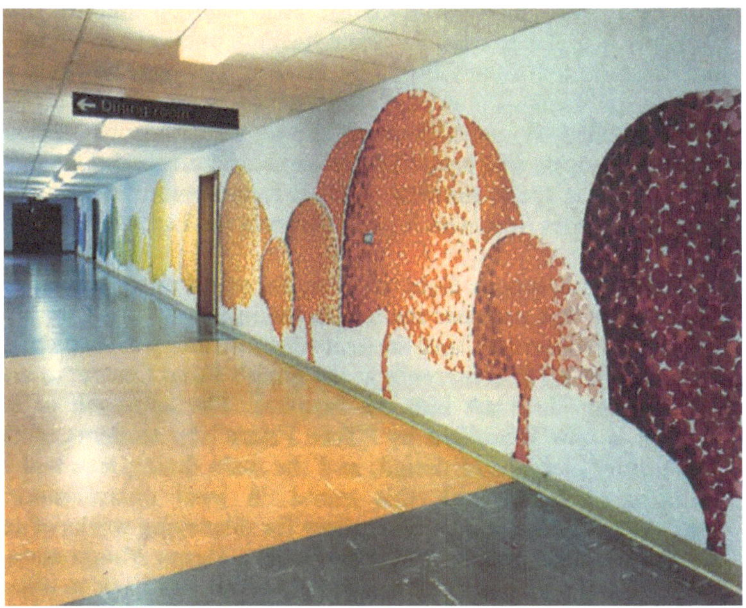

Figure 3.2 'Tree Frieze' by students of the Southampton faculty of art and design, Southampton General Hospital, found in Jeremy Hugh Baron and Lesie Greene, 'Art in Hospitals: Funding Works of Art in New Hospitals', BMJ, 22–29 December 1984), p. 1735. © Image reproduced with permission of the *British Medical Journal*. All rights reserved and permission to use this figure must be obtained from the copyright holder.

could offer an alternative, sometimes in a more evocative or abstract way that allowed people a form of distraction. In the same year, Hugh Baron and Lesley Greene argued strongly in the *BMJ* for greater investment in hospital arts for their humanistic potential and ability to evoke emotions.[76] In the light of these parallel trends, it is perhaps no coincidence that so many hospital arts programmes continued to represent scenes of nature.[77]

The conflation of high technology as 'dehumanising' and arts or nature as 'humanising' continued for many years. In 1993 Malcolm Miles wrote in *Hospital Development* that, when researching examples of good practice in NHS hospitals, he was 'unable to find any high-tech area of clinical space in an NHS hospital in which the environment had been successfully humanised [...] For the patient, this means stepping over the threshold from an attractive and relaxing public area, into a stark clinical area which gives the message "the pain starts here"'.[78] He complained that treatment areas such as ITUs (Intensive Therapy Units) and scanner rooms needed more innovative and 'imaginative design solutions' to distract patients from the high-technology spaces, pointing to examples in the US where light fixtures had been used to create false windows or underwater scenes. Such installations are now relatively common in the NHS, but it is notable that for Miles a purely technological space was subject to dehumanisation, and that the proposed solution was natural imagery.

Due to the general goals of such artwork, of providing distraction from medicalised surroundings and lifting spirits, it remained rare to see challenging or abstract artworks advocated as humanising forces in these contexts. Writing in 1999 about a mural painted in 1976 in a Northampton psychiatric hospital, Sarah Hosking and Liz Haggard noted:

> [The artist's] work reflected his older generation to whom narrative, decorative and accessible mural painting was a worthy end in itself. He did not seek to 'emotionally challenge' or 'energetically engage' his audience, as contemporary 'art in hospital' schemes sometimes claim to do, but to amuse, enchant, and befriend his audience.[79]

This trend continued for some time. In 1990, Peter Senior wrote on arts and health in the NHS, observing that '[p]atients report that it is fun to enter a hospital and find themselves in a tropical garden, walking through a desert or rainforest or looking out over the Greek Islands or into a subterranean aquarium'.[80] In the same year, the hospital architect Richard Burton, writing on his work at St Mary's Hospital, equated human design in the ward with visual 'interest'.[81] He drew on cultural inspirations, such as Japanese meditation gardens, to provide patients with 'opportunities to divert their minds from their illness'.[82] Ideas about 'art as a humanising agent' thus need to be recognised as contingent, as not all visual art was perceived as such.

Representations of nature in hospital art followed many of the other trends in hospital colour and decorative schemes, moving from soothing natural landscapes in wall paintings of the 1960s

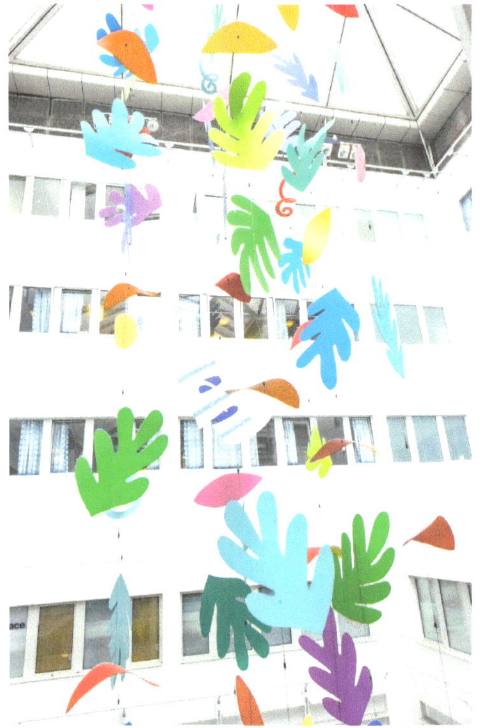

Figure 3.3 'Falling Leaves' (1993), Sian Tucker (1958–). © The artist. Image: Chelsea and Westminster Hospital NHS Trust. Reproduced with permission.

and 1970s, through to brighter, larger and more playful art interventions by the 1980s and 1990s. One well-known example of this trend is Sian Tucker's 'Falling Leaves', a large hanging mobile built into the atrium of Chelsea and Westminster Hospital when it opened in 1993. Such art helped to 'humanise' a space that was not otherwise at a human scale, by including a work that helped to make the space feel more proportionate and inviting.

I interviewed Sian Tucker and asked her what she remembers about her inspiration for this piece. She noted that much of the artwork was shaped by her personal feelings and her artistic training, but also noted how the specific requirements of the hospital shaped her work:

> I grew up in the countryside and my mother is from Wales by the sea, which is where we live now, and so it's always been a big part of me ... I'm happiest outside and I think it's funny how naturally I wanted to create and bring some of that outside into a hospital in that big atrium, like when you're looking up under a tree and you see all the leaves shimmering from underneath or looking out of a window at a tree, that's the kind of thing that I think I wanted to instinctively make for a hospital, because it was such a kind of building with lots of glass and rooms and no views of outside.[83]

When asked more about colour choices in her artwork, Tucker said 'I do like bright colours but not like really acidic colours, so it is much more like looking at a tree or the sea, there's so many different colours within that blue or what you perceive as green, isn't there? [...] when you're making something like a mobile, then you do have to have those counterbalance colours, those opposites to make it kind of work, I think'.[84] This important point – that something we often think of as one colour (such as the 'blue' sea) in nature is actually often multiple colours in balance – is crucial to understanding how colour operates in 'Falling Leaves'. In response to a further question about colour and shape, Tucker said,

> I do like simple shapes and I think definitely with the mobile, I do love Matisse and was obviously inspired and influenced by his cut-outs and they're the perfect simple shape to represent all those kind of things that I wanted to portray. I'm really not very three-dimensional, I do like a flat surface, so that's about as good as you're going to get, isn't it? To make them all float.[85]

Similar comments were made by retired NHS arts coordinator Anne Greer in discussions about her work in hospitals in the 1990s, in which she emphasised that 'natural' colours are not necessarily clichéd ideas of 'blue' and 'green': 'I look at flowers, I look at things that work in nature so that you can get the proportion of the strong colour with a weak colour or an upsetting colour and move things around'.[86] Tucker and Greer both emphasise that, in their work, 'natural' colours were not simply about adding blue or green, but about representing the balance and complexity found in natural colour schemes.

Tucker's use of a mobile to represent the movement of natural forms is reminiscent of some other important hospital projects. One example is an exhibition of Kenneth Martin's abstract mobiles in a London children's hospital ward in 1953. This was an unusual exhibition in many ways, typically discussed by scholars as part of histories of art, post-war modern architecture and constructionism. The mobiles were relatively unusual for a children's hospital, and a hospital in general, in their simple and abstract modern forms. Even these mobiles, though, had been designed to evoke some of the feelings, colours, and sensory experiences of engaging with nature. Martin noted that 'we lie on our backs and contemplate the ceiling' and that 'in the summer, in the open, we lie and watch the leaves of a tree, or the clouds', including reflected lights, the balance between dark ominous clouds and the white cumulus, 'so my black disc reflects orange on to the white above it, while this sets blue upon the next white, for my forms are two faced and, like the leaf, are not the same on both sides'.[87] The colour of nature here was not green but rather dynamic shades of light/dark that moved, changed, and interacted with light. These abstract mobiles were unusual in allowing for natural themes such as darkening clouds and rain, alongside the balance of other forms of weather such as the warm orange of the sun. As with Tucker and Greer cited above, artists working in hospitals have long embraced the complexity and variety of natural colour palettes. This variety is part of the specific intervention that artworks have been able to make in hospitals, as opposed to some of the 'flat' colour palettes that interior decorating can require for walls. Nature was evoked not by literal representations of landscapes but by colours, shapes, movement, and the expected position of the viewer (imagined here lying down, watching clouds). Sam Gathercole, writing on this exhibition, notes that children engaged with the mobiles and brought them to life in a range of ways, not always seeing 'nature' in their shapes and colours.[88] However, as Gathercole notes, the act of lying down and seeing shapes and stories in the mobile did actually – implicitly – do what Martin had intended in emulating the ways that children imaginatively watch clouds.

As hospitals increasingly commissioned bespoke artwork, where affordable, there was an increasing emphasis on representations of place that also reflected local surroundings. Colour schemes and images were selected to give a patient, visitor, or staff member a sense of belonging, and avoid the strange sense of dislocation that can come with a prolonged period in an anonymous or interchangeable medical building. Art no longer sought to transport people imaginatively to distant or abstract landscapes; many artworks focused instead on familiar places, which could include cityscapes as well as landscapes. In an interview with Guy Eades, I asked: 'I did notice the nature theme in a lot of the artworks as I was walking around earlier and that some of them, or quite a lot of them, seemed to speak to the local landscape. Was that a deliberate strategy?' Eades answered,

> Yes, it was, yes because I mean, also we tried to use ... artists who lived and performers who lived on the Isle of Wight so it was informed by that, yes. I think it's all – it's always informed by that ... I went to lots of other hospitals and every other hospital has its own ... aesthetic. So if you go to UCL or if you go to Manchester, they're all different because they reflect the particular community that lives there.[89]

Figure 3.4 shows just one of many examples of this kind of locally informed artwork. Such projects link to the way that, to quote Ann Rippin and Sheena J. Vachani, 'craft has long since been considered part of identity-making projects involving socially connective activities'.[90] The piece did not offer nature as a generic landscape; it was, instead, embedded in a specific location and hand-made by local people.

The collective nature of this project was representative of a more general shift towards collaborative, consultative, and participatory approaches to artwork in hospitals at this time: to quote Jane Willis of hospital arts consultancy Willis Newson, 'the idea of doing with, not doing to, is critical'.[91] Willis also discussed the importance of having a 'sense of place' in healthcare arts. One of the developments she has observed since the 2010s is the flourishing of wall vinyls using stock imagery. Willis warns that these need to be used with care, hinting at the dangers of a postmodern aesthetic that lacks authenticity: 'rather than creating a sense of place, it creates a sense of nowhereness!'[92] These examples add another important layer to the discussion of colour, arts, nature, and 'humanisation', emphasising that representations of nature have increasingly needed to be meaningful to be seen as 'humanistic'. They (ideally) represented the colour palettes and textures of the world outside, rather than reproducing the aesthetic qualities of a healthcare institution with a wipe-down,

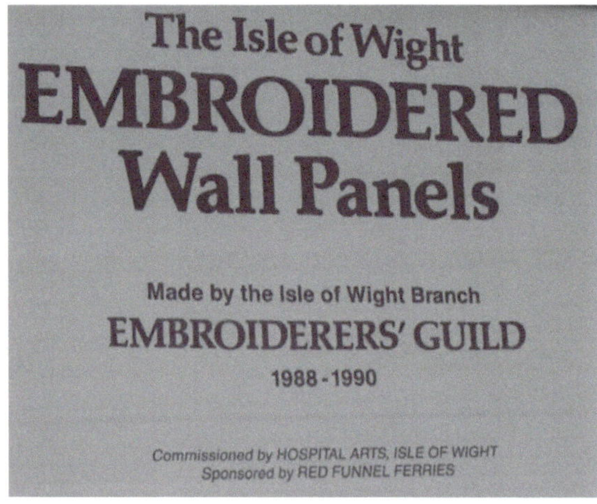

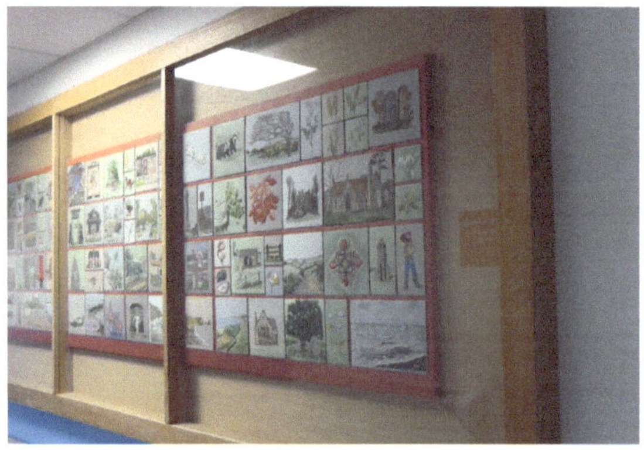

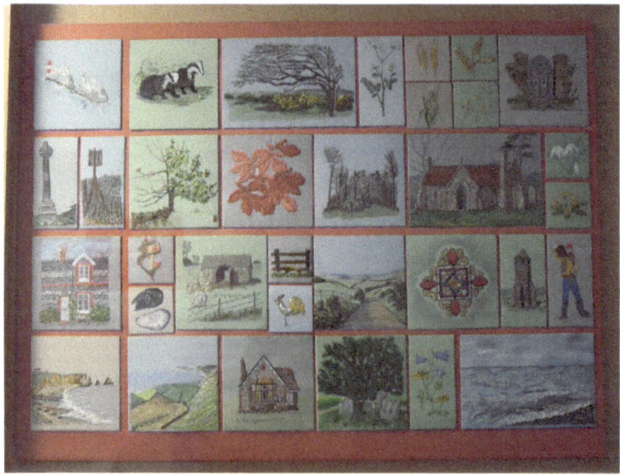

Figure 3.4 The Isle of Wight embroidered wall panels, Embroiderers' Guild, 1988–90. © The artists. Image: Victoria Bates.

mass-produced version of nature. Bespoke, collaborative, artist-led artworks have increasingly been seen as desirable but have not always been affordable for NHS hospitals.

In *Constellations: Reflections from Life*, Sinéad Gleeson remarks that '[h]ospitals are not unlike galleries. Interactive spaces; a large-scale installation of sound and colour'.[93] Gleeson's comments are a world apart from how people would have described hospitals a century – or even half a century – earlier. By the end of the century, some of the hospitals with flourishing arts programmes were indeed like galleries; they were designed to be public art spaces, often with a focus on contemporary and site-specific art. In other ways, though, hospital art was very specific. Its 'humanising' goal meant that, from the start, it typically veered away from being political or challenging, though it could be provocative in its own way. The most common theme in hospital arts has always been the natural world, understood and represented as calming and therapeutic. This is not to say that they were uninventive; quite the opposite. Hospital arts allowed for a more complex and sometimes more abstract exploration of the colours of the natural world than broad palettes such as 'pastel' blue and green; they recognised the depth and variety of colours found in nature, and brought them into hospitals in a way that went far beyond landscape paintings.

In many ways, the 'humanisation' of hospitals through artwork is better seen as a care practice than a design or medical one. To quote Annmarie Mol, Ingunn Moser, and Jeannette Pols,

> during the twentieth century it was commonly argued that *care* was other to *technology*. Care had to do with warmth and love while technology, by contrast, was instrumental. Care overflowed and was impossible to calculate, technology was effective and efficient. Care was a gift, technology made interventions.[94]

Hospital artworks aligned with this vision of 'care' in modern healthcare, even if the technology/human and technology/care division was largely rhetorical. The traditional perception of care work and its gendered dimensions may be relevant here, as – with a few notable exceptions from the early years of hospital arts – male arts coordinators or artists working in hospitals have been a minority.[95] Humanisation and care alike were more than simple design interventions, but were ongoing, culturally constructed, and relational practices.

Scale: corridors and navigation

Many large and distinctive artworks were important spatial markers in hospitals, with an overlooked role in navigation.[96] For old and new buildings alike, 'wayfinding' has remained a challenge throughout the existence of the NHS. Old hospitals were typically difficult to navigate. The post-war addition of new wards or extensions to existing sites often created counter-intuitive ways of ordering space. Newer buildings put 'user journeys' into building design, or were easier to understand by default, for example when built as towers, but came with problems of scale. By the 1970s leading architects were turning back towards low- or mid-rise hospitals, for example using a 'village' model.[97] However, the trend towards bigger District General Hospitals made it difficult to build to a 'human scale' or to ensure ease of navigation. Many such hospitals were also built in rural sites or on the outskirts of towns or cities, meaning that the difficulties of navigation could start at a bus stop, car park, or even at home.[98] Artwork and colour design could be an important part of making such buildings feel as though they were human in scale, with entrances that were easier to find and corridors that were less complex to navigate. Such design practices were particularly important when rebuilding was not possible, or buildings were particularly large. They became significant at the end of the twentieth century, when the idea of signposting expanded to 'wayfinding' in the NHS.

A 'beyond signage' approach was taken by many architects, artists, and interior designers throughout the post-war years. Many of these actors recognised the potential value of colour for marking out and distinguishing different spaces in hospitals, for old and new buildings alike, but had not formally branded their work as 'wayfinding'.[99] Some early work in this area was conceptualised, instead, as inclusive design. Colour and texture could help people to navigate to and within hospitals, most famously the green line painted from Old Street tube station to Moorfields hospital to help people with visual impairments.[100] Disability rights activists were also vocal and organised from the 1960s onwards, in advocating inclusive design as part of the social model of disability.[101] Early high-profile publications focused on specific issues such as dropped curbs for wheelchair users, rather than on colour, but such advocacy helped to fuel a broader interest in inclusive design.[102] Long before official NHS guidance on 'wayfinding', hospitals were using colours, arts, flooring, and more to support accessibility and inclusivity.

'Wayfinding' emerged as a named entity at the end of the century. A number of US publications from the 1980s – by J. R. Carpman, M. A. Grant, and D. A. Simmons – are commonly cited as the high-profile 'early' research on the subject.[103] It was really in the 1990s, though, that the concept took hold in British hospitals. This decade brought formal recognition of the importance of wayfinding strategies in hospitals, with standardised NHS checklists and surveys for people to evaluate their sites. In 1995, Stephen Nicoll wrote a piece for *Hospital Development* magazine called 'The Art of Good Signage' in which he noted that '[i]ncreasingly the word "signposting" is being replaced in the literature by the more generic term, "wayfinding", particularly in publications of US origin'.[104] There were corresponding shifts in NHS literature: in 1984, NHS guidance focused on 'signs' and offered a coherent brown-and-white system; in 1991, NHS Trusts were created and the guidance allowed for more local variation, but this tended to lead to a focus on 'corporate identity, colours and logo … rather than legibility'; in 1999, *Wayfinding* guidance was published with an emphasis that 'wayfinding is not just signs'.[105] Wayfinding strategies also continued to be shaped by research into disabilities, and the growing understanding that navigation – including accessibility considerations – often started long before people reached hospital.

Wayfinding was a multi-sensory concept, and colour was just one navigation strategy. The 1999 NHS *Wayfinding* guidance even noted that '[r]esearch has found that two out of three people did not notice colour-coding at healthcare sites with a colour-coding system' and that 'people can remember no more than five colours before they find it difficult to differentiate'.[106] The guidance noted that perception of colour distinctions often diminished with age, and that there were practical considerations that limited the value of colour-coding, such as conflation with 'safety colours' or the tendency for bright colours to fade. Stephen Nicoll noted that colour-coding spaces could be problematic for people who are 'captive' in them, including staff: 'nobody would advocate an exclusively red, orange or purple "prison"'.[107] The growing use of colour as part of wayfinding strategies had to be approached with care, and was not always necessarily effective for everyone in hospitals. It did, though, change the spatial organisation of colour in hospitals, and the way that people experienced hospital colour schemes.

Many wayfinding initiatives focused on the hospital corridor. The (white) hospital corridor has often been a shorthand for a feeling of never-ending wandering and looking, and consequently a focus of many efforts to help improve navigation.[108] As Roger Luckhurst argues, the hospital 'link corridor' originated in the late nineteenth century, but by the late twentieth century it was bound up with ideas about dehumanisation and the large institution:

> In 1967, medic Mayer Spivack published a study called 'Sensory Distortion in Tunnels and Corridors', suggesting that corridors that reached over a mile might actively induce mental illness rather than rationalise its treatment. Monster hospitals fell out of favour, denounced as 'total institutions', or what were later termed 'sick buildings.' Anti-psychiatry proved to be an anti-corridic movement.[109]

Corridors were seen as features of 'gloomy' inherited Victorian workhouses or wartime buildings, which often had a 'long enclosed corridor' either built in or to connect different buildings.[110] It was common to find post-war publications bemoaning 'an internal labyrinth of shiny corridors' or 'the walk down that endless corridor', to indicate the sense of overwhelm and confusion that navigating a large hospital could involve.[111] In a 1984 article called 'How to Beautify Your Old Hospital', J. H. Baron paid attention to the particular problem posed by corridors in inherited old buildings:

> Long main corridors are often [...] the most aesthetically depressing part of a British hospital. The visitor's heart sinks as he sees a gloomy prospect with the end scarcely in view. This will often be in a grubby decorative state but will still be gloomy when freshly painted in a single drab colour.[112]

Such comments continued to arise over the years. An article in *Hospital Development* from 1994 complained about 'the typical disorientating maze of bland functional rooms and corridors that spells "modern hospital"'.[113] High-rise buildings, common under the 1962 Hospital Plan for England and Wales, typically had shorter corridors but have continued to co-exist with older sites. As one recent article in *The Architectural Review* reflected,

> [i]t was not until the 1980s that an exploration really began of what makes for a better sensory experience for people, such as the quality of space, light, acoustics and finishes and how we can reduce stress through making buildings pleasant to approach and easier to navigate, in contrast with the notorious anomie of endless hospital corridors.[114]

Sometimes comments about 'endless' corridors seemed rhetorical, but they were also accurate for many locations: some single corridors were almost a mile long, with interconnected corridors running much further.[115] Efforts to redesign and rethink hospital corridors were, like many other design and architectural initiatives, fundamentally an attempt to rethink what the modern hospital was or could be.

Signage alone was not necessarily a solution, and could be overwhelming in itself. As Baron noted, simply repainting corridors in another monotonous colour did not help with the sense that they were 'endless'. Carefully designed colour schemes and artworks offered a subtle and apparently more 'humanistic' way to guide people gently around buildings, or hospital 'villages', without bombarding them with information to do so. The corridor was not the only space for this kind of intervention, but it has become an important one both for its genuine practical significance in navigation and its metaphor or role as maze, threshold, and space of movement or transition.[116] Corridors have become significant locations for artworks that support navigation. Many such interventions predated the official language of 'wayfinding'. As one publication on interior design for hospitals noted in the mid-1970s, colour and patterns could help to reduce the sense of scale of long hospital corridors:

> It is probably desirable to make the entrance to [a] department easily identifiable from a distance down the corridor. This may be done by introducing a strong pattern or colours in the corridor at this point and when it is continued into the reception it will form a bold visual break in the length of the corridor.[117]

It is significant that this publication pointed out the role of colour in offering a 'visual break' in long corridors as well as marking out particular departments and supporting navigation.

Corridors represented the problems of scale faced in hospitals. Colour use could be important in dividing space and helping to make hospital corridors feel less overwhelming. This effect could apparently be achieved by lighting, colour, wallpaper, or artwork, and often the lines between the three were blurred. Flooring could also be important. Geriatrician John Agate noted the value of using patterns with colour blocks at right angles, to help people to recognise their location and to 'break up' the perception of length so that people did not feel that they were going down 'a long, straight corridor … further and further away from the known world outside'; he also noted, though, the importance of avoiding diagonal lines, which could disorient patients or send them 'tottering sideways'.[118] Not all decorative schemes for hospital corridors were supported. In 1989, a number of staff members wrote to the hospital newsletter *Bedpost* about local efforts to enhance a corridor at Leicester General Hospital with paint and some floral decorations: one commentator noted 'what a difference a lick of paint and a few plants can make', but another complained that the hospital had 'any number of things higher on the list of priorities than artificial hanging plants' and bemoaned wasted resources.[119] The idea of decoration as a luxury, particularly when the NHS was struggling for money, was a repeated feature of discussion about colour schemes and hospital arts.

In line with the general histories of both 'wayfinding' and hospital arts, arts schemes became increasingly important in the 1980s and 1990s for supporting navigation. When arts were folded into 'wayfinding' in this way, they could be more easily justified (and financed) as part of the essential function of hospital buildings. Many corridor artworks also represented – or were inspired by – the colour schemes of nature, meaning that they were thought to 'humanise' space in multiple ways. In 1994, for example, a project in Manchester used 'tapestry-like hangings to enliven interminable hospital corridors' for people with dementia.[120] These were spaced twelve feet apart, meaning that they helped with the sense of scale and length of the corridors, but were also designed to evoke natural colour schemes: 'a transition from earthy shades of brown, tan and orange, blending up into sea and sky tones of ink and pale blue'.[121] Bridget Riley completed two pieces involving bright coloured horizontal stripes for hospital corridors in the 1980s: in 1983 at the Royal Hospital in Liverpool, and in 1987 at St Mary's Hospital in London. Originally Riley was commissioned to install her works on floors 8 and 9 of the St Mary's QEQM building, and was later (in 2014) invited to add floor 10 (Figures 3.5 and 3.6); the Liverpool pieces no longer survive. In both sites, the artworks were carefully

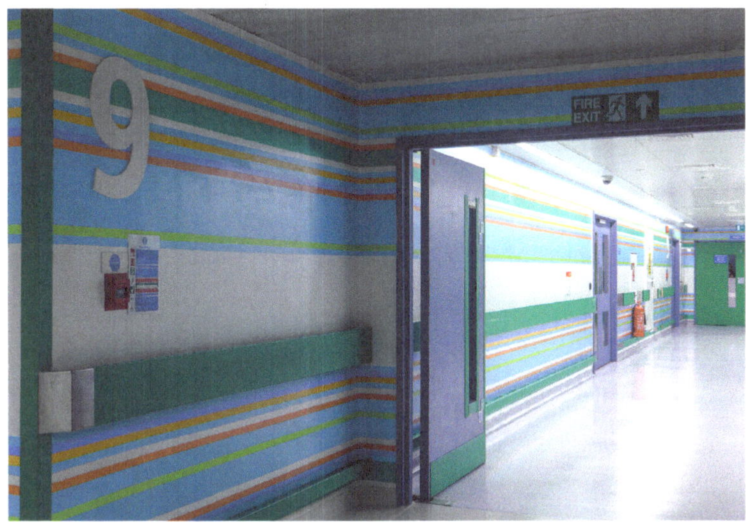

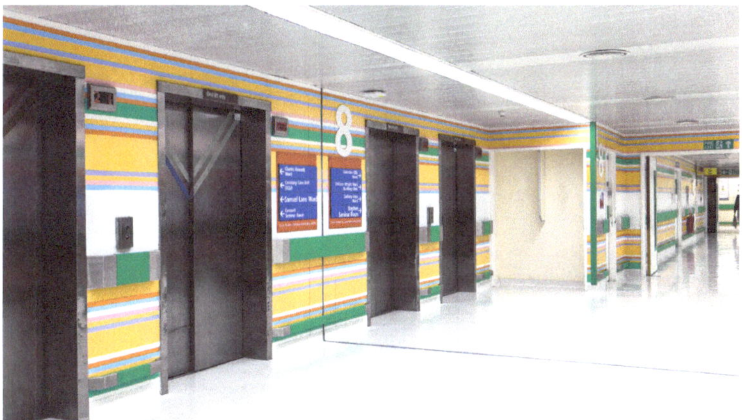

Figure 3.5 Installation view of mural commission, 1987, Bridget Riley, St Mary's Hospital, London © The artist. Image: Peter Cook, courtesy of Imperial Health Charity

designed to include fixtures and fittings as part of the colour scheme, supporting not only navigation through distinctive colour palettes for the three floors, but also the 'humanisation' of those spaces by hiding features such as wall buffers, which just appear as stripes. It may be relevant that John Weeks, a pioneer of 'humanistic' hospital

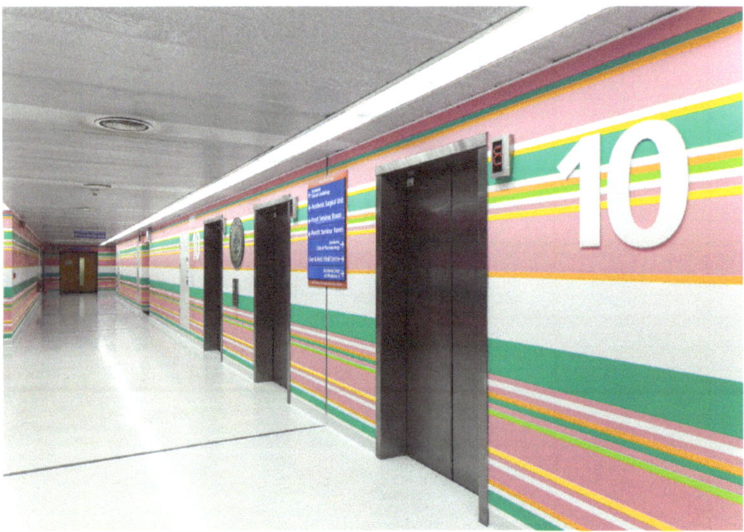

Figure 3.6 Installation view of mural commission, 2014, Bridget Riley, St Mary's Hospital, London. © The artist. Image: Peter Cook, courtesy of Imperial Health Charity. All rights reserved and permission to use this figure must be obtained from the copyright holder.

architecture and 'human scale' architecture, was the architect for the London building and commissioned Riley's work.[122] Despite being a high-rise building, such works helped to make each floor feel contained and reduce the perception of scale, as well as hiding 'medicalised' features of hospital corridors.

The use of different colour schemes on each floor was, in part, to make the spaces distinct and recognisable. In other ways, though, the installations were grounded in similar ideas and were all inspired by a trip that Riley took to Egypt in 1981. She drew on a colour palette found in ancient Egyptian underground tomb paintings, noting how they brought the feeling of light to dark spaces. In Riley's words, the colour schemes were intended to bring 'feelings of light and sun and all the pleasurable sensations associated with them'.[123] These colour palettes were, then, intended to evoke feelings about the natural world without representing a landscape or the sun. They were intended as multi-sensory, spatial art installations.

Their placement in the corridor was also part of this design, as Riley noted that people engaged with such artwork in specific ways.[124] The lines were painted as part of a dialogue with the rhythm of walking in corridors. The lines were, then, simultaneously a navigating mechanism, an effort to bring the multi-sensory feeling of light and warmth into dark clinical spaces, and a way of recognising the specific nature of movement around hospitals.

This emphasis on movement was important not only for patients, but for people who spent their days navigating hospitals and walking their corridors, such as hospital porters. People embodied the act of looking in specific ways when artworks were painted in corridors, or part of 'passive' navigation. As Mark Paterson notes, the ways that walking and looking are choreographed are 'mostly ignored in favour of that [...] curatorial imperative for bodies to remain immobile in front of paintings or artefacts'.[125] He argues, though, that there are particular 'social and spatial "bodily techniques" involved in ambulatory viewing, rhythms that respond to the spatial setting and the presence of other visitors that accrue over time'.[126] This emphasis on 'rhythms' and the particular nature of ambulatory engagement very closely aligns with Riley's ways of thinking about her artworks. They were designed – to further quote Paterson, writing on mosaic tiles – to be 'negotiated through movement, scanned with the eyes ... and in some form synchronized through previous proprioceptive experience in order to obtain some form of narrative immersion'.[127] An artwork such as Riley's was a similar form of multi-sensory 'immersion' and represented a way of guiding people through space, rather than being designed for the viewer to 'remain immobile'. People also, of course, moved through spaces in a range of ways and experienced this 'immersion' differently depending on their mode of transport: walking or moving independently, for example, would have offered opportunities to pause in a way that being pushed on a chair or trolley did not; each of these different modes of movement would also change the height from which a corridor artwork has been encountered, the 'rhythm' of the movement, the angle of engagement, and more.

Corridors were important for navigation, both literally and symbolically, but were not the only location for artworks that supported wayfinding. In his *Hospital Development* piece on signage

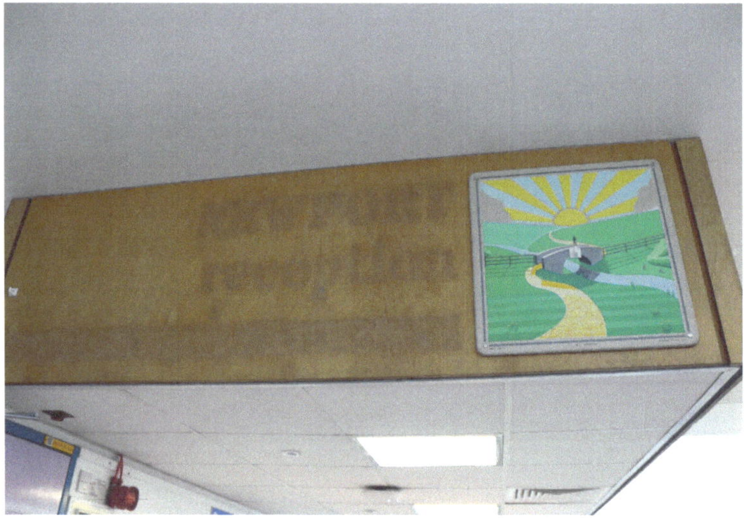

Figure 3.7 Wayfinding at St Mary's Hospital, Isle of Wight. © The artist. Image: Victoria Bates.

Stephen Nicoll noted that a single memorable mural could be a helpful 'wayfinding landmark', especially when sited in key public areas.[128] Artwork could also be integrated into signage schemes, for example through wordless signs. Nicoll himself designed 'six colour coded designs' for St Mary's Hospital on the Isle of Wight, only one of which now remains, at an old reception desk (Figure 3.7).

Nicoll wrote about the picture in Figure 3.7 in his article on signage in *Hospital Development*, noting that 'the yellow/green sign [...] co-ordinates with the colours of the staff-base desk, ceiling, door and frame, and with bedspreads and curtains designed by Sian Tucker'.[129] This wayfinding work was relatively subtle and achieved through a range of different colour-based artworks, from bed curtains (discussed more in Chapter 4) to furniture and signs, differentiating it from more traditional approaches to 'signage' or 'signposting'. The goal was to use a combination of colour and pattern to make a space implicitly recognisable, without creating an overwhelming 'prison' of any single colour or bombarding people with information. To quote Nicoll further, writing in 1995:

> A review of recent projects suggests that artworks have a dual function: to provide a source of introspection and calm to busy or troubled people; and to 'light the way'. A corner passed on an outward journey, remembered by its mural, banner or sculpture, is easier to pick out on the return trip. Hospitals are a mass of corridors and waiting areas and the principle aim of 'wayfinding' is to help the traveller in a witty and visually enriching manner.

The 'arts' in such schemes overlapped extensively with interior design, graphic design, and more, but many such schemes were grounded in the belief that artwork had a specific value. Artwork was thought to offer both a 'humanising' influence, and to be more memorable than words for people who were feeling troubled or overwhelmed. Similar projects can be found in other local hospital records from the 1990s. For example, the NHS Trust responsible for Conquest Hospital in Hastings appointed an artist to work with the design team – including architects Powell & Moya – to integrate artworks into its second phase and to incorporate them into a wayfinding strategy.[130] Their proposal included 'landmark' artworks such as a neon sculpture behind reception, and the integration of artworks into flooring, including board games in children's areas.

Not all wayfinding schemes endured. The faded legacy of the original Isle of Wight wayfinding scheme (Figure 3.7) also illustrates this point. As hospitals evolved and their personnel changed, original wayfinding schemes could be lost. Wayfinding schemes could be abandoned for a range of reasons. Some were replaced by a new interior design strategy or branding exercise. In other hospitals, wayfinding was commissioned as a single event, rather than an ongoing process, for example as part of architects' design of a new site. This could mean that the original strategy was forgotten or lost over time. In some places, hospital growth and flexibility simply meant that schemes were no longer fit for purpose, such that many hospitals came to contain 'ghost' wayfinding, in the form of artworks to direct people to a place that no longer existed.

The role of arts in helping people to navigate hospitals has shifted subtly. Early examples typically involved single distinctive artworks intended to be memorable and aid navigation. Over time, such artworks remained, but the introduction of 'wayfinding' meant that they were increasingly part of more coherent strategies that included more 'immersive' artworks in corridors, integrated colour schemes in new-build hospitals to differentiate areas and support accessibility, and the deliberate design of artwork to coordinate with colour schemes of specific wards. In line with the broader history of colour in hospitals, in the early 2000s, colour and wayfinding also became linked to commercial models. Artworks remained important in such schemes, but they were often part of wayfinding – and colour – strategies that emulated other spaces, such as airports, to help people to navigate.[131] As hospital spaces got larger, for example with the rise of atriums, hospital artworks also grew in scale to make the spaces feel more proportionate and offer notable spatial markers. Throughout these schemes, with their many different manifestations, artwork was used consistently to try to help to make large hospitals feel more 'human' in scale.

Conclusions

The backdrop of 'humanisation' is key to understanding the flourishing of hospital arts in the post-war years, and the nature of that art. Though hospital arts have always been diverse, they cannot be understood without recognising the widespread idea – sometimes explicit, sometimes unspoken – that they were there to counter-balance high-technology, biomedical, large institutions. As Tim Ingold notes, 'art is commonly regarded as one of the hallmarks of humanity' and distinguished from science as a 'specific historical achievement of the Western world'.[132] There have, also, been changes over time in what 'humanisation' meant and how it manifested in the arts. Since the 1960s there has been a shift from a model of democratising hospital arts, achieved through providing access to quite traditional artworks, to the use of more commission-based and participatory models of including patients and staff in artwork selection, design, and even sometimes the making of an installation. As with other colour trends, artworks became larger, bolder, and brighter over time.[133] New hospitals have provided opportunities to help with 'wayfinding' or to fill large spaces such as atriums with integrated artwork to make them feel more 'human' in scale. In other ways, there has been a lot of consistency, with the use of nature as a key theme and the integration of ideas about biophilia into arts strategies.

In colour terms, then, artwork has been varied but has tended to act as a form of balance, offering an alternative to or distracting from the 'white wall' with its apparently institutional implications.

'Humanisation' remained influential as a concept and practice until the end of the century, and beyond. One evaluation of the King's Fund 'Enhancing the Healing Environment Programme', launched in 2000, noted that a common feature of all of the projects was 'humanising the hospital environment by making places that are welcoming and uplifting'.[134] In 2005, the South Tees Acute Hospitals NHS Trust published a study of the 'art and science of creating environments that prevent illness, speed healing and promote well-being'.[135] *Designing for Health*, this publication argued, necessitated 'humanis[ing] the "inhospitable" hospital' in a range of ways, including providing a sense of control, external views, positive acoustics, natural light, pleasant fragrances, bodily comfort, varied colour and private space. The length of this list indicates the wide range of different design features considered to humanise a space, and how the term is often used as an umbrella to include anything that makes a hospital less 'inhospitable'. Colour was, then, by no means the only way to 'humanise' a hospital. It was, though, seen as important. To quote a *Hospital Development* article on interiors from 1988: '[w]ell thought out and co-ordinated colour schemes are able to provide solace, exhilaration and satisfaction. Above all, they can humanise a building, infusing an often soulless and impersonal environment with life'.[136] Colour was seen as important, in part, because it could combine so many of the other aspects of 'humanisation' such as the arts, nature, and making large institutions feel more 'human scale'.

Many features of humanistic design were not revolutionary, but were thought to serve a new purpose in counterbalancing high-technology, scientific, and institutional medical practice. The 'humanistic' hospital, as an ideal, operated as a symbol for wider social concerns about the loss – or decentring – of patients in modern medical practice. The term is not value-free; it carries with it assumptions about the dehumanisation of modern medicine, and has often been built on implicit binaries between the human and the technological. Understanding the meanings and influence of 'humanisation' in the late twentieth century is a crucial part of understanding some of the architecture, design, and colour palettes of the NHS hospital.

Notes

1 Part of this opening paragraph and elements of the first section of this chapter are reproduced from Victoria Bates, '"Humanizing" Healthcare Environments: Architecture, Art and Design in Modern Hospitals', *Design for Health*, 2 (2018), pp. 5–19.
2 Julie Willis, Philip Goad, and Cameron Logan, *Architecture and the Modern Hospital: Nosokomeion to Hygeia* (Routledge, 2019), p. 226.
3 Stephen Verderber and David J. Fine, *Healthcare Architecture in an Era of Radical Transformation* (Yale University Press, 2000), p. 52; Hughes, '"The "Matchbox on a Muffin": The Design of Hospitals in the Early NHS', *Medical History*, 44 (2000), pp. 21–56.
4 Sarah Hosking and Liz Haggard, *Healing the Hospital Environment: Design, Management and Maintenance of Healthcare Premises* (E. & F. N. Spon, 1999), p. 15.
5 D. Bardon, 'No Place Like Home?', *BMJ*, June 1981, p. 2052.
6 'Viewpoint', *Hospital Development*, 11 (1983), p. 6.
7 Anne Nardin (ed.), *L'humanisation de l'hôpital: Mode d'emploi* (Musée de l'Assistance publique, 2009). Hôpitaux de Paris. Nardin traces this trend back to early twentieth-century France, although notes that it became a newly pressing issue for government in the post-war period. The AP-HP archive and Archives Nationales in Paris also both hold extensive papers that show the ongoing interest of the government in 'humanizing' hospitals in the decades following this circular. A lot of this material focuses on care, but some relates to the design of humanistic environments; as this book shows, the two issues were never truly separable.
8 James Falick, 'Humanistic Design Sells Your Hospital', *Hospitals*, 1 February 1981, pp. 68–74.
9 Ian C. Lewis, 'Humanizing Paediatric Care', *Child Abuse & Neglect*, 7 (1983), pp. 413–19; Chizuru Misago, Takusei Umenai, Daisuke Onuki, Kiyoshi Haneda, and Marsden Wagner, 'Humanised Maternity Care', *The Lancet*, 16 October 1999, pp. 1391–2; O. M. B. Santos and E. R. C. Siebert, 'The Humanization of Birth Experience at the University of Santa Catarina Maternity Hospital', *International Journal of Gynecology & Obstetrics*, 75 (2001), pp. S73–9.

10 Elizabeth Bromley, 'Building Patient-Centeredness: Hospital Design as an Interpretive Act', *Social Science & Medicine*, 75 (2012), pp. 1057–66; Wil Gesler, Morag Bell, Sarah Curtis, Phil Hubbard, and Susan Francis, 'Therapy by Design: Evaluating the UK Hospital Building Program', *Health & Place*, 10 (2004), pp. 117–28.

11 Kenneth A. Penman and Samuel H. Adams, 'Humane, Humanities, Humanitarian, Humanism', *The Clearing House*, 55 (1982), pp. 308–10; Loretta M. Kopelman, 'Values and Virtues: How Should They Be Taught?', *Academic Medicine*, 74 (1999), pp. 1307–10.

12 Joanna Bourke, *What It Means to Be Human: Reflections from 1791 to the Present* (Virago, 2011).

13 As Megan H. Glick argues, 'imperialist ideologies have long used the figure of the animal to imagine non-western, non-white subjects as bestial subhumans without access to rational empirical thought'; Megan H. Glick, 'Of Sodomy and Cannibalism: Dehumanisation, Embodiment and the Rhetorics of Same-Sex and Cross-Species Contagion', *Gender & History*, 23 (2011), p. 267. The exact processes of 'dehumanisation' and hierarchies of the 'human' differed between contexts, but it was a common tool of colonialism. On the broad history and philosophy of dehumanisation and the construction of 'animalistic', 'beastly' or 'less than human' Others see David Livingstone Smith, *Less than Human: Why We Demean, Enslave, and Exterminate Others* (St. Martin's Press, 2011).

14 Michael Adas, *Machines as the Measure of Men: Science, Technology, and Ideologies of Western Dominance* (Cornell University Press, 2018).

15 Clare Hickman, 'Cheerful Prospects and Tranquil Restoration: The Visual Experience of Landscape as Part of the Therapeutic Regime of the British Asylum, 1800–60', *History of Psychiatry*, 20 (2009), pp. 425–41.

16 'The Chorlton Pauper Hospital', *The Lancet*, October 1866, pp. 421–2.

17 Those who advocated 'humanisation' sometimes emphasised that they were *not* criticising the existing health service. For example, Minister of Health Enoch Powell emphasised in a 1962 speech: 'Let me at the outset dispose of any notion that the emphasis which I have placed on the "humanisation" of the hospital service, and shall continue to place on it as long as I remain Minister of Health, implies that the service or those who work in it are either "inhuman" or "inhumane"'; Enoch Powell, 'Humanisation of Hospital Service', 19 October 1962, http://enochpowell.info/wp-content/uploads/Speeches/1962–1963.pdf [accessed: 15 October 2024]. However, it was more common for 'humanisation' to be presented as a solution to a problem when politics was not at play.

18 Corbett Lyons, 'Generational Design', in Kate Copeland (ed.), *Australian Healthcare Design 2000–2015: A Critical Review of the Design and Build of Healthcare Infrastructure in Australia* (International Academy for Design and Health, 2013), p. 54.
19 Many of these debates about modernity and individualism were longstanding within international sociology of the nineteenth and twentieth centuries, in the work of Durkheim, among others. See Peter Kivisto (ed.), *Key Ideas in Sociology* (Sage, 2010).
20 Ivan Illich, *Medical Nemesis: The Expropriation of Health* (Calder and Boyars, 1975).
21 Gerald P. Turner and Joseph Mapa, *Humanizing Hospital Care* (McGraw-Hill Ryerson, 1979).
22 Erving Goffman, *Asylums: Essays on the Social Situation of Mental Patients and Other Inmates* (Doubleday, 1961); Michel Foucault, *The Birth of the Clinic: An Archaeology of Medical Perception*, trans. Alan Sheridan (Tavistock Publications, 1973 [1963]).
23 Keith Petrie and Simon Wessely, 'Modern Worries, New Technology and Medicine', *BMJ* (March 2002), p. 324; Amelia Bonea, Melissa Dickson, Sally Shuttleworth, and Jennifer Wallis. *Anxious Times: Medicine and Modernity in Nineteenth-Century Britain* (University of Pittsburgh Press, 2019).
24 The emphasis on perception is important here, as a number of historians note that late twentieth-century critiques of the loss of holism do not entirely stand up to scrutiny; see, for example, Christopher Lawrence and George Weisz (eds), *Greater than the Parts: Holism in Biomedicine, 1920–1950* (Oxford University Press, 1998).
25 B. M. Korsch, 'Issues in Humanizing Care for Children', *American Journal of Public Health,* 68 (1978), pp. 831–2.
26 Jan Howard *et al.*, 'Humanizing Health Care: The Implications of Technology, Centralization, and Self-Care', *Medical Care*, 15 (1977), pp. 11–26.
27 *Ibid.*
28 See Victoria Bates, 'Yesterday's Doctors: The Human Aspects of Medical Education in Britain, 1957–93', *Medical History*, 61 (2017), pp. 48–65.
29 Elizabeth Kimball, 'Interior Design as Healing Agent', *Canadian Medical Association Journal*, 130 (1984), pp. 1364–72.
30 This section references recommendations from a range of colleagues; many thanks to those who responded to my request on social media for reading on experience and architecture.
31 Sigrid de Jong 'Experiencing Architectural Space', in Caroline van Eck and Sigrid de Jong (eds), *Companion to Eighteenth-Century Architecture* (Chichester, 2017), pp. 192–230. Quotes are taken from

the chapter abstract, see https://onlinelibrary.wiley.com/doi/10.1002/9781118887226.wbcha038 [accessed: 15 February 2024].

32 Edward Gillin and H. Horatio Joyce, 'Introduction', in Edward Gillin and H. Horatio Joyce (eds), *Experiencing Architecture in the Nineteenth Century: Buildings and Society in the Modern Age* (Bloomsbury, 2019), p. 1.

33 *Ibid.*

34 See, for example, this write-up of the conference 'Architecture, Citizenship, Space: British Architecture from the 1920s to the 1970s', https://picturesforschools.wordpress.com/2017/06/17/reflections-on-architecture-citizenship-space-british-architecture-from-the-1920s-to-the-1970s/ [accessed: 15 February 2024]; Michael W. Farr, 'James Stirling and Architectural Colour' (PhD Dissertation: University of Manchester, 2013), pp. 192–3.

35 For example, Clare Cooper conducted surveys on housing in 1970s and shared guidelines with architects, and Margaret Willis was a sociologist for London County Council. For scholarship on this trend, see Jon Lawrence, 'Class, "Affluence" and the Study of Everyday life in Britain, c. 1930–64', *Cultural and Social History*, 10 (2013), pp. 273–99.

36 Catherine Burke and Ian Grosvenor, *School* (Reaktion Books, 2008), pp. 103–4.

37 David Armstrong, 'Decline of the Hospital: Reconstructing Institutional Dangers', *Sociology of Health & Illness*, 20 (1998), pp. 445–57.

38 *Ibid.*

39 Many of these reports were published and can be seen in the online King's Fund digital archive, https://archive.kingsfund.org.uk. Original survey responses are also available at London Metropolitan Archives, see the series A/KE/.

40 Farr, 'James Stirling and Architectural Colour', p. 191.

41 *Ibid.*, p. 192.

42 *Ibid.*, p. 191.

43 Hugh Baron, 'A History of Art in British Hospitals', in Susan Loppert and Duncan Haldane (eds), *The Arts in Healthcare* (King's Fund, 1999), p. 11.

44 Ruth Nitkiewicz, 'Art in Hospitals', https://www.kingsfund.org.uk/insight-and-analysis/blogs/art-in-hospitals [accessed: 16 February 2024]; see also Richard Cork, *The Healing Presence of Art* (Yale University Press, 2012).

45 Baron, 'A History of Art in British Hospitals', p. 11.

46 Some examples are given here, but this is not a comprehensive timeline, and there were also many local or regional initiatives; see, for example,

the 'Timeline of London's Creative Health Sector Development', in Rebecca Gordon-Nesbitt, *Understanding Creative Health in London: The Scale, Character, and Maturity of the Sector* (Greater London Authority, 2024), pp. 32–3.

47 Historic England, 'Public Art 1945–95: Introduction to Heritage Assets', p. 3, https://historicengland.org.uk/images-books/publications/iha-public-art-1945-95/heag089-public-art-1945-95/] [accessed: 16 February 2024]. The history of hospital art is also entwined with public art in other countries, though in a slightly different way. For example, in the US, hospital murals were often produced as part of the early twentieth-century New Deal Federal Art Project. Examples can be seen at 'Living New Deal', https://livingnewdeal.org/locations/bellevue-hospital-new-york-ny/ [accessed: 16 February 2024]; original records are available at Archives of American Art e.g., see 'Federal Art Project, Photographic Division collection, circa 1920–1965, bulk 1935–1942'.

48 For example, see Christopher Tipping interviewed by Victoria Bates, 25 March 2023.

49 Paintings in Hospitals, 'Our History', https://www.paintingsinhospitals.org.uk/Blogs/collection [accessed: 16 February 2024].

50 Thomas Walshaw, 'The Healing Presence of Art', *Journal of EAHIL*, 15 (2019), p. 32.

51 *Ibid.*

52 Paintings in Hospitals do not have a formal or catalogued archive, but I was kindly given permission to see files that contain borrowing requests and agreements for paintings; it is on this basis that I make this claim.

53 Wellcome Library, ART/AFH/A/9/9.

54 Barclay, 'When It's Not the Main Game', p. 35.

55 This claim is, in large part, based on my many visits to hospitals and conversations with people working in such roles. There is also a wealth of literature on sensory work in OT. For example, see Anke Jakob and Lesley Collier, 'Sensory Enrichment for People Living with Dementia: Increasing the Benefits of Multisensory Environments in Dementia Care Through Design', *Design for Health*, 1 (2017), pp. 115–33.

56 In 2022–23 I conducted a series of interviews, including with many hospital arts coordinators, which showed that these jobs remain uneven. For example, many are funded by hospital charities, and are often part-time roles. See Victoria Bates, 'Sensing Spaces of Healthcare' interviews, published December 2024, https://doi.org/10.5523/bris.3b8eg2be3ecw52vt38l7nq9kah

57 For example, see Guy Eades interviewed by Victoria Bates, 13 March 2023: 'the National Network for Arts and Health ... morphed into the National Alliance and then that's morphed again into the Culture, Health and Wellbeing one. So it's always sort of kind of gone forward, but it's sort of kind of changed emphasis'. Victoria Bates, 'Sensing Spaces of Healthcare' interviews, published December 2024, https://doi.org/10.5523/bris.3b8eg2be3ecw52vt38l7nq9kah

58 Anne Greer interviewed by Victoria Bates, 14 April 2023. Victoria Bates, 'Sensing Spaces of Healthcare' interviews, published December 2024, https://doi.org/10.5523/bris.3b8eg2be3ecw52vt38l7nq9kah

59 Paintings in Hospitals, 'Collection Highlight: Julian Trevelyan', https://www.paintingsinhospitals.org.uk/blog/collection-highlight-julian-trevelyan [accessed: 16 February 2024].

60 Art UK, 'Gillian Ayres', https://artuk.org/discover/artists/ayres-gillian-19302018 [accessed: 16 February 2024].

61 Paintings in Hospitals, 'Landscape Art', https://www.paintingsinhospitals.org.uk/l-landscape-art [accessed: 16 February 2024].

62 Though I have resisted the temptation to put 'nature' in inverted commas throughout this book, it is important to recognise that the idea of 'nature' as encountered in and from hospitals has always been a construction.

63 This 'return to nature' or imbuing of nature with 'spirit' differed from ideas about the ways that humans needed to be separate from, or 'conquer' nature. See Carolyn Merchant, *The Death of Nature: Women, Ecology, and the Scientific Revolution* (Harper & Row, 1980). On how the Romantics offered an 'alternative vision, affirming the inherent value of the non-human world', see Kevin Hutchings, 'Eco-criticism in British Romantic Studies', *Literature Compass*, 4 (2007), p. 185.

64 Victoria Bates, *Making Noise in the Modern Hospital* (Cambridge University Press, 2021), p. 38.

65 Thrive, 'A Brief History of STH', https://www.thrive.org.uk/how-we-help/what-we-do/new-and-updates/a-brief-history-of-sth [accessed: 16 February 2024].

66 Constance Classen, *The Museum of the Senses: Experiencing Art and Collections* (Bloomsbury, 2017), p. 132; on the way that 'scent-less' works of art can be experienced through smell, see also Anette Stenslund, 'The Harsh Smell of Scentless Art: On the Synaesthetic Gesture of Hospital Atmosphere', in Sara Asu Schroer and Susanne Schmitt (eds), *Exploring Atmospheres Ethnographically* (Routledge, 2018), pp. 153–71.

67 For examples see Eugene Rosenberg and Richard Cork, *Architect's Choice: Art in Architecture in Great Britain since 1945* (Thames & Hudson Ltd, 1992), pp. 108–21.

68 *Kunst Rigshospitalets Forhal: En guide til udvalgte vaerker.* Thank you to Jacob Gyldenløve Aaen, Press Consultant, for sharing and translating this guide for me.

69 Peter Coles, 'Draft MS for Handbook for Art for Public Places', November 1985 in Wellcome, ART/AFH/A/12/3: box 75 'Landscape and Healthcare'.

70 Professor Penny Sparke, 'Say Aloe to my Little Frond', *99 Percent Invisible,* https://99percentinvisible.org/episode/say-aloe-to-my-little-frond/transcript/ [accessed: 16 February 2024]; see also Sparke's *Nature Inside: Plants and Flowers in the Modern Interior* (Yale University Press, 2021).

71 Clare Hickman, *Therapeutic Landscapes: A History of English Hospital Gardens since 1800* (Manchester University Press, 2013), p. 212.

72 Jeremy Hugh Baron and Lesley Greene, 'Art in Hospitals: Funding Works of Art in New Hospitals', *BMJ* (December 1984), pp. 1731–6.

73 John Gage, *Colour in Arts* (Thames & Hudson Ltd, 2006), p. 34.

74 Roger Ulrich, 'View Through a Window May Influence Recovery', *Science*, 224 (1984), pp. 224–5. The impact of this article is discussed further in the final chapter of this book, which concerns glass and windows.

75 Eades interview.

76 Baron and Greene, 'Art in Hospitals'.

77 The popularity of natural themes in art is also, of course, not limited to hospitals and there is a long and ongoing art history here. In 1995, two Russian artists launched a project called 'The Most Wanted Paintings' to identify and make a true 'people's art. It is perhaps unsurprising to find that they created a landscape, with hills, water, stags, and a couple of people walking gently. See 'Komar + Melamid: *The Most Wanted Paintings*', https://www.diaart.org/exhibition/exhibitions-projects/komar-melamid-the-most-wanted-paintings-web-project [accessed: 16 February 2024].

78 Malcolm Miles, 'Behind Closed Doors', *Hospital Development*, 24 (1993), p. 35.

79 Sarah Hosking and Liz Haggard, *Healing the Hospital Environment: Design, Management and Maintenance of Healthcare Premises* (E. & F. N. Spon, 1999), p. 63.

80 Wellcome Library, ART/AFH/A/5/2, Peter Senior, 'Art for Health's Sake', *Hospital Development* (1990), p. 30.

81 Richard Burton, 'St Mary's Hospital, Isle of Wight: A Suitable Background for Caring', *BMJ* (December 1990), p. 1423.

82 Burton, 'St Mary's Hospital, Isle of Wight', p. 1423.
83 Sian Tucker interview.
84 *Ibid.*
85 *Ibid.*
86 Anne Greer interviewed by Victoria Bates, 14 April 2023. Victoria Bates, 'Sensing Spaces of Healthcare' interviews, published December 2024, https://doi.org/10.5523/bris.3b8eg2be3ecw52vt38l7nq9kah
87 Cited in Sam Gathercole, 'The Expressive Unit of Constructionism: Kenneth Martin at Whittington Hospital', *British Art Studies*, 24 (2023), https://doi.org/10.17658/issn.2058-5462/issue-24/sgathercole.
88 Gathercole, 'The Expressive Unit of Constructionism'.
89 Eades interview.
90 They also, though, argue that crafting practices can offer forms of resistance and should not just be seen as a 'romantic' practice in this way; Ann Rippin and Sheena J. Vachhani, 'Craft as Resistance: A Conversation about Craftivism, Embodied Inquiry, and Craft-based Methodologies', in Emma Bell, Gianluigi Mangia, Scott Taylor, and Maria Laura Toraldo (eds), *The Organization of Craft Work: Identities, Meanings, and Materiality* (Routledge, 2018), Chapter 11.
91 Jane Willis interviewed by Victoria Bates, 21 February 2023; a very similar comment about the shift from 'done to' to 'done with' in his own work, since the early 2000s was also made independently by Guy Noble interviewed by Victoria Bates, 12 May 2023. Victoria Bates, 'Sensing Spaces of Healthcare' interviews, published December 2024, https://doi.org/10.5523/bris.3b8eg2be3ecw52vt38l7nq9kah
92 Willis interview.
93 Sinéad Gleeson, *Constellations: Reflections from Life* (Picador, 2019), p. 109.
94 Annemarie Mol, Ingunn Moser, and Jeannette Pols, 'Care: Putting Practice into Theory', in Annemarie Mol, Ingunn Moser, and Jeannette Pols (eds), *Care in Practice: On Tinkering in Clinics, Homes and Farms* (transcript Verlag), pp. 7–26, p. 14. Emphasis in original.
95 It is also racialised, see Naomi Gerstel, 'The Third Shift: Gender and Care Work Outside the Home', *Qualitative Sociology*, 23 (2000), pp. 467–83; Mary Phillips and Alice Willatt, 'Embodiment, Care and Practice in a Community Kitchen', *Gender, Work & Organization*, 27 (2020), pp. 198–217; Bill Hughes, Linda McKie, Debra Hopkins, and Nick Watson, 'Love's Labours Lost? Feminism, the Disabled People's Movement and an Ethic of Care', *Sociology* 39(2) (2005), pp. 259–275; Peta Bowden, *Caring: Gender-Sensitive Ethics* (Routledge, 1997). Christopher Tipping also observed this trend: 'the catalyst for my involvement in most projects is usually a woman, working in a

hospital environment in the capacity of an art consultant or an arts manager in some way and I'm really intensely grateful for that because out of all the projects I've worked on the NHS, I think only two of them have been driven by men in that capacity as the art manager', interviewed by Victoria Bates, 25 March 2023.

96 See Vicky Casey interviewed by Victoria Bates, 20 January 2023: 'if we can actually design a really vibrant public space and place a big piece of art either at an entrance point or whatever else – then people intuitively say, "Oh, I'll meet you by the three monkeys," or, "I'll meet you by the lion," or, "I'll meet you by the hoops" or whatever else'.

97 On the idea of the human scale see Victoria Bates, '"Humanizing" Healthcare Environments: Architecture, Art and Design in Modern Hospitals', *Design for Health*, 2 (2018), pp. 5–19.

98 On car parks and bus routes and the perception of care, see John Launer, 'Care Pathways', *Postgraduate Medical Journal*, 84 (2008), p. 392.

99 '*HD* Installations: Colour Co-ordination', *Hospital Development*, 16 (1988) p. 51.

100 I have been unable to verify exactly when the line was drawn, though this British Library blog states 1947: 'A visit to the Joint Library of Ophthalmology at Moorfields Eye Hospital', https://blogs.bl.uk/science/2019/02/a-visit-to-the-joint-library-of-ophthalmology-at-moorfields-eye-hospital.html#:~:text=In%201947%20the%20hospital%20merged,sighted%20people%20find%20their%20way [accessed: 16 February 2024].

101 For a summary of some of this history and its impact on formal design standards see Itab Shuayb, *Inclusive University Built Environments: The Impact of Approved Document M for Architects, Designers, and Engineers* (Springer, 2020), pp. 7–62. This book focuses on the growing emphasis on inclusive education and its impact on university design, but its claims can equally be applied to hospitals, and many of the design standards it outlines applied across different building types.

102 'Inventing the Dropped Curb', *The Bartlett*, https://www.ucl.ac.uk/bartlett/ideas/inventing-dropped-curb [accessed: 30 April 2024].

103 J. R. Carpman, M. A. Grant, and D. A. Simmons, *Design that Cares: Planning Health Facilities for Patients and Visitors* (American Hospital Publishing, 1986); J. R. Carpman, M. A. Grant, and D. A. Simmons, 'Wayfinding in the Hospital Environment: The Impact of Various Floor Numbering Alternatives', *Journal of Environmental Systems*, 13 (1984), pp. 353–64; referenced in Ann Sloan Devlin, 'Wayfinding in Healthcare Facilities: Contributions from Environmental Psychology', *Behavioral Sciences*, 4 (2014), pp. 423–36.

104 Stephen Nicoll, 'The Art of Good Signage', *Hospital Development*, 26 (1995), p. 24.
105 Colette Miller and David Lewis, *Wayfinding: Effective Wayfinding and Signing Systems. Guidance for Healthcare Facilities* (Stationery Office, 1999), p. 10.
106 Miller and Lewis, *Wayfinding*, p. 36.
107 Nicoll, 'The Art of Good Signage', p. 24.
108 For example, 'wayfinding' is primarily read as an issue of hallways and corridors in Julie Zook and Kerstin Sailer, *The Covert Life of Hospital Architecture* (UCL Press, 2022).
109 Roger Luckhurst 'Corridors' in The Hospital Senses Collective, 'Corridors', https://hospitalsenses.co.uk/corridors-2/ [accessed: 16 February 2024].
110 B. S. Platt, T. P. Eddy, and P. L. Pellett, *Food in Hospitals: A Study of Feeding Arrangements and the Nutritional Value of Meals in Hospitals* (Oxford University Press, 1963), pp. 116–25.
111 C. B. Denne, 'Bright Ideas for Interiors', *Hospital Development*, 16 (1988), p. 19; Bill Murray, 'Changing the Face of Patient Care', *Hospital Development*, 16 (1988), p. 23.
112 J. H. Baron, 'How to Beautify Your Old Hospital', *BMJ*, 29 September 1984, p. 809.
113 Peter Scher, 'All Systems Go', *Hospital Development*, 25 (1994), p. 35.
114 Sunand Prasad, 'Typology Quarterly: Hospitals', *The Architectural Review*, 27 April 2012, http://www.architectural-review.com/essays/typology-quarterly-hospitals/8629443.article [accessed: 16 February 2024].
115 On Withington Hospital near Manchester, one person wrote that 'we are the only A and E Dept with a four-mile corridor from one end to the other'; Roger Sim and Helen Kitchen, *More than a Place of Healing: An Anthology of Memories, Memorabilia and Anecdotes of Withington Hospital* (Hospital Arts, 1999), p. 118. In the 'Voices of Our NHS' interviews, one interviewee noted that he worked at Llandough Hospital, which had the longest corridor in Europe and that one junior doctor used to travel along it on a skateboard for urgent calls. As this corridor is almost 1 km in length, it seems that the Withington example refers to multiple connected corridors, and the 'longest corridor' claim to a single hallway. British Library Sounds, C1887/767, Peter Welsh interviewed by James McSharry, January 2018, Voices of Our National Health Service © University of Manchester.
116 See also Kirsi Heimonen and Sari Kuuva, 'A Corridor That Moves: Corporeal Encounters with Materiality in a Mental Hospital', in Monika

Ankele and Benoit Majerus (eds), *Material Cultures of Psychiatry* (Transcript Verlag, 2020), pp. 334–53.

117 The National Archives, MH166/1136, Harness Interiors produced by the interior designers from the Regional Health Authorities and the Department of Health & Social Security, part of the papers of the 'Technical Design Group' 1973–75, MH166/1136, p. 25.

118 Wellcome Library, ART/AFH/A/9/9; John Agate, 'Colour in Hospital', *World Medicine*, May 1969, pp. 13–17.

119 Record Office for Leicestershire, Leicester and Rutland, SP-2-B, December 1989, *Bedpost*, p. 8.

120 John Harding and David Jolley, 'Design for Dementia', *Hospital Development*, 25 (1994), p. 23.

121 *Ibid.*

122 Imperial Health Charity, 'Charity Celebrates 30th Anniversary of Bridget Riley Murals at St Mary's', 7 August 2017, https://www.imperialcharity.org.uk/news-and-stories/news/charity-celebrates-30th-annivesary-of-bridget-riley-murals-at-st-marys [accessed: 16 February 2024].

123 Chinati, 'Bridget Riley: Royal Liverpool University Hospital, 1983', https://chinati.org/exhibitions/bridget-riley/ [accessed: 16 February 2024].

124 Imperial Health Charity, 'Charity Celebrates'.

125 Mark Paterson, 'Architecture of Sensation: Affect, Motility and the Oculomotor', *Body & Society*, 23 (2017), p. 28.

126 *Ibid.*

127 *Ibid.*

128 Nicoll, 'The Art of Good Signage', p. 24.

129 *Ibid.*, p. 25.

130 Wellcome Library, ART/AFH/A/2/1, 'Conquest Hospital Phase II Arts Strategy'.

131 The Brunel Building of Southmead Hospital in Bristol even uses 'gates' to help people to navigate; see Vicky Casey interviewed by Victoria Bates, 20 January 2023.

132 Ingold argues against some aspects of this claim, including the idea that art predominantly 'represent[s] experience', but this does not make the cultural power of this idea any less significant. Tim Ingold, *The Perception of the Environment: Essays on Livelihood, Dwelling and Skill* (Routledge, 2000), p. 11.

133 On more recent examples of the vibrant use of colour in hospital arts, see Fiona McLachlan, *Colour Beyond the Surface: Art in Architecture* (Lund Humphries, 2022), pp. 119–24, 132, 141, 158–9.

134 The King's Fund, *Celebrating Achievement: Enhancing the Healing Environment Programme 2003–2005* (TSO, 2006), p. 6.

135 Jane Macnaughton, Peter Collins, Simon Coleman, Peter Kellett, Geoffrey Purves, Anu Soukas, Mike White, and Karen Taylor, *Designing for Health: Architecture, Art and Design at the James Cook University Hospital* (NHS Estates, 2005).
136 C. B. Denne, 'Bright Ideas for Interiors', *Hospital Development*, 16 (1988), p, 19.

4

Patterns: homeliness in the hospital

When the first patient arrived at the new Northwick Park hospital in 1970, she commented on how 'homely' she found its window curtains.[1] Almost twenty years later, *Hospital Development* magazine published 'Bright Ideas for Interiors' by C. B. Denne, Director of Works and Estates, Mid-Staffordshire Health Authority. Denne declared '[t]he institutional is dead, long live the homely!'[2] The idea that hospitals needed to be more 'homely' was quickly accepted. Echoing the umbrella concept of 'humanisation' under which it sat, homeliness was in 'full bloom' by the 1980s.[3] The concept became so influential that there was even some concern about the conflation of hospital and home. To quote one estates project officer in 1999, '[a] lot of companies are trying to bring the home into hospital, but it's going too far sometimes. If patients have had a bad time in hospital, they may then associate that with a "domestic" environment, and bring it back home with them'.[4] Denne was evidently right in declaring a victory of 'the homely' over 'the institutional' by the late twentieth century.

Homeliness was a broad and complex concept, with a long history in relation to healthcare settings and ever-shifting meanings. As Kieran Richards and Rebecca McLaughlan note, '[o]ne of the main barriers to implementing homeliness in care environments is its conceptual ambiguity'.[5] By unpicking some of the many meanings and manifestations of the ambiguous concept of 'homeliness' in late twentieth-century hospitals, it becomes possible to see the uses of colour, patterns, and textiles in making hospitals 'homely'. However, the idea that homeliness was produced entirely through material changes or design can be critiqued. As explored here, homeliness was also brought into the hospital through practices of 'everyday' design, in which people brought their own objects with them or made spaces more comfortable. The colour palettes of 'everyday' design were unpredictable and personal, and it was precisely these variable qualities that made them 'homely'.

Homely: the post-war return of an ideal

There is still very little understanding of what 'homely' meant in post-war Britain, either in theory or in practice. This ambiguity is, in part, because of the complexity of the concept of 'home'. Some historians have been interested in the material home, for example examining post-war reconstruction or how the concept of 'privacy' was built into British architecture.[6] Others have been more interested in the idea of 'home' and its construction in relation to factors such as age, gender, race, family, economics, politics, nationhood, and more.[7] As Martin Moore notes, 'ideas of the domestic had important political overtones in the immediate post-war period, with the family considered the ideal unit through which totalitarian regimes could be resisted and democratic citizens made'.[8] Homeliness and domesticity were, among other things, key to the post-war welfare state and the making of social democracy. It is perhaps unsurprising, given the richness of the concept of home and its importance in understanding post-war Britain, that it has drawn the extensive attention of scholars.

Post-war philosophers were also very interested in interrogating the concept of 'home', including how it overlapped and differed from, or felt different from, a house.[9] This distinction is particularly important for understanding 'homeliness' in hospitals. To quote Kieran Richards and Rebecca McLaughlan: 'actual physical homes do not always inform approaches to homeliness in care environments'.[10] Examples of hospital design in which homeliness has been interpreted purely in material terms, such as building streets or 'houses', are very rare.[11] Even when 'homely' design in hospitals did emulate houses, it was grounded in a somewhat nostalgic, cosy vision of middle-class white domesticity, which did not include everyone. As Melisa Duque *et al.* also note, for many people the link between house and home has also been broken by factors ranging from migration to divorce, and it is more productive to focus on the 'feeling of home, which is related to material, technological and sensory affordances as well as social relations with wellbeing implications'.[12] Their work relates to current-day healthcare contexts but is equally applicable to the historical ones considered here. Claire Langhamer's work on the meanings of 'home' in post-war Britain shows that

> home-centredness was never a uniform experience: the significant numbers who lacked homes of their own even at the end of the 1950s attest to this. As we have seen, significant numbers of households entered the 1960s without the privacy, comfort or labour-saving consumer durables which have become characteristic of the 'affluent' society.[13]

Ideas such as 'privacy' and 'comfort' that imbued healthcare models of 'homeliness' at the same time must not, then, be taken as representative of people's real living circumstances. In many healthcare contexts, homeliness was an anti-institutional concept, rather than a specific design intervention that emulated 'the house'. As healthcare architect Ronald Weeks noted in an article for *The Architectural Review* in 1980, the idea that medicine should underpin all design decisions 'produces an institutional effect and carries the patient one more step away from that impression of everyday life that he is craving', including the home.[14] The idea of 'home' was, then, about counter-balancing 'institutional' design, rather than emulating houses in a literal way. As one recent commentator noted in *The Architectural Review*,

> The supposed domesticity is questionable on two fronts: on the one hand it dilutes the reality of domesticity, turning it into a banal generality, a shallow symbol of comfort that can hardly convince. On the other hand it avoids the atmosphere of purity and danger so aptly conveyed by the Modernist hospital.[15]

Homeliness was seen as sensorially and conceptually soft: the essence of 'homely' design was natural materials, contrasting colours, patterns, art, textiles and soft furnishings, music, and muted lighting.[16] For example, in 1975 *Hospital Development* magazine reported on a new unit for the elderly at North Tees General Hospital, as follows:

> To complement the already established homely environment, attractive patterns of vinyl wallpaper are to be found in such areas as day spaces, reception areas and on all bed-head walls. The remainder of

> the décor is in silk finish emulsion paint of different colours. The floors to the wards, day spaces, staff bases, reception areas are all laid with carpet.[17]

This echoed some international literature on the subject. In an American publication on *Color in the Health Care Environment* in 1978, for example, Thomas R. C. Sisson wrote of

> the delight of patients to find hospital surroundings 'home-like' [...] the meaning is clear – the surroundings offer the *visual* contrast in colo[u]r, furnishings, and textures found in a home. Equally important is the use of light to enhance colo[u]rs and contrasts. Few homes are brightly lighted [sic] from above.[18]

In some ways, at first glance, such writing sought to bring elements of domestic design into the hospital in a literal way. However, it is important also to contextualise these design trends. In British literature, there were references to the 'homely' in contexts ranging from garden design to the ways that doctors interacted with patients to make a 'homely' atmosphere.[19] Often this literature made no real attempt to define the concept or link it explicitly to the material features of housing design, and – as argued above – it is important not to take these examples as straightforward evidence that hospital design was seeking to emulate the house directly. Even Sisson, who listed many elements of sensory design that made a hospital 'home-like' emphasised that 'of course, this is a misnomer, but the meaning is clear'.[20] The emphasis, then, was on the 'meaning' rather than on the 'home' itself.

Homeliness was a variable concept that shifted in meaning depending on context. In the early NHS, the term 'homely' was used extensively but loosely. The desire to make healthcare environments more 'homelike' was evident in a range of contexts, including General Practice (GP) surgeries and care environments.[21] Hospital design must be understood as part of this wider system, as part of – and potentially the end point of – a flow through other 'domestic' medical spaces. Homeliness was brought into the hospital in a range of ways, including care practices and daily routines. In 1961, for example, hospital authorities reviewed the pattern of in-patients' days in response to a Standing Nursing Advisory Committee report that recommended 'allowing patients to sleep longer and enjoy a day organised more nearly in accordance with that to which they were accustomed in their own homes'.[22] This example fits with other trends, such as the expansion of visiting hours, attempting to make hospitals more accommodating and flexible. Material changes, such as the use of domestic scale and 'homely' design, were an important part of this story but must be situated in this context. 'Homeliness' was not simply a matter of putting up wallpaper, but part of a complex and bigger picture of cultural change in the health service.

The colour palette of the 'homely' hospital was typically vague, but broadly non-institutional. In 1951, for example, *The Hospital* reported on the waiting hall for new physiotherapy and dental departments at Selly Oak Hospital as follows:

> A light and homely atmosphere has been maintained with a colour scheme of shell grey walls, tor grey doors, lacquer red frames, and [a] dusty red ceiling. Plant life has been introduced [...] while a focal point of interest for waiting patients is created by an abstract mural painting.[23]

It is unclear which aspect of this design was considered 'homely', and the colour palette did not obviously align with any interior design trends.[24] Other hospitals more clearly emulated homely colour interiors: for example, much hospital design literature advocated wallpaper in non-sterile areas. At this time there was little detail on recommended colours or patterns. Denne was unusually specific in 1988 about the value of 'small print wallpaper with neat flowery friezes and borders' for making hospitals 'homely'.[25] This claim might have related to trends in interior design and fashion, as patterns and floral prints were relatively popular in the 1980s; or it might, equally, have been something seem as timeless, or non-institutional because of the natural imagery.[26] Similar trends were also evident elsewhere. In the US. For example, David Charles Sloane and Beverlie Conant Sloane note that 'the functionalism of the post-World War II machine-medicine hospital has given way to brighter, more accessible, patient-centred designs', and that bringing in 'elements' of 'the home' was part of this trend.[27] In terms of colour, these elements could involve wallpaper or patterned fabrics, though 'homeliness' cannot be reduced to any one feature of design or decoration. It is difficult to tease out some of the principles underpinning 'homely' colour palettes and patterns when an explanation was so rarely given. It is necessary to dig deeper into the material, sensory, and emotional aspects of 'homely' design, to get beyond the generalisations and ambiguities of contemporary sources.

Advocates of 'homeliness' pointed to historical precedents, just as they had done with 'humanisation' more broadly. Florence Nightingale was, again, repeatedly quoted or referenced in appeals to a lost past apparently full of colour and shaped by homely ideals.[28] Homeliness had indeed been a guiding principle in Nightingale's work.[29] Scholars have also written on the role of domesticity, including material culture from furnishings to plants, in other Victorian long-stay institutions such as asylums and convalescent homes.[30] 'Modernity' incorporated such ideas into its many layers, combining tradition with novelty, and updating 'homeliness' in relation to the specific connotations of the 'home' in post-war Britain and the 'institution' against which it was situated. Appeals to history were, though, also selective and at times romanticised the past. They were part of a wider backlash against modern healthcare, and a reimagining of what it looked and felt like.

The complicated nature of 'homeliness' was evident in its colour schemes, or rather lack thereof. It was a more chaotic concept in colour terms. Though there were some broad, common design features, as outlined above, in practice the design of 'homeliness' was often localised and depended on the patient group. Examples in *Hospital Development* alone include, in 1976, a 'geriatric hospital', where a 'sense of home and family' was created by small bays, 'décor in light colours and large window areas', the texture of carpets, televisions and services such as hairdressing and food menus.[31] In the same year, in a very different context, it reported that a hospital for people with learning disabilities had 'bright colours and the walls hung with modern abstract paintings in the living area', which 'gives an impression of a home rather than a hospital'.[32] In colour terms, here there are two very different examples of home-like design: one 'light' as part of a traditional decorative scheme, and one 'bright' in combination with abstract art. The first implicitly linked home to family, and the second to a non-institutional aesthetic; these overlap, of course, but are not synonymous. Other examples from around the same time offer subtly different examples of 'homely' colour schemes: an article about the new North Wing of St Thomas' Hospital in 1977 noted that 'colourful doors and fittings ... contribute to a light and pleasant homely atmosphere'.[33] In this example, seemingly the emphasis was on colour contrast and again avoiding the institutional feeling of single colour palettes, rather than on any particular colour. As Jean Symons argued in 1973 in *Improving Existing Hospital Buildings for Long-Stay Residents*, 'matching colour schemes – e.g. everything in shades of blue in one day room, orange in the next, and green in another – do not produce a home-like environment'.[34] It is important, then, not to fall into neat generalisations about what constituted 'homely' design at this time.

If homeliness is best understood as a feeling rather than a specific design intervention, it is more useful to look at how the term 'homely' was used in publications, and the feelings with which it was associated, rather than trying to pin down its design or colour schemes. For some, such as the example cited above, the home was linked with family. Other examples provide different feelings, both emotional and sensory. For example, in a 1978 article on 'interior design on a restricted budget', Mary Wragg wrote that '[c]olour is particularly important to the schemes illustrated … because both are geriatric hospitals, demanding as far as possible, a warm, homely atmosphere for the well-being of patients, visitors and staff'.[35] In 1977, *Hospital Development* reported on a continuing care unit for cancer patients that offered a 'comfortable, cheerful and homely environment'.[36] Both articles were echoed in a later piece that referred to architects' efforts to create 'a cheerful, homely ambience' and 'a warm, domestic appearance'.[37] In 1988, in a piece called 'Home from Home', another *Hospital Development* contributor used the language 'warm and homely'.[38] The repeated connections between 'homely' and notions of warmth and cheerfulness speak to the emotional and sensory feelings that 'homeliness' sought to evoke, rather than to specific design interventions. The actual colours that aligned with ideas of 'warmth' or 'cheer' or even 'brightness' evolved over time, and were thought to vary according to patients' needs, so it is perhaps unsurprising to find that 'homeliness' had no simple, single colour palette. The few examples that exist for staff used some similar language but also noted the particular requirements of staff spaces. Reporting in 1983 on plans for the new Bournemouth General Hospital, for example, *Hospital Development* noted that the use of 'warm red brickwork' sought to create a 'familiar domestic vernacular' for the staff residences to distinguish work from – in this case a more literal – home.[39] This warmth was tied to the way that 'home' represented many of the qualities that people wanted in a hospital, such as safety, security, comfort, and care.

The home is often associated with dwelling, but this is not the only function of the 'homely'. Ian Ewart and Rachael Luck argue, drawing on conversations with older people, that 'an important aspect of "homeliness" is the capacity for the home to act as somewhere you leave, and not only somewhere to reside'.[40] Similar arguments were made implicitly in the late twentieth century. For example, in 1977, a *Hospital Development* article noted that

> facilities are aimed at encouraging out-patients on discharge to seek the company and comradeship available in old age pensioners clubs and local day centres. It is for these reasons that the architects and interior designers have made efforts to make rooms homely with pictures and warm colours.[41]

This article indicates that rooms were made 'homely' precisely in order to encourage older people to feel able to leave them. This model of 'homeliness' might help us to understand why many manifestations of hospital 'homeliness' did not directly emulate a house. They pointed instead to the prospect of recovery, and operated as a kind of liminal 'homeliness' between the institution and a person's real place of residence. This was not always the case, though, as 'homeliness' or 'home-making' was also a key feature of hospice design and care.[42] It is important, then, to recognise that homeliness had many different forms in healthcare and care settings. Different 'feelings' of homeliness were more important for certain spaces, or in relation to specific groups of patients.

The qualities of 'homeliness' were historically contingent. The idea of a safe home was particularly important after a World War and under a welfare state that was prioritising housing as a human right. Ideas of neighbourliness and privacy played out in social interactions and the spatial design of hospitals.[43] It is still useful to engage with histories of homes and housing, then, to understand some of the trends in 'homely' design, but with a focus on feelings and atmospheres, rather than on the materiality of houses. Even this history of ideas must be approached with some caution. Historical ideas of 'homeliness' cannot be directly transferred to healthcare settings. As with the 'human' discussed in Chapter 3, the hospital model of 'homeliness' always – and *only* – existed in relation to the institution that it was trying to counter-balance. Implicitly, 'homeliness' in hospitals was always as much about what it was *not*, as about what it was.

Anti-institutional sentiment was not in complete opposition to modernity. It might be more useful to think of humanisation and homeliness as new forms of modernity, particularly in terms of patient-centred design and the physical manifestation of patients having more control over their surroundings. 'Homeliness' was largely a patient-centred concept, whereas the term 'homely' was rarely used in the context of actual homes in hospitals, such as staff residences. Instead, it was entwined with a growing emphasis on patients' experiences of healthcare. By 1994, an article in *Hospital Development* explicitly listed it as part of 'components of patient centred care' as follows: '1. Patient Centred design (eg [sic] home-like environment, defensible space, attractive outlook, good lighting and signposting, facilities for visitors, decoration)'.[44] In practice, as Louise Hide notes, 'homeliness' was not always the benign and patient-centred intervention it appeared. In mid-century wards, some 'homely effects were intended to have a "civilizing" influence on patients' behavio[u]r'.[45] That said, for many working to improve hospitals at this time, the 'homely' was seen as a route to the 'human'.

Modern homeliness embodied a specific form of modernity in which people's rights were being renegotiated, both in healthcare and modern Britain more generally, and in which patients' comfort and control were seen as increasingly important. It was therefore a development from more paternalistic (and indeed maternalistic) models of 'homely' institutions found in the nineteenth century. That said, patients' voices were not yet at the forefront of decision-making in post-war British hospital design. Early efforts to 'humanise' spaces by making them more 'homely' seemingly involved little patient consultation, whether in new builds by architects or more localised renovations. Many early efforts to make spaces 'homely' were grounded in the ideas of different professionals (from architects to nursing staff) about what 'homeliness' meant. Later, more consultative models of 'experience' came to be significant forces in healthcare, but until that point personalisation was achieved largely through objects and small-scale, short-term decoration. Patients were still agents in making homeliness throughout this period, sometimes as part of negotiating rights or as acts of subversion. Over time, they did so increasingly with permission as part of a deliberate choice by hospitals to hand over some control.

Though the rise of 'homeliness' tended to focus on patients over staff, it did overlap with wider shifts in modern workplace design in the post-war years. Vicky Long's work on inter-war factories notes that the 'homely' factory was intended to 'connote a sense of coziness and to evoke the atmosphere of the domestic home' as part of efforts to 'reconcile modernity with tradition'.[46] Many of the same statements could be made for post-war Britain more broadly. It is crucial to remember that wards were workplaces as much as they were spaces of treatment and recuperation. Decisions made for the benefit of patient experience were also made for the apparent benefit of the institution as a whole, and in the early post-war years in particular, efforts to improve patient experience were always bound up with questions about work and the function of the hospital. Hospitals were, of course, not factories. However, there are clear overlaps in efforts to 'reconcile modernity with tradition', and trying to find new forms of modern institution at this time.

The concept of 'homeliness' has been shaped, and reshaped, by trends in NHS work and care. Particularly in the early years of the NHS, people could spend prolonged periods of time in bed recuperating. In 1948 it was not uncommon for people to spend two weeks in hospital after giving birth or even following a simple operation, such as repairing a hernia. The length of stay fell over the course of the late twentieth century, but it is significant that 'homeliness' took hold when the duration of stay was still relatively long. Over time, boundaries between hospital and home have become increasingly blurred. The number of hospital beds declined from the 1960s onwards, with conscious efforts made for certain patient groups – particularly long-stay elderly patients – to receive care at home.[47] This involved moving medical equipment and hospital beds into people's private spaces. The shift towards hospital-based childbirth also slowed, with the rise of a 'natural childbirth' and home birth movement. Some of these shifts were political and economic, others social, and some simply because the technology is now available for managing long-term health conditions at home. As 'homeliness' became entrenched in the hospital, the hospital was also moving more and more into the home. Recent studies have shown that 'adaptations and technology impact feelings of at-homeness' in the house, as much as anti-technology interventions have impacted feelings of 'hospital-ness' in the institution.[48]

The idea of 'home' has always been complex. It is no surprise that untangling it has been a focus of so much academic work, yet there remains no clear answer as to what home 'means' and why. It is a contingent and relational concept. In the hospital, in the post-war years, it served a particular function. Like the 'humanisation' umbrella under which it sat, 'homely' spaces sought to evoke feelings and atmospheric qualities that were explicitly anti-institutional. The modern and modernist hospital was not in opposition to humanistic values or notions of care and comfort, but this juxtaposition was rhetorically helpful. To return to the opening quote: 'the institutional is dead, long live the homely!' There were shifts over time, with gradual movement towards a more experience-centred model of 'homeliness' that allowed patient agency and in which power and control were as important as care and anti-institutional design. By the end of the century, the boundaries between home and hospital were increasingly blurred, but the goal of 'homeliness' still carried weight as a form of NHS value system.

Designing homeliness: televisions and textiles

'Homeliness' was an important way in which patient-centred values were built into the material environment. However, it is often difficult to grasp what the aesthetics of 'homeliness' were in the hospital, and why specific decisions were made. This section digs further into homeliness, its meanings, and its manifestations by examining the idea from an object-based approach. It explores the history of colour televisions and hospital curtains and their role in 'homeliness', showing the importance of televisions for community, and curtains for privacy and personalisation. Each of these different forms of 'homeliness' had its own colour palette, which was always designed and negotiated in relation to very specific ideas of the 'homely' and associated feelings.

It is impossible to reduce 'homeliness', as a complex and dynamic affective atmosphere, to any one design feature. That said, certain aspects of 'homely' design served specific functions, or sought to evoke particular feelings. The case study of televisions reveals how 'homeliness' was manifested through, or in relation to, one object. David Howes and Constance Classen note that 'for many hospital patients the one bright spot, the one homey element, and the one avenue of escape from their overwhelmingly disengaging environment, is the television set on the wall of their room'.[49] As far back as the 1960s, commentators made similar comments about the role of television sets in homely atmospheres. Reporting on a visit to a Stockholm Hospital, the Group Secretary of Gloucester, Stroud and Forest Hospital Management Committee wrote in July 1963 that

> I was struck by the very real effort at this hospital to identify the patient as a 'person' and not as a 'case'. As an example, in the ward units a day room is provided where patients and staff can gather in the evening to watch television and have coffee etc. This is encouraged and is said to create a pleasant homely atmosphere.[50]

Television sets were increasingly common in hospitals at this time, and there was a shift over the course of the late twentieth century from televisions in communal 'day rooms' to private sets with headphones, and from black-and-white to colour televisions. The space of television-watching also shifted from the day room to the ward, from the chair to the bed, and eventually to personal technologies. Television programmes were increasingly vibrant and colourful, whether in the form of sports, nature shows, or comedy. In this sense they provided a unique form of colour in hospitals, in the form of a non-medical moving screen.

In social history terms, this growing emphasis on television as a way of making spaces 'homely' aligned with the rise of television in homes, and the domestication of certain technologies.[51] As David Morley notes, drawing on anthropological approaches, the 'TV set' is 'a meaningful "visible object" in the symbolic field of the home, as much as a visual medium'.[52] He notes the 'journey' of the TV set in homes from a 'singular "stranger", allowed only into the most public/formal space of the house (in the living room), through the development of the multi-set household and TV's gradual penetration of the more intimate spaces of our kitchens and bedrooms'.[53] This trend almost exactly aligns with the broad story told above about how the television was integrated into hospitals, and moved from more communal to individual spaces. In that sense, what was *on* the television was less important than the presence of the TV set itself and the way it emulated the role of television in homes. Returning to an earlier point, 'homeliness' was also always about more than emulating the material conditions of the house. The television set was as much a signifier as it was a transplantation of the 'house' into the hospital. It offered the *feel* of 'homeliness', such as a sense of community in the early days, and later some sense of control over visual and auditory surroundings.

The meaning of the television also shifted in relation to its aesthetic. As Deborah Chambers notes, TV sets shifted between the 1930s and 1960s from 'wooden cabinets [designed] as family furniture to the shaping of portable sets as symbols of progress'.[54] It may also be relevant, then, that wooden or laminate furniture and fittings were also often deemed to be 'home-like' or 'homely' in post-war hospitals.[55] Chambers notes that 2.5 million British households had television sets by 1953, and this number grew exponentially over subsequent decades.[56] These televisions – and particularly the newer, shiny, portable televisions – signified progress and modernity for many people.[57] The television, then, was a modern technology in the home, but a 'homely' technology in the hospital; its meanings were contingent, and context-specific. As discussed, 'homeliness' was never the neat opposite to 'modernity' that it is so often supposed to be. Rather, homeliness was a new form of modernity.

The role of televisions in making hospitals 'homely' is also complicated when they are considered as part of practice, rather than static design features. In her work on televisions in 'long-stay psychiatric and "mental handicap" wards, 1950s–1980s', Louise Hide considers how television-viewing operated in the making of space and place. She shows that

> the real therapeutic benefits of television were believed to be gained not through the direct interaction between a patient and the TV screen but through a triadic relationship between patient, television, and staff involving activities and interactions based on programs they had watched together.[58]

On the surface, this appears to be a valuable form of care or community-building, as people gathered in day rooms to watch television together. In practice, patients had little control over when or what they watched. As Hide notes, sometimes 'television was a convenient way of trying to keep patients occupied with as little effort as possible'.[59] Some patients were 'left in front of it for hours on end, thus maintaining the appearance that they were doing something'.[60] Interviewees for the 'Voices of Our NHS' project made similar observations about televisions in wards, noting that elderly people were 'bored' and 'isolated', 'sitting beside their beds' facing walls 'painted white' and a 'piddly little television set'.[61]

It is, then, important not to assume that the experience of watching television was always 'homely'. Television did bring visual change, and increasingly a new form of moving technological, colourful, bright images from the outside world into hospital spaces in a way that superficially deinstitutionalised the space. It offered a new kind of shared viewing experience comparable with the 'living room' at home. In practice, though, televisions could also be ways to reinscribe institutional power relations. The impact of bright colour or moving images in the pursuit of 'homeliness' should not be taken at face value. Televisions are offered here as examples of 'homely' objects that changed the aesthetic and colour palette of hospital spaces, but that complicate the idea of 'homeliness' on closer examination.

Similar arguments can be made about other objects, such as hospital bed curtains, which are rarely closely interrogated. To understand the role of bed curtains in making 'homeliness', it is important to return to the history of the NHS and its architecture. The NHS inherited a significant number of hospitals that still had so-called 'Nightingale' wards. These open-plan wards were viewed largely unfavourably in the early NHS. As miasma theory gradually fell out of fashion, and hospitals invested in antibacterial cleaning, there was less concern about the need for natural air flow to remove 'bad' air. Researchers interested in how to improve NHS hospitals, particularly for patients, identified open-plan wards as problems, for reasons ranging from the lack of privacy to noise. *Studies in the Function and Design of Hospitals* (1955) recommended that new hospitals should build bays instead of open-plan wards.[62] In this context, fewer beds (if well designed) could indicate a better hospital experience: they were more 'homely' and 'comfortable'.[63] However, at this time there were very few new hospitals under construction. Most NHS sites focused on the repair and renovation of existing spaces. In this context, hospitals needed to create the feeling of smaller wards in larger ones. Curtains often provided a way to achieve this.

In some hospitals such curtains were already commonplace. For example, a postcard from the London Hospital, thought to be from the early twentieth century, shows curtains that could be pulled around each bed for privacy.[64] In many others, though, the wards were left completely open and curtains were added as part of post-war upgrades. Southmead Hospital in Bristol, for example, 'upgraded' its Nightingale wards in 1955 by improving its lighting and putting curtains around each bed.[65] At this stage, the function of curtains was largely practical in many hospitals; they helped to create visual and some acoustic privacy, and could help with temperature-related issues caused by draughts in large wards. It is difficult to know from black-and-white archive photographs exactly what colour they were, but most appear to be plain. In 1982, Susan Black wrote in *Hospital Development* of progress in hospital interior design, comparing it to older beds and fabrics; twenty years ago, she argued, patients were faced with 'decidedly unpleasant curtains and bedspread[s], dark brown or green courted floor[s] of indeterminate composition, and a "stack" in the centre bearing weary flowers and curling X-rays'.[66] If Black was writing about the early 1960s, it seems that early attempts at homeliness paid more attention to the spatial effects of curtains (creating smaller spaces, and more privacy) than to their design. However, her description of curtains does not reveal anything specific about the patterns or colour schemes deemed 'unpleasant'. It might be significant that this post-war trend was at a time when privacy was an increasingly important part of the concept (and design) of homes. As Andrew Seaton notes, the use of curtains also allowed for the communalism embraced by 'social democracy' at this time, and curtains represented a careful balance between social interaction and privacy.[67] As with television sets, though, ideals and practice did not always correlate. Some patients found the experience of being surrounded by curtains isolating, rather than feeling a sense of privacy or homeliness; older patients, in particular, seemed to prefer a sense of community on wards.[68]

Some hospitals, in what seems to have been a local practice driven by individuals, used curtains from the start to contribute to the atmosphere of wards rather than to create privacy. These sites paid much more attention to colour when creating cubicles. Peter Horrocks, for example, notes that, when he worked as a consultant of geriatrics in Hull (appointed in 1969),

> We did cubicalise some wards to provide bays of four beds and so on, that's true, but mostly it was in terms of making the wards more homely and giving good visual clues about where people's beds were, where the toilets were, which were the bathrooms and that sort of thing … we introduced duvets, the cubicle curtains were all of different colours and were in sort of domestic designs rather than hospital plain colours … you don't have to have very plain environments or threatening environments to do good medicine … more human.[69]

Horrocks treated design as an active part of making the affective qualities of hospitals, positioning 'sterile' hospitals in opposition to the 'human' qualities of soft and patterned furnishings. His attitude to 'cubicalising' wards was attuned to the feel of the ward and the potential role of curtains in creating a 'domestic' feel. It is likely no coincidence that Horrocks's discussion of 'making the wards more homely' and giving 'good visual clues' related to geriatric medicine. For Horrocks, the 'domestic' was made through a combination of soft textures and 'designs', as opposed to the hospital that was 'plain', 'shiny', and 'sterile'. It is notable that he also talked about 'domestic designs' that would have been familiar, rather than more modern designs that could have been confusing or alienating to older people. Horrocks's reference to the use of different colours to help people to recognise their cubicles was also symbolically about more than wayfinding. It was a way of personalising spaces in a broadly impersonal, large ward: just as rooms in a house had different paint or wallpaper, different hospital cubicles had visual identity. This trend became more visible over time; hospital curtains were no longer required just to cubicalise or create 'human scale' and privacy in newer hospitals, and their role in 'homeliness' became more about colour and pattern. As one report on a Derbyshire paediatric ward noted in 1993, 'all the bedding and curtains are different, i.e. as at home'.[70] It was not just colour and pattern, then, but the sense of personal and identifiable patterns for curtains and bedding that made a space 'homely'.

One set of hospital curtains survives in physical form in the Wellcome Library archive, which allows for a closer examination of the objects and their multi-sensory qualities. The curtains were commissioned in the late 1980s by Healing Arts at St Mary's Hospital (Isle of Wight) as part of their 'Design for Health' strategy, and designed by artist Sian Tucker. Tucker worked across several hospital sites, including most famously on the 'Falling Leaves' atrium installation at Chelsea & Westminster (1993) discussed in Chapter 3. The cubical curtains were printed by Skopos Fabrics and featured geometric shapes, wavy lines, dots, dashes, and other stimulating patterns. The prints were not in a regular pattern and therefore were designed to be stimulating for the eye without being sensorially overwhelming. Despite the use of patterns for healthcare that – to quote the company that made the fabric – evoke 'warmth, relaxation and the familiarity associated with home', these products are still materially clinical with regard to specific treatments and washing methods.[71] The curtains do feel relatively soft, but not like curtains from the home; in material terms, they were a hygiene–homeliness hybrid (Figure 4.1).[72]

The choice of colours was different for each level of the hospital, again assisting with wayfinding and a sense of ward identity. Level A curtains were blue, grey, green, and yellow; Level B curtains were blue, grey, turquoise, and yellow; and Level C curtains were pink, grey, green, and coral.[73] Guy Eades, who was director of Healing Arts at the time, saw them as part of exploring 'how the arts could be sort of integrated' into the hospital in a 'not too obvious way'.[74] They were, then, in his mind very much part of the arts scheme rather than furniture, tying in closely with the 'humanisation' agenda discussed in Chapter 3. From interviews with both Eades and Sian Tucker, it is clear that they were a collaborative project. Tucker notes that she provided the design but did not select the fabric, and also noted that the curtains were designed to coordinate with other parts of the design: 'they would have given me paint colours of the corridors and floors and wall colour'.[75] Tucker and Eades also separately recalled that hospital staff were given a range of options and gave feedback on early designs, including moderating some of the colours. To quote Tucker:

> I did one [set of curtains] and then I did samples of different colourways and they went on the walls in some corridor and then people could make comments on them and then I adjusted to the comments – and the comments were I had to calm it down a bit, because of people not feeling very well after they come around after anaesthetic and

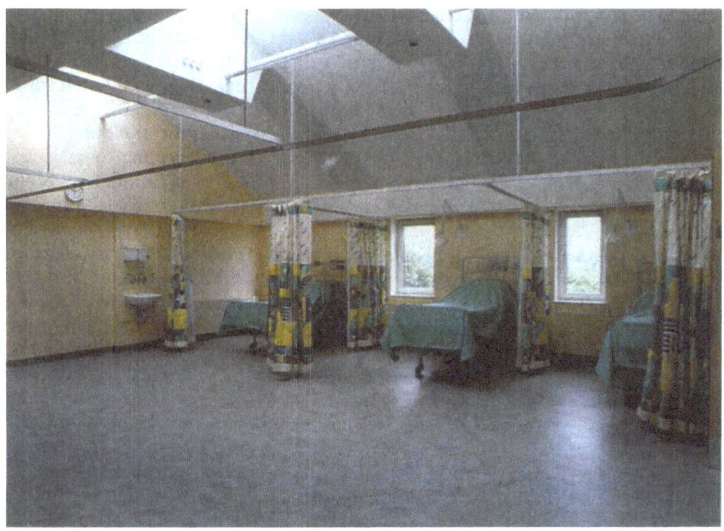

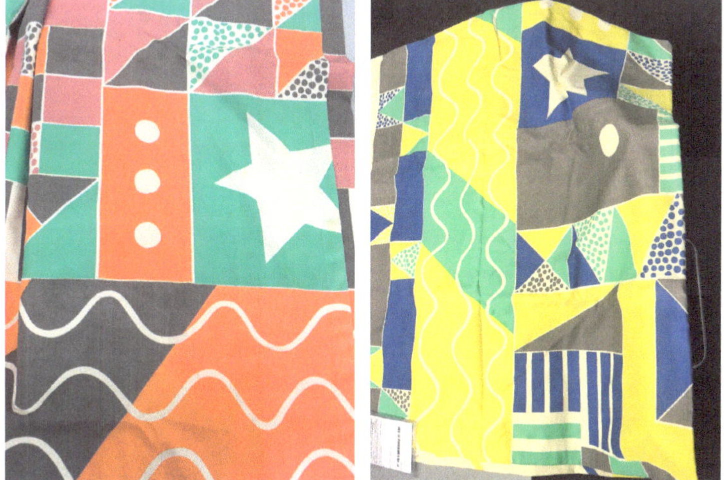

Figure 4.1 Richard Burton, 'St Mary's Hospital, Isle of Wight', *BMJ*, 22–29 December, 1990, p. 1423, photograph by Terry Grimwood. Every effort has been made to trace the copyright holders and obtain permission to reproduce this material. Please do get in touch with any enquiries or information about this image or the rights holder. Wellcome Library, ART/IOW/F/1-4. Sian Tucker, design of ward curtains at St Mary's Hospital, 1987–89, reproduced with permission of Sian Tucker and the Isle of Wight NHS Trust.

> also think about the colours that elderly people might prefer: more muted and more pastel colours ... in my own memory I really, really toned it down. It would have been really much brighter, like that peachy colour would have been red probably.[76]

These interviews offer a rare but important insight into the different, often invisible, processes involved in hospital art and design. Tucker noted that the sea was also an important influence on the design, particularly the shapes that evoked sails and waves, indicating that they were intended to be meaningful and closely linked to the hospital's island geography. On the basis of these interviews, it would be an overstatement to argue that 'homeliness' was the driving force in the design of these curtains; neither Tucker nor Eades used the term in our interviews. However, they did speak of seeking to evoke many of the feelings associated with homeliness: privacy, personalisation, and a non-institutional feel.

Artist-designed curtains were never widespread in the NHS, but Skopos was a major NHS supplier and patterns in general were increasingly common. Figure 4.2 shows some fabrics from a different supplier – Gradus – contained in a 2006 'toolkit' for Gloucestershire Hospitals, in a box called 'fabrics' that stated 'well-chosen fabrics can enhance and humanise hospital areas'.[77] Chapter 1 argued that sometimes whiteness and texture was used to create the illusion that spaces were cleaner than they really were, indicating that hygiene was desirable. Such curtains offer the opposite: their design and materiality tried to hide the fact that they were a hygienic, medical object. In certain contexts at least – the bed, the ward, recovery – people no longer felt the need to be surrounded by the material signs of sterility.

The two objects discussed in this section are very different. In the broadest of terms they were both ways of bringing the 'home' into the hospital and used bright colour in order to do so: the colour television in a vibrant, digital form, and the bed curtain in non-institutional patterns. They also, though, signified distinct aspects of 'homeliness' and served specific functions. Both objects changed in form, materiality, meaning, and role in the hospital over time, and brought different dimensions of the 'home' into the hospital. Some of these features of 'homeliness' appeared contradictory at first glance, such as community and privacy. In taking two different

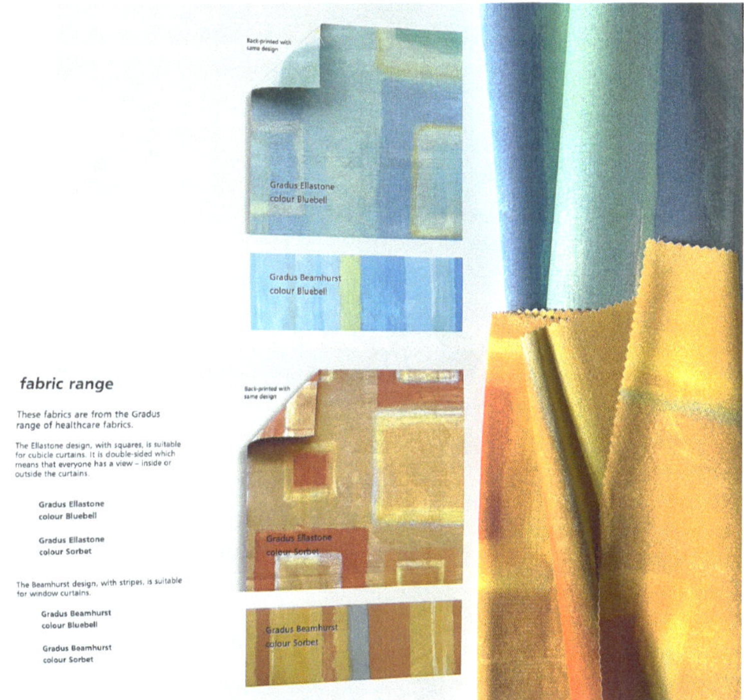

Figure 4.2 Page and fabrics from Gloucestershire Hospitals Toolkit '5: Fabric'. © Anne Greer, photographs by Victoria Bates. With thanks to Anne Greer for permission to publish. All rights reserved and permission to use this figure must be obtained from the copyright holder.

objects in this way, it is possible to show that the 'homely' was actually a multifaceted concept in hospitals and could mean different things in different settings, or in relation to particular elements of hospital design.

Making homeliness: person-centred design

There is only so much value in broad generalisations about 'homeliness' as a shared feeling or type of care. It is ultimately more productive to recognise that the 'homely' has always been context-specific and relational. Moving from an object-based approach to a person-based approach, this section shows that 'homeliness' could also mean different things to specific groups of people. Taking the examples of childbirth spaces and design for children, it is possible to see how an assemblage of different design features and human behaviours were thought to make spaces 'homely' and 'welcoming'. These two case studies also emphasise that not all hospital spaces or groups of people in hospital are comparable or equivalent.

The post-war years and the early NHS marked a general period of the negotiation of patients' rights and the roots of patient-centred care. Childbirth spaces were particularly important examples of this.[78] Childbirth was one of the few events in hospitals that would not necessarily involve sickness or medical intervention, especially as childbirth was no longer seen typically as a life-threatening event but as a formative experience for all involved. As Julian Ashley noted in *Anatomy of a Hospital* in 1987, writing about a fictionalised and generic teaching hospital that drew upon his 30 years of real-life experience in hospital work:

> Unlike the other departments [...] [the Maternity Wing] is associated with normal, healthy, happy human activity and this is reflected in the pleasant and informal atmosphere and the colourful and attractive furnishings which are more suggestive of an hotel than a hospital.[79]

As noted elsewhere, there was often some blurring of concepts such as 'home-like' and 'hotel-like' at this time, as both spoke broadly to pleasant, welcoming, and comfortable anti-institutional design. This design aesthetic seemed more appropriate in a space where people anticipated health and happiness, with a 'carpeted' entrance lobby containing 'potted ferns'.[80]

There were also practical reasons for the focus on maternity wards in efforts to make hospitals more 'homely'. Maternity wards were one of the key areas of investment in the early NHS, and were a focus of efforts to expand bed numbers even as reductions were made elsewhere for the sake of efficiency.[81] As Angela Davis notes, there was a 'dramatic shift from 1965 to 1975', with around a third of births taking place at home between the late 1940s and mid-1960s, but fewer than 5 per cent of births taking place at home by 1975.[82] There was therefore an opportunity to consider what a 'good' maternity ward or childbirth space looked or felt like, and whose experience should be central to designing such spaces. At the same time, childbirth was an obvious focal point for activist groups, ranging from feminists who sought to challenge the power imbalances experienced by women in the healthcare system, to new groups invested in protecting the sanctity of the 'birth experience' in hospital spaces. Perhaps the most prominent such group was the National Childbirth Trust, launched in 1956 as the Natural Childbirth Trust (NCT). Those giving birth and their families also put forward their views of 'good' and 'bad' childbirth experiences, though often through mediated forms such as surveys, complaints, and activist groups. Such efforts to make maternity spaces 'home-like' or 'domestic' were also international.[83]

This context is crucial to understanding why maternity wards were a focal point for post-war efforts to make hospitals more 'homely', including through colour. In 1951 *The Hospital* magazine reported on careful colour choices in maternity wards to 'infuse a feeling of confidence and restfulness in the expectant mothers'.[84] *Hospital Development* magazine also reported on new maternity units in the 1960s and 1970s, showing that architects paid careful attention to sensory design.[85] In 1965 the *Nursing Times* gave an example of a 'modern maternity department' that used 'restful pastel shades' in the theatre and had a colourful day room with 'bright furnishings' to help 'mothers to feel at home and at ease'.[86] This article also noted how 'individuality' was created in wards by 'different wall colouring around the beds, and the bright uniforms of the nursing staff complement the carefully planned colour scheme'.[87] This maternity ward was used as a case study to support claims made elsewhere in the article about how to make day rooms, particularly for people in geriatric and maternity wards, feel 'as like home as possible' using features such as wallpaper and carpets.[88] The example is interesting for a range of reasons. Firstly, it shows how certain spaces were thought to be more appropriate for 'homely' design than others, particularly day rooms, communal spaces, and non-sterile spaces. Secondly, it suggested a subtle distinction between the 'restful' colours required for theatre and 'bright' colours for more homely spaces, indicating that 'bright' colours were thought to evoke warmth and cheer. Finally, it brought in a sense of individuality and identity within wards – created by a combination of decoration and uniforms.

Well into the 1980s, maternity colour schemes continued to draw on older recommendations of colour theorists such as Faber Birren, who suggested that maternity wards should have 'warm colours, tones of peach, pink, fawn, soft yellow'.[89] Though some sites moved towards brighter colours for specific spaces such as day rooms, as in the *Nursing Times* example given above, pastel colours dominated maternity wards for decades.[90] In general, there was also a tendency to use very gendered colour palettes for maternity design. Princess Mary Hospital in Newcastle in 1988, for example, used a 'soft pink colour scheme'.[91] It is often unclear how far such decisions were based on patient or service user consultation.[92] There is an extensive literature on the ways that hospital design can feel hostile to queer and gender non-conforming people; heteronormative models of the 'family' and 'home' alongside such culturally gendered colour schemes may have unintentionally contributed to such issues.[93] Recent research for the 'Sensing Spaces of Healthcare' project has also shown that – with time – such pastel colours have actually themselves become seen as institutional, and many maternity service users want more vibrant decorative schemes.[94] The 'home' could never be universal, and some efforts to create welcoming or comfortable patient-centred spaces may have been counter-productive.

Homely maternity care was often seen as part of modern healthcare, rather than in opposition to it. East Riding Archives holds a report from August 1988 on new maternity facilities opened in Beverley in Yorkshire, which implicitly conceptualised the 'home environment' as a modern idea by noting that 'old ideas and values were dismissed in favour of providing a "home environment" within a hospital'.[95] It noted that such a space could be created through 'home decor, wallpaper and carpets' as well as facilities to give people control such as 'tea making ... so mum could now brew up when she wanted'.[96] Alongside such design choices, the 'modern maternity hospital' kept '"high-tech" equipment ... readily available' but 'subtly removed from view'.[97] Overall, this hospital combined discrete technology, decorations such as wallpaper, and some element of personal control, in making its modern 'homely' maternity space. Such models of homeliness implicitly rejected the more nostalgic rhetoric of some contemporaries, and there was no romanticisation of the Victorian hospital that the new building replaced. For contemporary commentators, the 'homely' was a modern concept as much as a historical one. Reporting on this site, the local health services magazine *Healthview* also wrote that 'technology has been combined with modern comforts to create a "home from home" atmosphere'.[98] It noted that 'every effort is being made to give the unit as domestic and "non-hospital" an atmosphere as possible'.[99] As I have argued elsewhere, writing with Jennifer Crane and Maria Fannin on the history of the birthing pool, 'modern maternity … was able to hold together a number of ostensibly contradictory characteristics such as tradition and innovation, experience and safety, nature and science, and more'.[100] Modern maternity was being redefined in the late twentieth century through new design features, which held all of these tensions in a delicate balance.

The idea of homeliness in maternity services was complicated, increasingly, by activists and groups such as the NCT pushing for home births. Some advocates of home birth emphasised that real homeliness could never be achieved in the hospital, because of the absence of genuine control. An editorial in the Patients' Association magazine *Patient Voice* stated in 1980 that '[o]f course it may be possible to "humanise" the hospital by training the staff to have a more flexible approach and by the choice of more "homely" decorations: but a facelift would not alter the fact that when one is in hospital someone else is in charge'.[101] Such questions were particularly significant in maternity spaces, in which feminist activists had long pushed back against the traditional power dynamics of modern medicine. Though the concept of control and flexibility was folded into 'homeliness' elsewhere, feminists continued to question whether the patient or service user could ever truly be 'in charge' in a hospital.

Overall, then, the combination of 'homely' design, a sense of control, and staff 'attitudes' were perceived as key to childbirth. Colour, in theory, was actually one of the least flexible or adjustable aspects of a maternity space. However, it was closely connected to some other adjustable design features such as lighting. As one American physician noted in 1978, 'incandescent lamps' could provide a warmer light and give a more 'home-like atmosphere'.[102] Adjustable or dimmable lighting, warmer lighting, and lamps or sidelights all served to change the colours of walls and furnishings, making them feel softer, warmer, and more 'homely'. Researchers working on contemporary lighting design have shown that 'it all came down to trying to create a "home-like, cosy feeling" in the delivery room', and that 'midwifery lighting practices … of also tuning and attuning to saturated spectral compositions of lighting throughout the birthing process' were part of producing this 'feeling'.[103] This quote is from research conducted in contemporary Copenhagen but its findings fit broadly with modern British history. Midwives in the NHS also played a key role in adapting birthspaces to make them feel more 'homely', often using colour, light, and decorative elements to do so, and increasingly inviting people to personalise spaces; such interventions could be light touch, for example adding potted plants next to birthing pools.[104] Though there were ongoing debates about who was truly 'in charge' in such situations, there is evidence that midwives attempted to create a sense of control or personalisation of colour, lighting, and other sensory aspects of hospital births.

Overall, the idea of 'home' had particular social and political connotations in post-war maternity care. Generic statements about post-war 'homely' colour palettes and decorative schemes are insufficient to understand the different ways that 'homeliness' operated in the hospital. While the examples of objects given above expressed ideas such as community and privacy, the example of maternity emphasises even more strongly the idea of de-medicalisation and of home as a space of control and personalisation. These different meanings of 'homeliness' were as much about the negotiation of patients' and service users' rights as they were about decorative schemes.

Other groups, such as children, were also a focal point of efforts to make hospitals 'homely'. In the early 1970s, interior designers from the Regional Health Authorities and the Department of Health & Social Security recommended that '[t]he atmosphere of the children's department should be friendly and home-like in scale and character to put children and relatives completely at ease. Colourful furniture, fabrics and carpet will contribute to pleasant surroundings'.[105] This point was also illustrated (Figure 4.3) with a waiting area that included books, magazines, toys, a television, plants, patterned cushions, stripy wallpaper, soft chairs, hanging non-institutional lighting, and more. This broad emphasis on colour, fabric, and texture was commonplace throughout 'homely' design.

Some elements of 'homely' design were specific to children, particularly the idea that a 'home' included elements of play. This conflation between home and play was also expressed by parents.

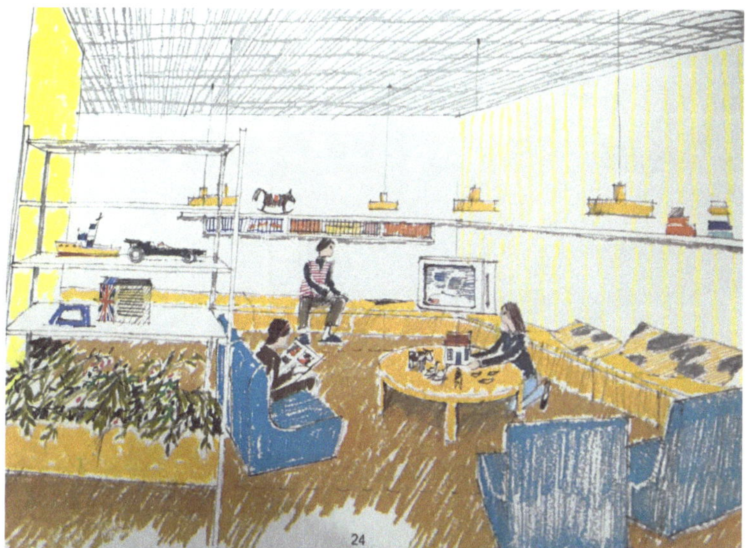

Figure 4.3 National Archives, MH 166/1136, Harness Interiors produced by the interior designers from the Regional Health Authorities and the Department of Health & Social Security, part of the papers of the 'Technical Design Group', 1973–75, p. 12. Representation of a children's ward. © Crown Copyright. All rights reserved and permission to use this figure must be obtained from the copyright holder.

For example, in one outpatient department survey at Great Ormond Street Hospital from 1963, someone noted that '[m]y little girl felt quite at home with all the toys about'.[106] There was also often a blurring of lines in contemporary texts between home and school as sites of play and learning. There was extensive discussion about bringing 'home' into school, and bringing school and home into the hospital. In 1984, for example, the Department of Education and Science Architects and Building Group wrote of both in relation to 'the experience of continuing familiar play and learning activities in "non-clinical" surroundings' to reduce the trauma of hospital visits.[107] 'Many hospitals', they went on,

> recognising this, have gone to great lengths to create a home-like atmosphere on the wards and other areas where children are treated. Similarly, many of the schoolrooms and playrooms in hospitals have been designed to look as much like schools or nurseries as possible.[108]

This trend towards bringing school and play into the hospital is discussed more in Chapter 5 on 'bright' colours. For now, it is worth noting the conflation between school and home as sites of 'non-clinical' and 'familiar' play and learning activities. In the light of this emphasis on play and learning, design for 'homeliness' in children's hospitals took on a very specific meaning that does not have an equivalent in adult spaces.

Although patterns, artwork, and reassuring colour schemes were widespread in hospitals, they were thought to serve subtly different purposes depending on the needs of the patients. To quote a 1984 Health Building Note on 'Hospital Accommodation for Children', the 'effects of separation from home and family' were a particular concern for children because of their age, and designers were thought to have an important role in creating an 'interior which is comfortable and pleasant to look at in order to reassure and simulate the children'.[109] This building note recommended 'light colours combined with a carefully balanced selection of patterns' and 'suitable artwork on walls and ceilings' to 'attract the child's attention and help to lessen anxiety'.[110] Using colours, patterns, and 'homely' design to reduce anxiety and reassure patients was not limited to children. However, compared with writing on adults, there was more explicit concern about children being separated from the home and family support structures. This was even more the case for long-stay inpatients, or children who needed to move through rehabilitation or transitional spaces during recovery.[111]

As with maternity wards, the shift to 'homeliness' in children's hospitals and wards took place against a background of growing political interest in children's rights. When a new Health Building Note on 'Hospital Accommodation for Children' was introduced in 1984, to replace one from 1964, the first page noted that 'in the past two decades, the greater knowledge of child development and the recognition of the fundamental emotional, as well as physical, needs of children has created a more enlightened attitude to the care of children in hospital'.[112] The role of 'homely' design in helping to rebalance hospital power relations was, of course, very different in relation to age rather than gender. However, the role of 'homeliness' in allowing for autonomy and personalisation was important in both contexts. The example of a new Hull Children's Unit in 1990 illustrates how central this concept became, and how it underpinned the rise of 'homely' hospital design. The Health Authority's Acting Director of Planning declared that '[w]e are putting the patients first and the whole concept of the design takes into account children's needs and aspirations regarding them as special people in their own right – not just as small adults'.[113] Yorkshire health service newspaper *Healthview* noted, in relation to the Hull project, that '[e]verything possible will be done to allow a patient to "personalise" their own area and make them feel immediately welcome'.[114] Again, these trends were particularly evident from the 1980s onwards, with the rise of interest in patients' 'experience' and the emergence of the patient-as-consumer. *Healthview* also noted that the unit would use 'modern' clinical practice and 'modern lighting, furnishing, fittings and design concepts' alongside emphasising the homely:

> Every effort will be made to help the hospital's youngest patients feel at home from the moment they first leave the lift to go onto the ward till the time they finally leave. The 'hospital atmosphere' will be lost as far as possible without interfering with treatments.[115]

A 'home-like' hospital was also, for maternity and children's units alike, anti-institutional but not anti-modern.

This section has taken the examples of maternity and children's units to show the nuances of 'homeliness' for different groups of people in hospital. Others could also be given as examples here, each with their own specific version of 'homeliness' and some shared characteristics with the others. People who were dying, for example, were also often a focus of efforts to make spaces 'homely' in hospitals and hospices. This was in part because of the fact that, to quote a *Report of a Committee of the Central Health Services Council* in 1976, 'a gradually increasing number of deaths is taking place in hospital' while 'it is often said that most people would prefer to die at home'.[116] For long-stay residents, particularly before the dramatic decline in such beds with 'community care' in the 1980s, the hospital often *was* their long-term living environment. Contemporary experts on built environments emphasised that 'all long-stay residents … need "home" rather than "institutional" surroundings'.[117] As *Hospital Development* magazine observed in 1986, 'greater emphasis is being placed on the domestic nature of the furniture and fittings and how these can work towards giving the [long-stay] resident an optimum degree of privacy and dignity: it is after all their "home"'.[118] For each of these groups of patients and service users there was some commonality in the 'homely', and the uses of colour, pattern, and texture in bringing it into being. For each, though, the 'home' also had a specific connotation and the 'homely' sought to evoke a particular feeling.

Homeliness was a heterogeneous concept, given meaning in relation to specific groups of people. It also shifted subtly in meaning and in colour schemes, as well as other design interventions, across time and place. The idea of what was 'homely' and why 'homeliness' was necessary was also a social and political one, and was increasingly informed over time by conversations about patients' rights, personhood, agency, and autonomy in hospitals. Homeliness was also always relational, brought into being by a combination of objects, people, care practices, colour schemes, architecture, and more. This is not to say that it was an entirely meaningless concept. There was a core to the idea of the 'homely', which was about crafting a new type of modern healthcare in which the person – rather than the institution – was the primary concern. Modern, homely hospitals were safe and included technology, but 'homely' healthcare prioritised feelings such as comfort, security, privacy, and community. In the early twentieth century, some of these 'humanistic' feelings – such as security and safety – were produced by visible hygiene and sterility. By the late twentieth-century, they were produced by 'warm' colours, textiles, and behaviours.

Creating homeliness: personal palettes

Over the course of the late twentieth century, the idea of 'homeliness' was increasingly entwined with the ability to adjust or personalise hospital surroundings. Some adjustable design was built into a space, for example in the form of light fittings. Other types of personalisation, though, were more informal. Patients, visitors, and even sometimes staff, brought their own objects into hospitals to make them more familiar, personal, and ultimately more homely. 'Homeliness' apparently meant permitting 'personal knick-knacks on mantelpieces, and corner tables' alongside more systematic decorative choices.[119] By the 1980s and 1990s this trend was explicitly advocated in hospital design literature, and the structures to support personalisation were built in, such as shelves for pictures. However, even outside such designed-in forms of permission, hospitals had been important sites of such so-called 'everyday design'.

There is a long history of patients making themselves 'at home' in large institutions, through a combination of actions and subtle material changes to environments.[120] Patients, visitors, and staff resisted the power structures of hospital spaces often before they were given official permission to do so. In colour terms, they brought a wide palette of personal colour that was meaningful to them, in forms ranging from clothing to toys, photographs, and food. The personalisation of hospitals was not entirely new. Susan Barclay notes that, in the late nineteenth century, '[d]espite the use of drab-coloured paints, prints and flowers installed by nurses transformed dull wards into pleasant environments'.[121] In 1890, an article in *The Hospital* noted 'the fine show of arum lilies and other blooms displayed on the centre table ... sent by residents in the neighbourhood' for the children's hospital.[122] The flow of objects between home and hospital was an important part of making the 'homely', amongst other things: to quote Sara Ahmed, 'emotions can move through the movement or circulation of objects'.[123] Graham Mooney has argued that, in relation to tuberculosis patients in Edwardian England, domestic design was part of the process of moral regulation: 'appropriation of domestic space transformed the sanatorium's "rules of health" into "rules for living"'.[124] However, domestic objects that people brought in, or which were sent by visitors, could also subvert some of the control inherent in other forms of 'domesticated' design.

In the late twentieth century, then, it was not entirely a new practice for patients to bring in their own objects. However, such practices took place against a new social and political backdrop, in which patients' rights were being negotiated in a new era of 'patient-centred' care. Personalising space was increasingly important in this context, which included complaints about the relative lack of input that patients and visitors had into design choices. The apparent failure of architects, for example, to consult people in maternity design was noted by contemporary activists. In 1964, a representative of the Association for Improvements in the Maternity Services (AIMS) wrote to *Architects' Journal*:

> at least in the case of maternity departments surely some discussion should take place between the architects and the mothers themselves, as well as with the midwives and obstetricians. Our organisation is in touch with the viewpoint of mothers in various ways, through questionnaires [...] meetings, talks and discussions.[125]

As noted above, maternity activists had a particular interest in power and representation, and it is crucial to recognise the gendered dimensions of 'everyday' design and its role as a form of agency and resistance.[126] Though midwives often helped to adjust the sensory qualities of maternity spaces, much 'formal' architecture and design was done by men in the post-war years, and women remain under-represented in architecture.[127] Bringing in objects and adapting space, in this social and political context, was an important way in which women could navigate a healthcare system in which they rarely otherwise had control.

Aligning with some of the trends outlined above, age was also an important factor in relation to personalisation and power. One article on interior design from *Hospital Development* in 1982, by Susan Black, is worth quoting at some length here:

> Many architects and designers are constantly frustrated by health service staff who consider they themselves not only far better qualified to decide on colour schemes and fabric patterns, but also to be the prime users within the hospital environment. 'We have to work here', and 'don't bother the patients, we know what they would want' are too often heard, one gathers. However, the designer himself can also fall into the trap of thinking that he is projecting himself into the minds of, say, a 75-year-old, or an 18-year-old, when he is in fact following his own aesthetic leanings. That rather amusing print of surrealistic daisies could seriously damage the health of the patient who lies opposite, counting and recounting each extravagant petal in his boredom, and in out-patients, a querulous juvenile could well occupy himself by doodling on the fetching pale gold hessian wall-covering with a felt-tip![128]

Black's comments are important for a few reasons. They raise ongoing concerns about the tendency to design *for* patients rather than to design *with* patients, and show some of the different groups who claimed to speak on their behalf. In particular, here, younger and older patients were likely to be incorrectly spoken *for*. Black also noted specifically some of the trends that might be considered conventional examples of 'homeliness' – such as introducing prints – and the ways in which they might fail to achieve their aim. Finally, Black introduces the human element and the ways in which people (here a 'querulous juvenile') have always been able to personalise, disrupt, repurpose, and adapt spaces even in the absence of permission to do so.

There is some scholarly literature on 'everyday designing' and 'homeliness' in healthcare settings, which shows the importance of the relationship between the two. One recent example is ethnographic work by Melisa Duque *et al.* who argue that 'homeliness can be constituted for instance by patients bringing significant possessions with them to a healthcare environment' and that more attention should also be given to 'the role of health care staff as everyday experts who articulate and constitute homeliness in relation to the contingencies of particular places of care and the people who occupy them'.[129] They offer visual design and the introduction of colour as one way in which staff adapt spaces for their patients. There is less discussion of such trends in historical context, though scattered around the literature – and photographs – is evidence that staff and patients were constantly subtly redesigning and remaking spaces. For example, in the early 1990s a report from Southern Derbyshire Community Health Council noted – in relation to parents' accommodation for a children's hospital – that '[e]fforts have been made to make the environment friendly with bed-side lamps and rugs etc … The staff really try to make a home from home atmosphere'.[130] They also bemoaned the fact that such efforts were being 'abused' by people stealing the objects.[131]

Patients also created 'homeliness' in relation to a range of sensory aspects of hospitals, from music to smell and most commonly food. To quote one study of British hospital catering from 1963:

> The patient provided a duck egg of her own to provide an egg sandwich for her tea. A milk pudding that was served looked nasty and sticky, and the sampled patient did not eat it, preferring her own bread and butter and a banana, which had been sent to her from her home.[132]

Some people personalised spaces by bringing in objects that represented their faith; for example, there were reports of Sikh patients bringing in food and cards during Diwali.[133] Colour was an important part of such home-making processes, in combination with other sensory 'everyday design', but in many ways the actual shade or hue was irrelevant.

Figure 4.4 shows images from the King's Fund publication from 1975, *Hospitals for People*, demonstrating how individuals adapted spaces (decorating a maternity bed with cards) and how staff made opportunities for them to do so (pinboards for children). As noted above, over time hospitals introduced more deliberate opportunities for personalisation. This came not just in the form of 'adaptable' design, but in space – or permission – to bring in personal possessions and display them. Some of the trends visible in Figure 4.4 were also evident in other hospitals over subsequent decades. In relation to St Mary's Hospital on the Isle of Wight, Richard Burton wrote that 'visual interest is sustained by specially designed curtains and by pin boards on to which patients can put cards, letters, family photographs'.[134] As John Berger noted in 1972, in relation to pinboards, they make all images on display 'equal' because 'they have been chosen in a highly personal way to match and express the experience of the room's inhabitant'[135]. Of course, these spaces were often strictly controlled and were not equivalent to having full freedom in one's own home. The introduction of pinboards might be seen as a way to take control of the more anarchic 'everyday designing' that was already happening, and to contain it in specific spaces, rather than as a genuine freedom. Whether such trends are interpreted as a form of freedom or another form of control, they did serve to make space for more personal colour palettes in hospitals.

Significantly, freedom for 'everyday' designing happened at a time when hospitals were bringing in arts and colour strategies. In some ways, the colourful chaos of 'homeliness' was disappearing at this time. As arts coordinator Penny Calvert, who started her work in Salisbury in 1999, recently observed in an interview:

> The first thing we did was establish a paint chart [...] the result of not having any kind of framework is that the place looks like a jumble sale and people pick whatever they fancy and forgetting that, well, it's not your living room, it's a public space and it would be nice if the building looked like it communicates with itself and it has some kind of professional thought out look overall.[136]

This interview echoes another that I conducted with a hospital estates manager in London, who said 'if you give NHS staff the

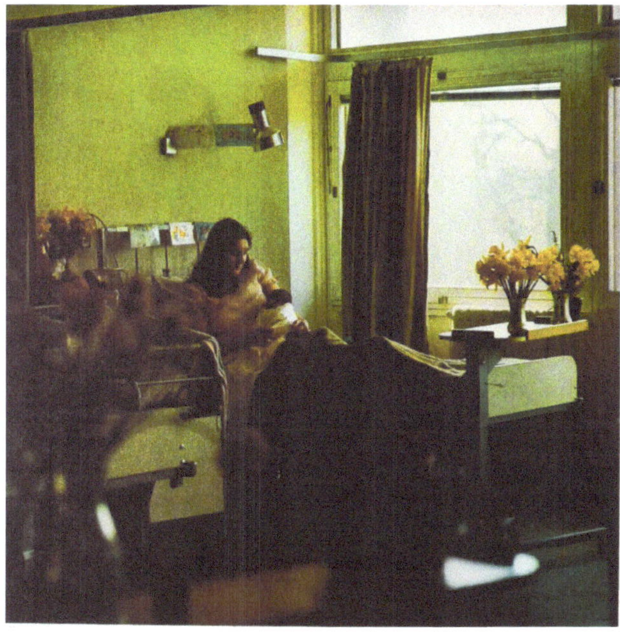

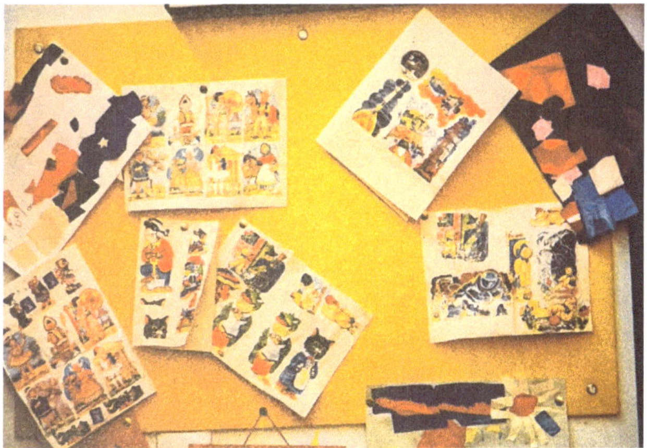

Figure 4.4 Maternity unit at St Peter's Hospital Chertsey and a pinboard in a children's ward at West Suffolk Hospital. James Calderhead, *Hospitals for People: A Look at Some New Buildings in England* (King Edward's Hospital Fund for London, 1975), pp. 52 and 54. Every effort has been made to trace the copyright holders and obtain permission to reproduce this material. Please do get in touch with any enquiries or information about this image or the rights holder. Images from the King's Fund Digital Archive.

Dulux colour chart, it is the equivalent of giving a hand grenade to a monkey!'[137] In line with this kind of thought, and the professionalisation of hospital arts and interiors outlined in the previous chapter, an increasing number of hospitals had arts and colour strategies by the end of the twentieth century. These strategies were informed by patient and staff consultation, and often included 'homeliness'. However, they approached colour in an increasingly controlled and consistent way, in line with branding and hospitals' visual identities across a site. This meant that 'everyday designing' was becoming the primary outlet for the colourful chaos of a home-like hospital, and an important way for people to express their agency.

The nature of what people wanted (and were permitted) to bring in varied widely depending on factors ranging from their demographic group to the nature of their illness. Long-stay patients were the most likely to be invited to personalise their spaces. Some long-stay elderly patients in non-sterile spaces were even allowed to 'bring in some domesticated pets, e.g. a budgerigar or tropical fish' in the 1970s alongside more traditional 'homely' features such as 'an attractive ledge for flowers, pot plants, and patients' cards or photographs'.[138] Pets were highly unusual, but this example (from North Tees) shows the range of non-human elements that could be brought into a space to make them more 'homely' and lively. Cards and photographs were much more commonplace, and introduced splashes of colour into spaces at a small but important scale. After the shift towards community care in the 1980s, there was an even stronger emphasis on the personalisation of long-stay healthcare spaces. In relation to one 'home from home' for young people with learning disabilities, for example, an article in *Hospital Development* noted that 'children will be encouraged to personalise the home with their own possessions'.[139] This trend was seemingly even stronger in the private sector. In 1985, for example, *Hospital Development* reported on a total care facility in Croydon, and noted that '[r]esidents will be encouraged to individualise their rooms, and will be able to bring their own furniture if they wish'.[140] Though it was extremely unusual to find equivalent examples in the NHS of people bringing their own furniture into hospitals, this example shows the general direction of travel in relation to the 'homely'. In this context, the trend was not just from design *for* to design *with*, but in many ways design *by* the patients. Allowing people to bring small items into hospitals was a budget-friendly way to achieve patient-centredness, which could otherwise be an expensive approach to interior design.

Clothing is also a notable example of change over time, and is an important subject from a colour history perspective. In the early years of the NHS, patients were often not permitted to keep or wear their own clothing. In the mid-1950s, a Yorkshire hospital patients' guide noted:

> In the ward you will be asked to go to bed until you have been examined by the doctor, and probably bed rest will form part of your treatment later on. Your clothes can, therefore, be given into the charge of the relative or friend who has accompanied you to the Hospital so that they can be taken home until you are ready to be discharged [...] as we have only a very limited [amount] of storage space.[141]

Local practices were often variable, and subject to the discretion of staff managing specific wards. In broad terms, though, there was a shift in the latter decades of the twentieth century towards encouraging patients and service users to bring more personal objects into hospital, including clothing. Such changes are often overlooked when discussing subjects such as the histories of hospital colour, but they would have had a dramatic impact on the colour palette of any hospital ward. Personal clothing meant that the colour palette of a ward was always shifting and dynamic, and it allowed patients to be more visible as people, rather than interchangeable bodies in beds. This trend was part of a shift away from bed rest, and towards the goal of getting patients up and moving more quickly. The culmination of this trend might be seen as the 2017 'End-PJ-Paralysis' campaign that sought to get patients up and out of bed, including getting them out of pyjamas and into clothes.[142] There is evidence that this trend even extended to staff in some contexts. One respondent to the Mass Observation 1997 Spring Directive reflected on her experience of psychiatric care and noted that in the 'large mental hospital' she attended in 1969 it was 'very strict and forbidding. The nurses wore uniforms and they didn't talk to you', but in a psychiatric ward in a local hospital in 1982 '[t]he nurses wore their own casual clothes [...] and used to spend a lot of time with me [...] It was very bright and cheerful'.[143] The different atmosphere of the 1982 example cannot be reduced to staff clothing alone, but for this respondent 'casual clothes' were an important part of making a space that felt more colourful, 'cheerful', and homely.

As with 'homeliness' more generally, children benefitted particularly from more liberal policies in hospitals. In 1980, a newspaper article on York District Hospital noted that, in children's hospitals only 30 years previously, 'each child, dressed in hospital clothes, was allowed perhaps one toy, not its own'.[144] Now, it noted, hospitals were 'more like home', with liberal visiting hours, large play areas, and more personal touches. In York, it noted, there was the 'cheerful disorder of an infants' school with bright paintings on the windows, childish drawings pinned on the walls and corridors, and children in their own clothes playing with their own beloved toys'.[145] Visitors could also treat the space 'like home', particularly when staying overnight, with spaces to make cups of tea or to smoke. Some of these trends were specific to children's needs, as they took place in the same context outlined above, of growing interest in child development. Some psychological theory at this time, for example, was particularly interested in the importance of objects (or 'object attachment') and the value of allowing children personal objects that reminded them of home.[146] The *BMJ* noted in 1982 the particular importance of children having their own toys with them, including for siblings of patients: 'Parents thought it important that siblings were made welcome, had a play area, and were allowed to bring a few of their own toys'.[147] As already noted, the tendency to talk about play, schools, and homes together was also a specific trend in children's wards.

There is little evidence that patients explicitly conceptualised their acts as forms of home-making, or described hospital spaces as 'homely' just because they brought in a few photographs from home. This label was largely imposed by hospital designers and architects. Very occasionally surveys showed that patients used the language of 'homeliness' in relation to hospitals, albeit in a range of contexts and not limited to colour, for example writing in relation to waiting room music that 'it makes a very homely atmosphere, not like hospitals years ago' (1962).[148] In 1997, reflecting on change over time in NHS hospitals, one Mass Observation respondent noted that '[m]y experience of hospitalisation is that wards are much more friendly and homely now'.[149] They seemingly used 'homely' in these contexts as shorthand for 'non-institutional'. In some ways this point echoes that made in the preceding sections: like architects and designers, it is important not to assume that patients conflated 'homely' with their actual homes. By extension, it seems unlikely that they were trying directly to emulate their homes when they adapted spaces or engaged in acts of 'everyday designing'. It is possible that the opposite was the case, and that objects from the home showed up the hospital as *un*homely. In relation to homely atmospheres, Tim Edensor and Shanti Sumartojo note that

> domestic atmospheres form part of the unnoticed background of everyday life that is maintained, stabilized and monitored through unreflexive habits that may only become apparent when disrupted by unusual affective or sensory intrusions or experienced after a period of absence.[150]

Going into hospital was a form of 'disruption' that may have actually shown up the differences between the healthcare setting and the 'domestic atmosphere' of home (and its objects). Bringing objects from home into the healthcare setting helped to 'stabilise' this atmospheric disruption, but not in a way that directly emulated a material living space.

Overall, the personal and 'everyday' aspects of hospital design are an important reminder that 'homeliness' was an unstable and relational concept. Though many hospitals sought to design the 'homely' into spaces, and there was an aesthetic that signified 'homeliness', in practice people also *made* homeliness in hospitals. This 'homeliness' was multi-faceted and multi-sensory, with personal colour palettes as one part of the assemblage of human and non-human elements that brought it into being. Walls could not be repainted, but 'homely' colour could be brought in via photographs, pictures, clothing, and sometimes pets. The 'homely' in hospitals was in some ways a type of care, articulated through design, and in other ways a form of resistance to the power structures and constraints of hospitals. Over time, there was more formal permission, as part of patient-centred care. Pinboards and shelves both invited patients and visitors to personalise a space and sought – not always successfully – to contain personalisation to specific spaces. Young people who 'doodled' on walls or fabrics arguably did as much as, if not more than, design interventions to make a space 'homely'.

Ideas such as 'homeliness' and 'humanisation' were not in tension with modernity. The new NHS was redefining 'modern' healthcare and constantly adding new layers of meaning to the concept. Homeliness was an older concept that was revived and folded into the concept of 'modern' healthcare in the late twentieth century. Everyday designing offered the 'familiarity or comfort' of home, but cleanliness, sterility, and even high-technology environments remained desirable for many people.[151]

Conclusions

In 1984, *Hospital Development* reported on a new psychiatric department at St Mary's Hospital in Paddington. It said that 'John Weeks, who designed the wing, believes that "hospitals are like huge houses for gigantic families" and he has been successful in creating a homelike and pleasant environment'.[152] This was a significant shift in tone from functionalist, early twentieth-century ideas of the hospital as a 'machine for healing'. Weeks was an important and influential figure in NHS hospital design, and had long advocated more 'human' approaches to hospitals. Making hospitals more 'homely' or 'homelike' was seen as an important practical way to 'humanise' them. However, the concept of 'homeliness' was left almost as ambiguous as 'humanisation'.

'Homeliness' had a range of meanings in the late twentieth-century hospital, expressed through colour schemes and coloured objects. There were some common threads between the different types or models of 'homeliness', particularly a broad attempt to reject what was thought of as a dehumanised modern institution and to balance out some of its power relations. Homeliness was both a nostalgic concept that pointed back to the lost 'homely' qualities of Victorian hospitals, and a distinctly modern one that folded in technology, patient-centredness, and other working principles of the new NHS. Terms like 'homely', 'home-like', 'at home', and 'homeliness' were used repeatedly but often indistinguishably and rarely defined. Their only common feature was that they sought to evoke the emotional qualities of 'home', rather than to emulate people's material living conditions.

'Homeliness' is best understood as a feeling, and as shorthand for the ideals that a 'home' represented. These ideals were context-specific and variable. For some, homeliness meant safety, comfort and security; for others, individuality, privacy, and control; and for yet others, homeliness was a more collective concept that represented family, community, and belonging. Many of these trends co-existed, and continue to be important today. In an interview in February 2023 with Jane Willis, I asked 'what does success look like, feel like, to you? How do you want people to feel in a hospital you've designed?' Jane replied:

> I want them to feel at home and I want them to feel that it's their hospital. I think that's really important. So, the idea of doing with, not doing to, is critical, and I want them to feel at home in the sense of [pause], well, [a] sense of belonging.[153]

This idea of feeling 'at home' as meaning a 'sense of belonging' and ownership is particularly important, and is perhaps the sense of 'home' that emerged most strongly in the late twentieth century. Most recently, hospital staff have been brought back into this picture. Jane Willis, for example, went on to say that 'I want them [staff] to feel proud of where they work' and emphasised that it was also important for them to have a sense of ownership.

Early post-war interventions had tended towards simple anti-institutional aesthetics, but over time the idea of making a 'home' increasingly meant ownership, control, and belonging. Such efforts were not necessarily successful; efforts to make 'most' people feel 'at home' could equate homeliness with a particular form of 'Britishness' that may have excluded historically marginalised groups or made spaces feel hostile. 'Homely' spaces were often imbued with class-based, gendered, and heteronormative assumptions about what a 'home' was and who would inhabit it. Though 'homeliness' typically meant a feeling, rather than a house, it was difficult to create a sense of belonging, familiarity, and ownership for everyone equally. However, growing interest in 'homeliness' did represent an increasing interest in – and support for – the principles and practices of patient-centred design.

Overall, 'homeliness' did not have a distinctive colour palette. It certainly had some trends, for example the use of pattern in combination with softer materials and textiles. Some of these aspects of homeliness were designed into hospital spaces, while others can be seen as acts of 'everyday design' by staff, patients, and visitors. Homeliness was marked less by any single design, and more by an acceptance of slightly disorderly multi-coloured schemes and space for personal, colourful objects such as pictures and clothing. Overall, then, 'homeliness' was not a specific palette, but an opportunity for people to bring colourful chaos into the hospital.

Notes

1 Quoted in Elain Harwood, *Space, Hope and Brutalism: English Architecture 1945–75* (Historic England, 2015), p. 295.
2 C. B. Denne, 'Bright Ideas for Interiors', *Hospital Development*, 16 (1988), p. 19.
3 'Viewpoint', *Hospital Development*, 11 (1983), p. 6.
4 'Nouvelle Cuisine', *Hospital Development*, 30 (1999), p. 25.
5 Kieran Richards and Rebecca McLaughlan, 'Beyond Homeliness: A Photo-Elicitation Study of the "Homely" Design Paradigm in Care Settings', *Health & Place*, 79 (2023), p. 2.
6 For example, Alistair Fair, 'Privacy, the Housing Research Unit at the University of Edinburgh and the Courtyard House, 1959–70', *Architectural History*, 65 (2022), pp. 327–58; Catherine Flinn, *Rebuilding Britain's Blitzed Cities: Hopeful Dreams, Stark Realities* (Bloomsbury, 2018).
7 For example, Claire Langhamer, 'The Meanings of Home in Postwar Britain', *Journal of Contemporary History*, 40 (2005) pp. 341–62; Gregory Salter, *Art and Masculinity in Post-War Britain: Reconstructing Home* (Routledge, 2020).
8 Martin D. Moore, '"Bright-While-You-Wait"? Waiting Rooms and the National Health Service, c. 1948–58', in Jennifer Crane and Jane Hand (eds), *Posters, Protests, and Prescriptions: Cultural Histories of the National Health Service in Britain* (Manchester University Press, 2022), p. 214.
9 Wim Dekkers, 'Dwelling, House and Home: Towards a Home-Led Perspective on Dementia Care', *Medicine, Health Care and Philosophy*, 14 (2011), pp. 291–300 looks at Heidegger, *Building Dwelling Thinking* (*Bauen Wohnen Denken*, 1954), Bollnow, *Lived-Space* (*Der erlebte Raum*, 1960), Bachelard, *The Poetics of Space* (*La poétique de l'espace*, 1957), and Levinas, *Totality and Infinity* (*Totalité et infini*, 1961).

On these theories see also Alison Blunt and Robyn Dowling, *Home* (Routledge, 2006).

10 Richards and McLaughlan, 'Beyond Homeliness', p. 2.

11 For a rare example of a more literal interpretation of 'homely' see 'Sensing Spaces of Healthcare' interview, Benedict Zucchi interviewed by Victoria Bates, 23 March 2023: 'in the context of a hospital, actually the house idea specifically has informed the scheme we're doing at Great Ormond Street which is we always describe it as houses and gardens. So the wards are organised as two houses which look like houses and on the street elevation they're expressed as houses with intervals, with balconies and gardens … Absolutely homely. I mean, that was key to it'; for an example of an approach that sought explicitly to 'mirror' homes in the private sector see also 'Elland Hospital', *Hospital Development*, 14 (1986), p. 45. Victoria Bates, 'Sensing Spaces of Healthcare' interviews, published December 2024, https://doi.org/10.5523/bris.3b8eg2be3ecw52vt3817nq9kah

12 Melisa Duque, Sarah Pink, Shanti Sumartojo, and Laurene Vaughan, 'Homeliness in Health Care: The Role of Everyday Designing', *Home Cultures*, 16 (2019), p. 215.

13 Langhamer, 'The Meanings of Home', p. 361.

14 Ronald Weeks, 'Interior Design: Hospitals', *The Architectural Review*, 1 July 1980, p. 46.

15 'Comment: The Hospital as Building Type', *The Architectural Review*, 1 March 2002, p. 43.

16 Francis J. Blaise, 'The Color Prism in Today's Hospital', *Hospital Management*, 89 (1960), p. 36. The association between lighting and homeliness was international, but also in some ways culturally specific – see, for example, the discussion of *hygge* in Mikkel Bille, *Homely Atmospheres and Lighting Technologies in Denmark: Living with Light* (Routledge, 2019).

17 'North Tees General Hospital: Harness Unit for the Elderly', *Hospital Development*, 3 (1975), p. 10.

18 Thomas R. C. Sisson, 'Some Relationships of Color and Light to Patient Care', in Brian C. Pierman (ed.), *Color in the Health Care Environment* (Department of Commerce/National Bureau of Standards Special Publication 516, 1978), pp. 23–4. Emphasis in original.

19 'New Nurses Home', *The Hospital*, June 1948, pp. 255–8; Department of Health and Social Security and Welsh Office, *The Organisation of the In-Patient's Day: Report of a Committee of the Central Health Services Council* (HMSO, 1976), p. 25.

20 Sisson, 'Some Relationships of Color and Light to Patient Care'.

21 Moore, '"Bright-While-You-Wait"', p. 214.

22 Department of Health and Social Security and Welsh Office, *The Organisation of the In-Patient's Day*, p. 1.
23 'Selly Oak Hospital: Design of Physiotherapy and Dental Departments', *The Hospital*, December 1951, p. 843.
24 *Good Housekeeping* magazine shows some use of pastels in 1950s houses, but in general its 'trends' show brighter homes with more extensive pattern and colour, including colours that were rarely seen in hospitals. For example, in 1955 one article said 'every year we are offered a "new" colour in decorating. This year it is lilac for pretty rooms, turquoise or orange for smart ones'; Harriet Reeder, 'Softer Shades are in the Fashion', *Good Housekeeping*, 67 (1955), pp. 78–81.
25 Denne, 'Bright Ideas for Interiors'.
26 Evidence for contemporary design trends for interiors can be found in the online collections of the Museum of Domestic Design & Architecture, https://moda.mdx.ac.uk.
27 David Charles Sloane and Beverlie Conant Sloane, *Medicine Moves to the Mall* (Johns Hopkins University Press, 2003), p. 87.
28 For example, see 'The Sound of Music', *Hospital Development*, 25 (1994), p. 37, which quoted Nightingale saying 'an air-like "Home, Sweet Home" … will sensibly soothe [the sick]'.
29 See 'homely institutions', in Paul Crawford, Anna Greenwood, Richard Bates, and Jonathan Memel, *Florence Nightingale at Home* (Palgrave, 2020), pp. 109–42.
30 For example, Eli Osterweil Anders, '"So Delightful a Temporary Home": The Material Culture of Domesticity in Late Nineteenth-Century English Convalescent Institutions', *Journal of the History of Medicine and Allied Sciences*, 76 (2021), pp. 264–93.
31 'Mini-Data. Hinchingbrooke Geriatric Hospital, Huntingdon', *Hospital Development*, 4 (1976), p. 24.
32 'Mini-Data. Manor Hospital Epson, Unit for the Somatically Ill', *Hospital Development*, 4 (1976), p. 14.
33 'News: St Thomas' Hospital Development', *Hospital Development*, 5 (1977), p. 8.
34 Jean Symons, *CEH Design Guide 1: Improving Existing Hospital Buildings for Long-Stay Residents* (CEH, 1973), p. 24.
35 Mary Wragg, 'Interior Design on a Restricted Budget', *Hospital Development*, 6 (1978), p. 27; on the link between geriatric hospitals, the rejection of 'modern' design and the focus on 'domesticity', see Edward Patrick DeVane, 'Building the NHS: Planning, Publics and Britain's New State Healthcare Facilities, 1945–74' (PhD Dissertation: University of Warwick, 2022), p. 256.

36 ‘Moorgreen Hospital, Southampton: Continuing Care Unit’, *Hospital Development*, 5 (1977), p. 19.
37 ‘Installations: Kingswood House, Bromley: Floor Tiles’, *Hospital Development*, 11 (1983), p. 12.
38 D. Westerman, ‘Home from Home’, *Hospital Development*, 16 (1988), p. 9.
39 ‘Bournemouth DGH’, *Hospital Development*, 11 (1983), p. 26.
40 I. Ewart and R. Luck, ‘Living from Home’, *Home Cultures*, 10 (2013), p. 25.
41 ‘NE Thames RHA. Geriatric Wards and Day Units’, *Hospital Development*, 5 (1977), p. 26.
42 Ken Worpole, ‘A Home at the End of Life: Changing Definitions of “Homeliness” in the Hospice Movement and End-of-Life Care in the UK’, in Bernike Pasveer, Oddgeir Synnes, and Ingunn Moser (eds), *Ways of Home Making in Care for Later Life* (Palgrave Macmillan, 2020), pp. 135–58.
43 This trend was also evident in relation to ‘noise’ control in hospitals. See Victoria Bates, *Making Noise in the Modern Hospital* (Cambridge University Press, 2021) which draws on some of the ideas in Karin Bijsterveld, ‘“The City of Din”: Decibels, Noise, and Neighbors in the Netherlands, 1910–1980’, *Osiris*, 18 (2003), pp. 173–93.
44 Peter Shearer and Jacquetta Gray, ‘Vehicle for Change’, *Hospital Development*, 25 (1994), pp. 13–15, p. 15.
45 Louise Hide, ‘The Uses and Misuses of Television in Long-Stay Psychiatric and “Mental Handicap” Wards, 1950s–1980s’, in Monika Ankele and Benoît Majerus (eds), *Material Cultures of Psychiatry* (Columbia University Press, 2020), p. 190; Jane Hamlett, *Home in the Institution: Material Life in Asylums, Lodging Houses and Schools in Victorian and Edwardian England* (Palgrave Macmillan, 2015).
46 Vicky Long, ‘Industrial Homes, Domestic Factories: The Convergence of Public and Private Space in Interwar Britain’, *Journal of British Studies*, 50 (2011), p. 434.
47 Agnes Arnold-Forster and Victoria Bates, ‘Care and Crisis: Making Beds in the National Health Service’, *Journal of British Studies* (2024), pp. 1–27.
48 Tracy Karen Mitchell, Lucy Bray, Lucy Blake, Annette Dickinson, and Bernie Carter, ‘“It Doesn’t Feel Like Our House Anymore”: The Impact of Medical Technology upon Life at Home for Families with a Medically Complex, Technology-Dependent Child’, *Health & Place*, 74 (2022), pp. 1–8.
49 David Howes and Constance Classen, *Ways of Sensing: Understanding the Senses in Society* (Routledge, 2014), p. 57.

50 N. H. B. Duncalfe, 'A Scandinavian Tour of Hospitals', *The Hospital*, July 1962, p. 446.
51 Helen Wheatley, 'Television in the Ideal Home', in Rachel Moseley, Helen Wheatley, and Helen Wood (eds), *Television for Women: New Directions* (Routledge, 2017), pp. 205–22. However, this wasn't a totally smooth or universal transition. See Helen Wood, 'Television – The Housewife's Choice? The 1949 Mass Observation Television Directive, Reluctance and Revision', *Media History*, 21 (2015), pp. 342–59.
52 David Morley, 'What's "Home" Got to do With it? Contradictory Dynamics in the Domestication of Technology and the Dislocation of Domesticity', in Thomas Berker, Maren Hartmann, Yves Punie, and Katie J. Ward (eds), *Domestication of Media and Technology* (Open University Press, 2006), p. 21.
53 Morley, 'What's "Home" Got to do With it?', p. 29.
54 Deborah Chambers, 'The Material Form of the Television Set: A Cultural History', *Media History*, 17 (2011), pp. 359–75.
55 'Steele Wing opens at Addison Gilbert Hospital – An American Project', *Hospital Development*, 1 (1973), p. 10; Norman J. Logan, 'Interior Design: Surfaces which Cut Operating Costs', *Hospital Development*, 1 (1973), p. 46.
56 Chambers, 'The Material Form of the Television Set'.
57 Tim O'Sullivan, 'Television Memories and Cultures of Viewing 1950–1965', in John Corner (ed.), *Popular Television* in *Britain* (BFI, 1991).
58 Hide, 'The Uses and Misuses of Television', p. 192.
59 *Ibid.*, p. 193.
60 *Ibid.*, p. 199.
61 British Library Sounds, C1887/659, Jilliane Norman interviewed by Carla Hennion, April 2019, Voices of Our National Health Service © University of Manchester.
62 Nuffield Provincial Hospitals Trust, *Studies in the Functions and Design of Hospitals* (Oxford University Press, 1955).
63 For example, 'a single-storey 25-bed unit … is expected to accept its first patients early this year and will provide a comfortable, cheerful and homely environment'; 'Moorgreen Hospital, Southampton: Continuing Care Unit', *Hospital Development,* 5 (1977), p. 19. See also Arnold-Forster and Bates, 'Care and Crisis'.
64 This postcard is shown in Chapter 5, as part of a discussion of red blankets (Figure 5.9).
65 Marian Summers and Sue Bowman, *Of Poor Law, Patients and Professionals …: A History of Bristol's Southmead Hospital* (self-published, 1995), p. 64.

66 Susan Black, 'Interior Design Trends', *Hospital Development*, 10 (1982), p. 24.
67 Andrew Seaton, *Our NHS: A History of Britain's Best-Loved Institution* (Yale University Press, 2023), p. 80.
68 For example, see British Library Sounds, C1887/294, Norman Sharp, interviewed by Debra Hearne, June 2019, Voices of Our National Health Service © University of Manchester.
69 British Library Sounds, C512/48, Dr Peter Horrocks interviewed by Margot Jefferys, Oral History of Geriatrics as a Medical Specialty © British Library.
70 Derbyshire Record Office, D6082/18/2/3, 'Southern Derbyshire Community Health Council visit to Derbyshire Royal Infirmary, 1993'.
71 'Healthcare: Care Homes, Hospitals, and Healthcare Environments', https://www.skoposfabrics.com/sectors/healthcare [accessed: 21 February 2024].
72 I took some time in the archive to feel these curtains, their weight and softness. I cannot make any claims for other – or past – people's physical encounters with them, but they were materially distinct both from the wipe-down disposable curtains that signify infection control and from the fabric of curtains in the home at this time.
73 Wellcome Library, ART/IOW/F/1–4, Sian Tucker, design of ward curtains at St Mary's Hospital, 1987–89.
74 Guy Eades interviewed by Victoria Bates, 13 March 2023. Victoria Bates, 'Sensing Spaces of Healthcare' interviews, published December 2024, https://doi.org/10.5523/bris.3b8eg2be3ecw52vt38l7nq9kah
75 Sian Tucker interviewed by Victoria Bates, 22 March 2022. Victoria Bates, 'Sensing Spaces of Healthcare' interviews, published December 2024, https://doi.org/10.5523/bris.3b8eg2be3ecw52vt38l7nq9kah
76 Eades interview, Tucker interview.
77 Thanks to Anne Greer for sharing this toolkit as part of our interview; Anne Greer interviewed by Victoria Bates, 14 April 2023. Victoria Bates, 'Sensing Spaces of Healthcare' interviews, published December 2024, https://doi.org/10.5523/bris.3b8eg2be3ecw52vt38l7nq9kah
78 This paragraph draws on Victoria Bates, Jennifer Crane, and Maria Fannin, 'The Construction and Politics of the "Birth Experience" in Britain, 1948–93', *Cultural History*, 13 (2024), pp. 100–23.
79 Julian Ashley, *Anatomy of a Hospital* (Oxford University Press, 1987), p. 88.
80 *Ibid.*
81 Arnold-Forster and Bates, 'Care and Crisis', pp. 1–27.
82 Angela Davis, 'Choice, Policy and Practice in Maternity Care since 1948', *History and Policy*, 30 May 2013, https://www.historyandpolicy.org/

policy-papers/papers/choice-policy-and-practice-in-maternity-care-since-1948 [accessed: 22 February 2024].

83 Annmarie Adams gives an example of this trend from the 1920s in Canada in Annmarie Adams, *Medicine by Design: The Architect and the Modern Hospital* (University of Minnesota Press, 2008), pp. 48–50. At this time, home births were still common and Adams notes that this design feature was partly a way to attract paying patients, who would stay for 10–12 days. On the rise of hospital births and its implications for maternity design in post-war Canada, which is a story more in line with that told here, see Whitney Wood, '"A Familiar, Not Fearful Place": Sensory Histories of Childbirth in Twentieth-Century North America', *Senses and Society* (2025), pp. 1–14, https://www.tandfonline.com/doi/full/10.1080/17458927.2024.2402966 .

84 'Colour Planning in Blackburn', *The Hospital*, April 1951, pp. 271–2.

85 'Mini-Data: Bishop Auckland General Hospital Maternity Department', *Hospital Development*, 3 (1975), p. 45; 'Mini-Data. Royal Lancaster Infirmary Maternity Unit', *Hospital Development*, 4 (1976), p. 24.

86 Wellcome Library, ART/AFH/A/9/9, Dorothy W. Strachan, 'Colour in Hospitals', *Nursing Times,* 61 (1965), pp. 627–9.

87 *Ibid.*

88 *Ibid.*

89 Dorset History Centre, D-PPY/A/4/3/8/1, Pilkington's, *Hospital Tiling* (nd).

90 See Chapter 6 on the rise of brighter shades by the 1980s and 1990s elsewhere.

91 'Installations: Primary Colours', *Hospital Development*, 16 (1988), p. 51.

92 I used the term 'service users' alongside 'patients' because in a number of healthcare contexts, the people accessing services do not see themselves as 'patients'. Maternity is one such example, because many people using maternity services are not unwell, and 'service user' is often used to signify this.

93 Benjamin Dalton, 'Paul B. Preciado's Queer Hospital: Healthcare Architectures for Pleasure, Transformation and Subversion', *The Senses and Society* (2024), pp. 1–14.

94 A1013 interviewed by Rebecka Fleetwood-Smith, 2022.

95 The precise author or context of this report is not provided, but it is held as part of archival records about the hospital. East Riding Archives, DDX1369/2/17, 'Maternity Unit – Westwood Hospital', August 1988.

96 *Ibid.*

97 *Ibid.*

98 East Riding Archives, JL/49/198/1988, 'Royal Day at New Wing', *Healthview [The newspaper for the Health Service in the Yorkshire Region]*, August 1988, p. 17.
99 East Riding Archives, JL/49/198/1988, 'Mums Get New Home from Home', *Healthview [The newspaper for the Health Service in the Yorkshire Region]*, April 1988, p. 9.
100 Victoria Bates, Jennifer Crane, and Maria Fannin, 'Fluid Modernities: The Birthing Pool in Late Twentieth-Century Britain', *Medical Humanities*, 50 (2024), pp. 312–21.
101 Wellcome Library, SA/PAT/F/1/6, 'Editorial', *Patient Voice*, 13 (1980), p. 2.
102 William C. Beck, 'Hospital Light and Color from the Physician's Standpoint', in Brian C. Pierman (ed.), *Color in the Health Care Environment* (Department of Commerce/National Bureau of Standards, 1978), p. 6.
103 Stine Louring Nielson, 'The Midwifery Feel of Light', in Shanti Sumartojo (ed.), *Lighting Design in Shared Public Spaces* (Routledge, 2022), p. 73.
104 See Bates, Crane, and Fannin, 'Fluid Modernities', p. 317.
105 The National Archives, MH166/1136, Harness Interiors produced by the interior designers from the Regional Health Authorities and the Department of Health & Social Security, part of the papers of the 'Technical Design Group', 1973–75.
106 Archive Service, Great Ormond Street Hospital for Children NHS Foundation Trust, GOS/15/314, OPD Survey 1963.
107 The National Archives, ED 173/63, Department of Education and Science Architects and Building Group, *Meeting the Educational Needs of Children in Hospital. Design Note 38* (Department of Education and Science, 1984), p. 2.
108 *Ibid.*
109 Department of Health and Social Security Welsh Office, *Hospital Accommodation for Children: Health Building Note 23* (HMSO, 1984), p. 11.
110 *Ibid.*
111 Great Ormond Street Archive, Kevin Telfer, *The Remarkable Story of Great Ormond Street Hospital* (Simon & Schuster UK, 2008), p. 188.
112 Department of Health and Social Security Welsh Office, *Hospital Accommodation for Children*, p. 1.
113 East Riding Archives, JL/49/1990/Healthview, 'Kids Rule OK', *Healthview [The newspaper for the Health Service in the Yorkshire Region]*, October 1990, p. 19.

114 *Ibid.*

115 *Ibid.*

116 Department of Health and Social Security and Welsh Office, *The Organisation of the In-Patient's Day*, p. 45.

117 Jean Symons, *CEH Design Guide 1: Improving Existing Hospital Buildings for Long-Stay Residents* (CEH, 1973), p. 5.

118 'Viewpoint: Shifting Trends', *Hospital Development*, 14 (1986), p. 5.

119 Denne, 'Bright Ideas for Interiors', p. 19.

120 See Cara Dobbing, 'Pauper Lunatics at Home in the Asylum, 1845–1906', in Joseph Harley, Vicky Holmes, and Laika Nevalainen (eds), *The Working Class at Home, 1790–1940* (Palgrave Macmillan, 2022), pp. 193–211; Jane Hamlett, *Home in the Institution: Material Life in Asylums, Lodging Houses and Schools in Victorian and Edwardian England* (Palgrave Macmillan, 2015).

121 Susan Barclay, 'When It's Not the Main Game: Art in Hospitals' (PhD Dissertation: University of Western Sydney, 2015), p. 89.

122 'The Children's Hospital, Birmingham', *The Hospital*, April 1890, p. 15.

123 Sara Ahmed, *The Cultural Politics of Emotion* (EUP, 2014 [2004]), p. 11.

124 Graham Mooney, 'The Material Consumptive: Domesticating the Tuberculosis Patient in Edwardian England', *Journal of Historical Geography*, 42 (2013), p. 165.

125 B. R. Wilson, 'Letters: Mothers in hospital', *Architects' Journal*, 4 March 1964, p. 510.

126 On activist groups and their interest in the 'birth experience' see Bates, Crane, and Fannin, 'The Construction and Politics of the "Birth Experience" in Britain, 1948–93'. On feminist health movements and their relationship to organisations such as the NCT see also Hilary Marland, '"Drowned in a Sea of Inhumanity": Natural Childbirth, Postnatal Depression and the National Childbirth Trust, 1956–80s', *Social History of Medicine*, 37 (2024), pp. 69–92.

127 See Naomi Stead (ed.), *Women, Practice, Architecture: 'Resigned accommodation' and 'Usurpatory Practice'* (Routledge, 2014).

128 Susan Black, 'Interior Design Trends', *Hospital Development*, 10 (1982), p. 24.

129 Duque, Pink, Sumartojo, and Vaughan, 'Homeliness in Health Care, p. 228.

130 Derbyshire Record Office, D6082/18/2/1, visits to Children's Hospital, 1980s–90s, quote from 15 June 1993.

131 *Ibid.*

132 B. S. Platt, T. P. Eddy, and P. L. Pellett, *Food in Hospitals* (Nuffield Provincial Hospitals Trust for Oxford University Press, 1963), p. 171.
133 Alix Henley, *Asians in Britain: Caring for Sikhs and their Families: Religious Aspects of Care* (National Extension College for the Health Education Council, DHSS, and the King Edward's Hospital Fund for London, 1983), p. 59.
134 Richard Burton, 'St Mary's Hospital, Isle of Wight: A Suitable Background for Caring', *BMJ* (December 1990), p. 1424.
135 John Berger, *Ways of Seeing* (Penguin, 1972), p. 30.
136 Penny Calvert interviewed by Victoria Bates, 27 February 2023.
137 Steve Eames interviewed by Victoria Bates, 26 April 2023.
138 'North Tees General Hospital: Harness Unit for the Elderly', *Hospital Development*, 3 (1975), p. 10.
139 'Home from Home', *Hospital Development*, 16 (1988), p. 9.
140 'Total Care in Croydon', *Hospital Development*, 13 (1985), p. 17.
141 East Riding Archives, DDX1497/7, *Beverley Westwood Hospital Patients' Guide*, c. 1957.
142 Amelia Crabtree, Tyler J. Lane, Lisa Mahon, Taryn Petch, and Christina L. Ekegren, 'The impact of an End-PJ-Paralysis Quality Improvement Intervention in Post-Acute Care: An Interrupted Time Series Analysis', *AIMS Medical Science*, 8 (2021), pp. 23–35.
143 Mass Observation Archive (University of Sussex), Replies to Spring 1997 directive [C1713].
144 Borthwick Institute, YDH 1/1/2, 'York District Hospital: This is Your Life!' Cuttings Book. Article from 18 June 1980 – newspaper name not provided.
145 Borthwick Institute, Cuttings Book.
146 On the history of attachment theory, see Inge Bretherton, 'The Origins of Attachment Theory: John Bowlby and Mary Ainsworth', *Development Psychology*, 28 (1992), pp. 759–75.
147 'Parents' Meetings in Two Neonatal Units: A Way of Increasing Support for Parents', *BMJ* (September 1982), p. 863.
148 London Metropolitan Archives, A/KE/I/01/001//017, Background Music in Hospitals: Completed Questionnaires, 1962.
149 Mass Observation Archive (University of Sussex), Replies to Spring 1997 directive [B26].
150 Tim Edensor and Shanti Sumartojo, 'Designing Atmospheres: Introduction to Special Issue', *Visual Communication*, 14 (2015), p. 260.
151 In a recent interview a designer spoke about how the idea of a 'spaceship' still dominates many people's preferences, alongside homeliness. Craig Wightman interviewed by Victoria Bates, 10 March 2023.

152 'Roundabout: St Mary's Hospital, Paddington', *Hospital Development*, 12 (1984), p. 6.

153 Jane Willis interviewed by Victoria Bates, 21 February 2023. Victoria Bates, 'Sensing Spaces of Healthcare' interviews, published December 2024, https://doi.org/10.5523/bris.3b8eg2be3ecw52vt38l7nq9kah

5

Red: risk and reward

In 1987, a new West Dorset County hospital 'shot [...] to fame in the world of NHS building'.[1] The reason was its 'lively details and bright materials', which were generally well received despite 'reservations about "excessive red paint" expressed by Prince Charles' (Figure 5.1).[2] This hospital marked an important shift in hospital design. As a report for the King's Fund Hospital Design Competition noted in 1994, '[w]hether one likes the external colour scheme [...] is ultimately a matter of personal choice [...] But this hospital is exciting and stimulating. It shows how new ideas can be introduced into NHS building'.[3] Vibrant colours such as red, which had previously been avoided as overstimulating or reminiscent of blood, started to become increasingly common. By the end of the century, the 'humanistic' hospital was playful and stimulating, rather than therapeutic and soothing. 'Bright' colours were an important part of this trend, as the meaning of the word subtly shifted from light to vibrant.

The roots of this brightening-up trend are found in the 1970s. However, it was really in the 1980s and 1990s that vibrant colours shifted from being seen as 'garish', or as only acceptable as accents in fixtures and fittings, to being embraced more extensively as markers of modernity. This trend was in part a consequence of broader changing ideas about colour and a lessening of the so-called chromophobia that previously characterised modern Britain, and by extension its architecture. It was also facilitated by changes in healthcare practices, as the late twentieth century was characterised by the decline of long-stay patients. Bright colour schemes supported the goal of 'stimulating' patients, increasing recovery rates and moving people through hospitals more quickly. Over the course of the late twentieth

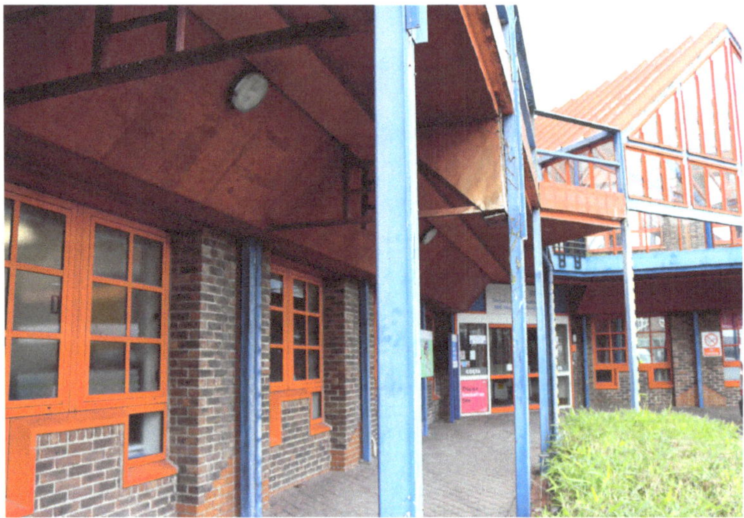

Figure 5.1 Dorset County Hospital, Dorchester (previously West Dorset County Hospital), 2023. © Image: Victoria Bates. Reproduced with kind permission of Dorset County Hospital NHS Foundation Trust.

century, the concept – and vibrant colour palette – of playfulness expanded beyond design for children.

Bright: vibrancy and vitality from the 1970s

'Brightness' had long been seen as a quality of modernity, particularly in built environments. To quote Mark M. Smith, modern cities were 'newly designed urban spaces with broad avenues, geometric thoroughfares, and generally bright – and, increasingly lighted – environments'.[4] In the post-war period, 'brightness' came increasingly to be articulated through colour and positioned in contrast to 'dreary' pre-war towns.[5] Similar rhetorical devices were used for hospitals, where post-war colour and lighting schemes were described in broad terms such as 'bright' and 'modern' to differentiate them from clinical and sterile pre-war hospitals. Those pre-war hospitals had, however, often also been described as bright and modern when they were built. The term 'bright' was thus associated with modernity in hospitals throughout the twentieth century, but it changed meaning.

As recent commentators have noted, brightness 'is a word which has been used particularly ambiguously in colour studies' to mean anything from a fully saturated vivid colour to something that is pale or well-lit.[6] This applies equally to historical uses of the term. Despite the difficulties of pinning down the meaning of 'bright' colour, at least until the more widespread use of colour photographs in architectural journals, all existing evidence shows that very vibrant colours were unusual in hospitals of the early-to-mid-twentieth century. Outside specific contexts such as children's wards, vibrant colours were only a feature of the modern hospital in the final decades of the twentieth century. The meaning of 'bright' must be read as socially contingent. In relation to hospitals, it often meant white and light in the early twentieth century; modern, pale, and fresh colours in the post-war years; and expanded to include more vibrant colour from the 1970s onwards. Some early and mid-century sources emphasise the link between 'brightness' and modernity, but leave the exact meaning of 'bright colours' unclear.[7] This often makes it difficult to know what exactly was meant by 'brightness', though it is possible to speculate based on context and knowledge of hospital colour schemes at the time.

Vibrant colour schemes were not widely apparent in the early NHS. However, they did have some early advocates, and were more common elsewhere. In the 1950s, a delegation from the Ministry of Health visited Scandinavia and observed the colour schemes in their hospitals, including careful use of bright colours and geometric shapes to promote rest.[8] However, contemporaries continued to articulate general concern about colours that were 'too intense', including the apparent risk that they would make patients look more unwell.[9] The specifically British post-war understanding of 'brightness' was grounded in an apparent national dislike of so-called *overly* vibrant colour palettes. In his 1951 article 'Colour in the Hospital', Arthur L. Hall cited the 'unaccountable British fear of clean, bright colour' as one of the factors limiting change.[10] Truly 'bright' colours, or 'non-natural shades', did not enter hospital palettes widely until the end of the century.[11]

The 'unaccountable' fear that bright colour was 'brash' was widespread in a range of contexts at this time. Sarah Street, for example, notes that this perception was common in relation to technicolour in the 1930s and 1940s, as 'it was associated with Hollywood and wider discourses about national difference' because of ideas 'that the British use of colour was somehow more tasteful than its application in the USA'.[12] Christine Slobogin quotes similar comments from a 1951 publication on *Colour Cinematography* about the 'antipathy to excessive use of vivid colour' because of its association with Hollywood.[13] The link between 'brash' American bright colours and 'muted', tasteful British colours in the post-war period was evidently widespread in culture, from cinema to hospitals. The artist David Batchelor – author of *Chromophobia* – notes the continued negative connotations of words such as 'lurid' or 'garish' in much of Western culture, even today, and comments that colour 'is often represented as feminine, or Oriental, or primitive, or infantile, rather than grown-up and philosophical and serious [...] and it's clearly indexed to issues of race, culture, class and gender'.[14] Though recent design trends have clearly started to challenge the fear of vibrant colours in public architecture, if not private properties, the continued fear of over-using vibrant colours might be grounded in such cultural concerns.

In the mid-twentieth century, colours such as vibrant red and yellow were still primarily used for warnings, the visual equivalent of an alarm; indeed, when more complex electronic communication systems were brought in during the post-war years, a flashing red light often came with a sound.[15] This association between bright colours and alarm was not new, nor was it specific to British hospitals. Red lights had long meant 'stop' or 'danger', with yellow or amber as warnings, for example in traffic systems.[16] Primary colours were also used as warning colours in systems from electrics to factories, largely because of their visibility against neutral backdrops. To return to Faber Birren's colour schemes from the 1950s discussed in Chapter 2, primary colours were still largely 'Safety and Identification' colours in the mid-century: he listed 'high visibility yellow', 'alert orange', 'fire protection red', 'safety green' and 'precaution blue'.[17] Reports of the evaluation of New Guy's House at Guy's Hospital in London in 1962 show that 'yellow and red lines' were used to mark sterile areas.[18] Such use fits with claims made widely in contemporary colour theory and international literature on colour in healthcare that there was a 'traditional and well-recognised' pairing of colour and meaning: 'yellow for "caution" and red for "stop"'.[19]

Red has traditionally been rare in hospital architecture and interior design outside the context of safety, because of its associations with blood and illness, though the following section shows it was more commonly found in objects. As David Howes and Constance Classen note, such associations have a long medical history, going back to humoral theory in which 'the colour of a patient's complexion might be taken to suggest an overabundance of a particular humour – a red complexion was associated with a surfeit of blood'.[20] The association between red and blood was obvious, common internationally, and difficult to move away from. In an article on hospital artwork in 1983, one commentator noted that 'the greatest care is needed [...] when selecting images for areas such as psychiatric wards – when the most innocent of imagery, such as a bunch of red flowers, could be interpreted as pools of blood'.[21] Even in relation to hospital design for children, where brighter colours were more widely used, one American publication by the National Institute of Mental Health in 1965 was simply titled '*Red is the Color of Hurting*'.[22] Some of these bright colours, such as red, indicated warning or alarm in a range of cultures, though of course the association between red and fire made it lucky in other countries such as China.[23] Such cultural nuances were, though, rarely taken into account in conversations around hospital design, though age and gender were usually considered. Decorative schemes were grounded in what might be considered 'Western' ideas about colour, but of course in practice people from a range of backgrounds inhabited those spaces and engaged with their colour schemes.

A danger of bright colour, as believed in mid-century, was over-stimulation. In 1950, influential colour theorist Faber Birren made the following assessment of red:

> Red is the most energetic colour. Biologically, it has been found to have the effect of increasing blood pressure and heart rate. In terms of its psychological effect, red equates to arousal and stimulation, it increases nervous tension and also helps to increase productivity.[24]

Birren's notion of red as 'exciting' was broadly unchallenged in the late twentieth century, but this quality was no longer considered dangerous. There was growing interest in the therapeutic potential of stimulation, entangled with concern about boredom and productivity, and recognition that 'calm' (associated with blues and greens) might not be the only emotional goal in hospitals.[25] Some of the earliest commentators to embrace colour in the late 1960s focused on the recovery or 'rehabilitation ward', where it was thought that a 'single bright red wall' could have a positive, 'electrifying effect'.[26] Stimulation was thought to be of value for staff and patients alike, at least at first. To quote the *BMJ* in 1962, hospital colour schemes had three main goals: '(1) To make the hospital a bright and cheerful place' for patients, '(2) To make the hospital a pleasant place in which staff can work', including supporting staff relations and efficiency, and '(3) To ensure that dirt can be seen'.[27] Consideration of staff in hospital design waned over the course of the century, but never disappeared.

In subsequent decades, there was more interest in the therapeutic potential of stimulation and a waning fear of the 'brash'. Bright colours were increasingly seen as 'modern', and as part of the colour palette of new architecture. In the early 1970s, for example, the interior designers from Regional Health Authorities and the Department of Health & Social Security collaborated on a publication on 'Harness Interiors' that – like the Harness scheme itself – promoted a more systematic and standardised approach to hospital design. Many of their recommendations echo those found in other documents already discussed, and in the work of colour theorists working on hospitals, but it is significant that this official booklet was produced for new British hospitals. Such literature moved colour theory and interior design away from narrow areas of interest found in medical or design journals, to core parts of the guidance provided by the DHSS. Few Harness hospitals were ever built, but such publications remain part of the history of ideas and their circulation in the NHS.[28] This document particularly advocated a hospital that echoed the 'atmosphere of an entrance and reception of a large comfortable hotel', a trend that predated the later rise of consumer models of hospital architecture and design. Their illustrations showed bright colours in communal areas (Figure 5.2), but stopped short of recommending specific colour schemes; the aim of this booklet was, seemingly, to recommend and illustrate ideal design, and to encourage incorporating the 'specialised skill' of interior designers into every project.

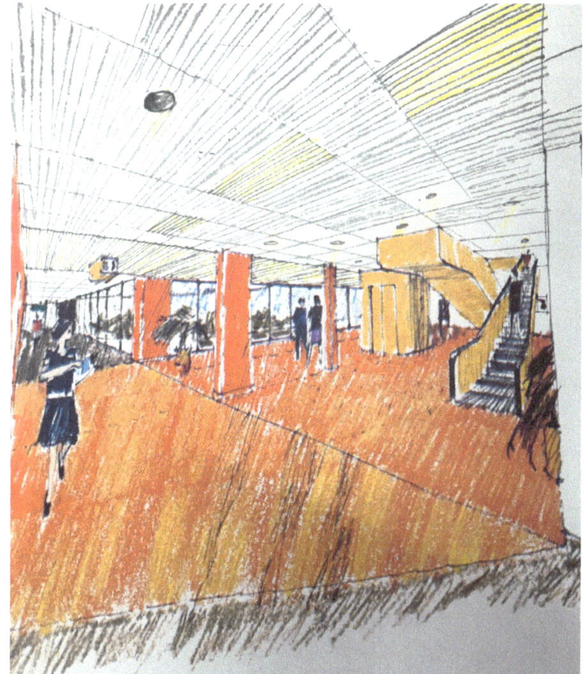

Figure 5.2 National Archives, MH 166/1136, Harness Interiors produced by the interior designers from the Regional Health Authorities and the Department of Health & Social Security, part of the papers of the 'Technical Design Group', p. 12. Representation of the 'Harness Zone' – a street to connect departments.

Increasingly, ideas about 'good' interior design also came from patients rather than just from professionals. It is difficult to date this shift, as there was no single turning point or intervention that marked this change, and patient surveys had been a feature of organisations such as the King's Fund throughout the post-war years. However, there was a subtle shift in the tone of published literature, and by the 1970s and 1980s greater space was being made for patients' opinions. Research into patients' preferences upturned some of the previous assumptions about colour schemes, showing more demand for bright colour among older adults than previously expected. As

Susan Black noted in an article on interior design trends in 1982, many designers thought elderly patients preferred 'restful blues, purples and browns' while those aged 17–30 'would go for lively yellows and reds'; research conducted in 1974, however, 'showed almost the reverse to be true'.[29] There was thus not only a growing interest in the potential value of stimulating colours for health, but greater research into and more nuanced understandings of the needs of different patients. New colour schemes did not just articulate or represent NHS principles such as patient-centred care, but also shaped and informed those principles through research that challenged assumptions about 'the patient' as a homogeneous group. Such research was part of a wider shift in patient-centred design from designing *for* an imagined patient, to consulting with and listening to patient voices.

At this time, brightness in hospital interiors was advocated on the page but not widely evident in practice. There were pioneering examples of colour use in mainland Europe that went far beyond anything seen in Britain at the time. Herlev Hospital in Copenhagen, for example, 'was one of the first polychrome hospitals in the world' when it was completed in 1976. One of its stand-out design features was vibrantly coloured walls (Figure 5.3).[30] This was an exceptional example even for Denmark, and illustrates what Tim Edensor describes as '[t]he affective and sensory potential that inheres in a radical encounter with vivid colo[u]r'.[31] The artist Poul Gernes was commissioned to add some art to the building and his role had expanded in line with his belief that 'architecture without colours is meagre'.[32] He considered himself a 'decorator' more than an artist, though it is clear that these two were entwined in his interiors. Though Gernes was unique at the time, he was influential; nearly fifty years later, the work still stands, as an example of how ambitious and vibrant hospital colour schemes could be.

No British hospital quite followed Gernes headfirst into the world of dizzying polychrome, but they did certainly brighten up and attempt to use colour to make hospitals feel more joyful over subsequent decades. Herlev inspired many British observers and commentators, one of whom wrote extensively in *The Architectural Review* in 1980 and complained that British '[h]ospital walls are rarely decorated by more than sparsely scattered reproduction prints or, more usually, by grim health warning posters'.[33] At this time,

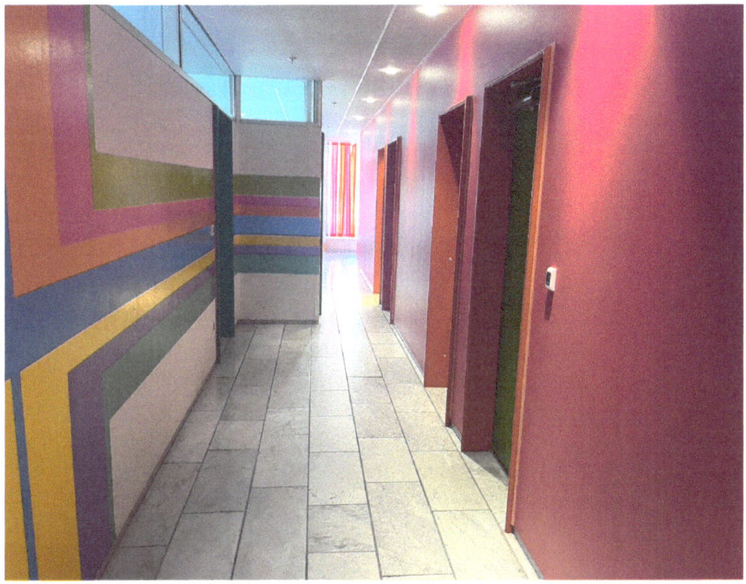

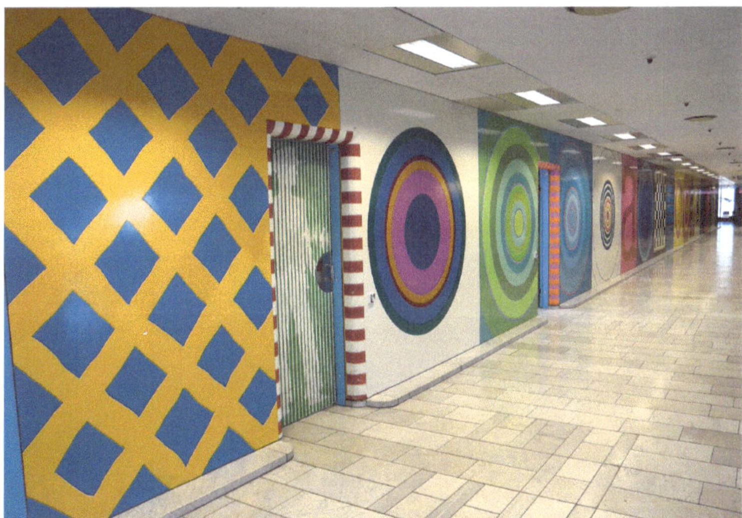

Figure 5.3 Poul Gernes, Herlev Hospital, Copenhagen, 2023. © The artist. Images Victoria Bates. Reproduced with kind permission of Klara Karolines Fond Stiftet af Aase & Poul Gernes.

there was a turn towards bolder interventions in British hospital colour schemes, in arts, architecture, and interiors.[34] In 1980, architects Faulkner Brown & Partners backed 'the Formalux elements' of the exterior canopy of the Royal Victoria Infirmary in Newcastle 'with red lining, and the plenum of the interior reception area was also painted red to add warmth to the lighting'.[35] Such use of red for cheerful or stimulating 'warmth', as part of a balanced colour scheme with 'cooler' calmer shades, was increasingly common. In Milton Keynes District General Hospital, discussed in *Hospital Development* in 1984, 'a feature of the corridors and common areas is the green-based colour scheme that gives way to tangerines and reds in other areas. The colour scheme is both bold and pleasing – and well coordinated'.[36] This trend, towards more extensive use of vibrant colour, was boosted by changes in how patients moved through hospitals. One commentator in 1980 noted that

> it is not usual practice nowadays to move patients from ward to ward (and hence different colour areas); to ensure therefore that patients are exposed to a suitable colour scheme, a variety of colours is required in each patient space.[37]

Changes in colour use and the distribution of colour in hospitals was interwoven with processes of patient care, including the ways that people moved – or did not move – through the building.

There was also growing interest in how white could reflect and enhance the potential of more vibrant colours; white was never replaced by such schemes, but rather was an integral part of them. When Richard Saxon wrote an 'Appraisal' piece in *Architects' Journal* in 1983 about leading hospital architects Powell and Moya's Maidstone design, he observed that 'Powell and Moya continue their memorable tradition of white space with accents from timber and from primary colour in furniture and wall painting'.[38] Vibrant blues, oranges, and greens used by Llewelyn-Davies Weeks for a new psychiatric wing for St Mary's Hospital in 1984 were similarly designed to 'reflect off the white walls of the corridors giving subtle nuances of colour'.[39] Vibrant colours were used, in balance, to 'enliven' spaces.

It was still rare for hospital exteriors to be as bright as West Dorset County Hospital, with its futuristic shades of yellow and red. However, other healthcare buildings in Dorset were also some

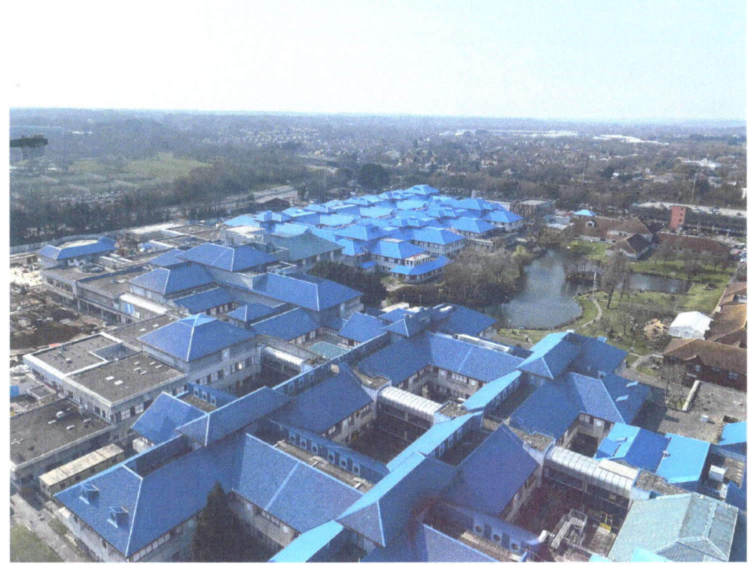

Figure 5.4 The blue roof of Royal Bournemouth General Hospital. © Image: University Hospitals Dorset NHS Foundation Trust. Reproduced with kind permission. All rights reserved and permission to use this figure must be obtained from the copyright holder.

of the brightest exteriors at this time, indicating some degree of geographical influence on the trend. Bournemouth General Hospital (1988/9, later renamed Royal Bournemouth General Hospital, see Figure 5.4) had an unusual bright blue roof on its nucleus hospital, and a new Community Health Clinic in Poole (1988) had a 'distinctive, red painted entrance porch'.[40] Peter Scher described the Royal Bournemouth General Hospital as the 'very pleasant visual equivalent of a good popular song [...] they have applied rich colour at every opportunity'.[41] Though led by different architectural firms, these projects shared an architect. West Dorset County Hospital's first phase was conducted by PTP Architects in collaboration with Barry Payne, regional architect of Wessex Regional Health Authority, and the changes to Bournemouth hospital were led by HLM, also in collaboration with Payne.[42]

Elsewhere, people were generally more reluctant to put bright colours on hospital exteriors than interiors, even on new-builds where more innovation was possible. Scher noted that the Bournemouth example was unusual even for a new hospital, which could often only afford 'sober, often dreary, brickwork and roof tiles'.[43] In part, this conservatism was because hospital exteriors were more difficult to change, and needed to be more weather-resistant, so bright colours were only possible in certain forms such as tiles and steels. Architects Powell and Moya, who were at the cutting edge of NHS hospital design with their 'humane modernism', considered but backed away from the use of red on the exterior of their Great Ormond Street Hospital redevelopment in the 1994 Variety Club Building (Figure 5.5).

As confidence grew about how, where, and why to use bright colours, they became more widespread and more fully integrated into buildings, rather than in removable or replaceable objects and furnishings. In November 1993, *Hospital Development*'s cover depicted a yellow, blue, green, and red tropical mural on a hospital wall, with the title 'Bright Ideas for Interiors'.[44] Such vibrant covers, with their attention to hospital interiors, had been unusual before this. The modern colour palettes that they depicted differed from more traditional shades, which tended to be richer, deeper colours such as 'crimson' rather than primary colours.[45]

Artworks were some of the first examples of bright colours in hospitals, as discussed in Chapter 3. They helped to normalise vibrancy, and to shift the language around such colours from 'over-stimulating' to providing 'interest'. This trend was also international. In an article published in 1984, the *BMJ* provided an image of a large red wall hanging from an Australian hospital (opened in 1978), alongside red carpet and chairs (Figure 5.6). The use of contemporary art alongside concrete in this context supports the argument that vibrant colours were increasingly the palettes of modernity. Susan Barclay also discusses this work in her thesis on art in hospitals, noting that the interior designer 'decided to push sedate colours aside and introduced a vibrant red palette which included red carpet and furniture'.[46] This designer had been influenced by the British arts and health movement, and the publication of this artwork in the *BMJ* helped to close the circle by feeding ideas about the potential value of bold colour schemes and contemporary art back to British readers. The snowballing of this vibrant colour trend was encouraged by international research and publications, and by the dialogue, travel, and enthusiasm of individual interior designers and artists.

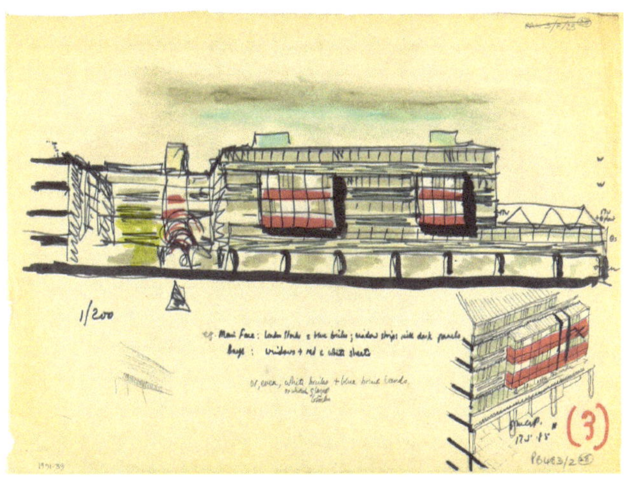

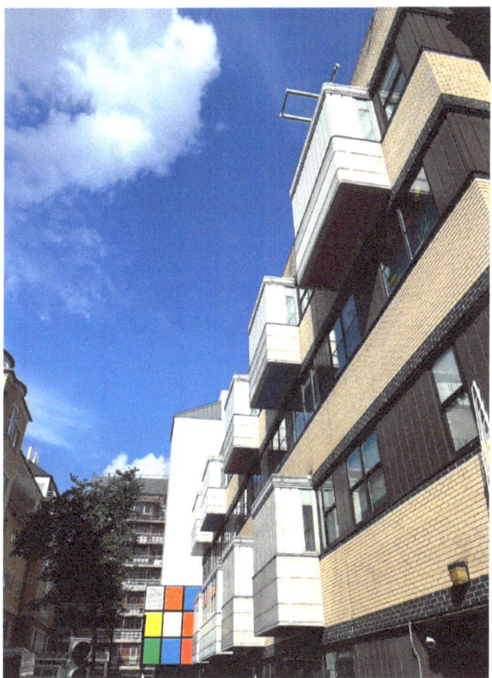

Figure 5.5 RIBA Collections, PB483/2(28), Powell & Moya, Great Ormond Street Hospital, perspective sketches. © RIBA Collections; Variety Club Building, Great Ormond Street Hospital 2023 © Image: Victoria Bates. The Rubik's Cube was added later, in 2013/14.

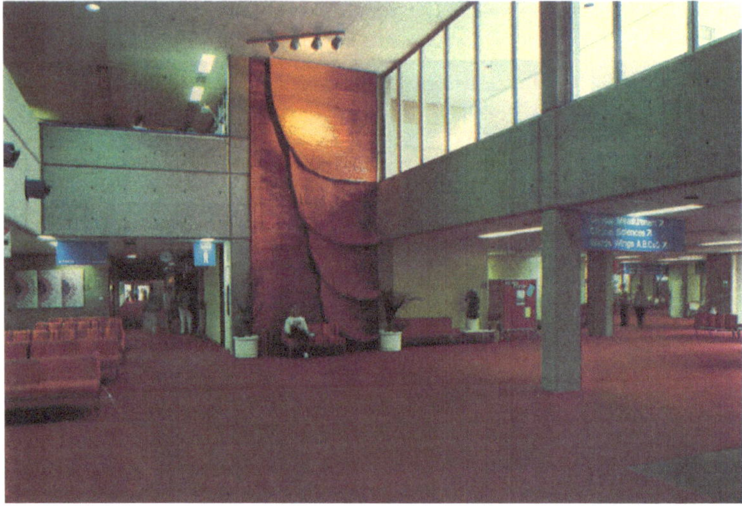

Figure 5.6 Jutta Fedderson wall hanging in Westmead Hospital. Jeremy Hugh Baron and Lesley Greene, 'Art in Hospitals: Funding Works of Art in New Hospitals', British Medical Journal, 22–29 December 1984), p. 1734. Image reproduced with permission of the *British Medical Journal*.

Such colour palettes came hand-in-hand with different materials, forms, and messages, which sought to encourage interaction, stimulation, and joy rather than calm. One contributor to *Hospital Development* in 1987, writing on 'The Healing Arts', commented that 'for young and old alike a carefully thought out mural offers a rich kaleidoscope of visual attention and interest'.[47] This language emphasised the value of stimulating positive emotions, rather than only providing a calming or therapeutic colour scheme, and brought with it a change to the traditional colour palettes of hospitals towards more vibrant 'warm' shades such as orange and even the previously shunned 'blood' red. Such schemes tended to be in areas such as waiting spaces to counteract boredom, or in artworks that people passed by so that there was no risk of over-stimulation. One article in *Architects' Journal* in 1974 observed that in one new hospital 'the entrance hall itself is a bustling lively place' with 'orange patterned carpet', but that 'carpeting on the floors stops here – from now on it is 2mm vinyl, white emulsion and the odd coloured wall'.[48] The use of colour in waiting areas could, then, be in stark difference to other parts of the hospital.

By the end of the century there was more discussion of creating positive atmospheres rather than just soothing ones. Such design goals were often conceptualised as a 'total environment' approach, of which colour was a part. In relation to Gloucestershire Royal NHS Trust, for example, arts coordinator Anne Greer wrote of a strategy to create 'a colourful, positive environment which lifts the spirits of staff, patients and visitors'[49]. An example of this trend is shown in Figure 5.7, in which bright complementary colours (vibrant orange and blue) were used alongside each other in a stairwell; the artwork explicitly gives the viewer permission to laugh or feel joy, even in the context of a hospital, with a simple and clear message to absorb as people passed it by on their way to or from appointments.

Such changing colour schemes did not necessarily mean a dramatic shifting of design principles, or the complete abandonment of 'humanisation' or 'homeliness'. Many architects, artists, and interior designers continued to use the home as a reference point, even when they brought in new, vibrant colours. In the Llewelyn-Davies Weeks psychiatric ward discussed above, the use of bright colours was part of a 'homelike' feel.[50] In 1987, the first purpose-built ward for the treatment of AIDS patients at The Middlesex Hospital used 'colours brighter than normally associated with wards' in combination with a reduction of the 'scale' of the wards, to enhance 'the "domestic" character'.[51] Over the subsequent decade, British hospitals increasingly incorporated American models of 'humanisation', influenced by contexts such as shopping centres, with bright colours that echoed commercial rather than domestic contexts.[52] However, these two approaches were never entirely mutually exclusive.

A trend towards brightness should not be confused with universal support for vibrant colour palettes. Writing in 1999, Greer acknowledged that the reception of very bright colour schemes and artworks was not universally positive, and that some 'sceptical staff and visitors' viewed vivid colours as 'visual disturbance'.[53] She acknowledged that one 'real mistake' was changed after feedback, but that in general 'most schemes win favour' over time and as a whole hospital strategy comes into being.[54] Most commentators continued to note that bright colours should be used carefully and

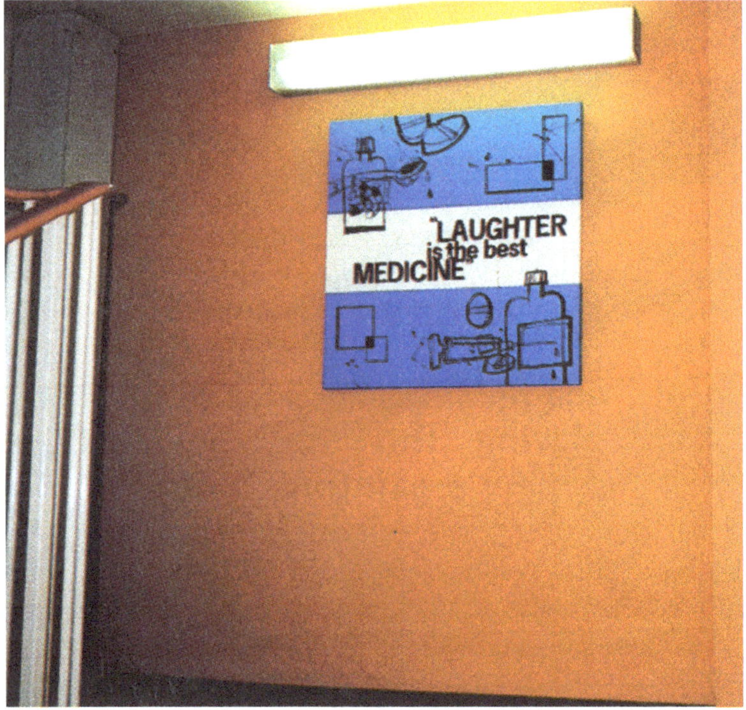

Figure 5.7 Panel by Richard Baldwin, depicted in Anne Greer, 'Colour Therapy', *Hospital Development*, 30 (1999), p. 20. © Image: The artist and Anne Greer, courtesy of RIBA Collections. Thanks to Anne Greer for permission to reproduce. All rights reserved and permission to use this figure must be obtained from the copyright holder.

in balance with others, rather than as dominant colour schemes. Correspondence held by the National Network for the Arts in Health, for example, which ran over the last two decades of the twentieth century, noted that colours such as purple and blue should not be used too extensively.[55]

There remain many hospitals, or specific areas within them, where colours such as red are avoided. For example, in 2003 an article in *Architects' Journal* suggested that 'red and "dense" orange' can raise anxiety levels in maternity spaces, although it also presented the idea that 'wearing orange can encourage the mother of a premature baby to lactate'.[56] Dalke *et al.* also note that

> In dermatology departments, orange is not recommended as a background colour. Staff in these units also reported that reds and oranges make patients feel itchy; yet orange was particularly popular for a maternity unit … In mental health wards, oranges and reds are disliked.[57]

They also note that some mental health patients cannot tolerate orange and red, and some autistic people also struggle with the intensity of such colours.[58] Such issues remain concerns for inclusivity and accessibility, including in the light of disability legislation.[59]

The changes outlined to this point were also, of course, not universal across NHS hospitals. Colours could be changed more rapidly than architecture, but in general new colour schemes often continued to sit alongside older ones; hospitals were rarely redecorated throughout, but rather in segments or by area, or new wards were built onto older buildings with fresh colour palettes. 'Brightening up' was typically a piecemeal process. In practice, in line with the rise of patient-centred care, most of the new, vibrant colour schemes outlined thus far were in patient-facing areas. Although there was a general understanding that such colour schemes also benefitted the staff, it is significant that few staff-facing areas were redecorated in the 1980s and 1990s. In his 1998 cancer memoir, John Diamond reflected that one hospital was a 'rather gloomy Victorian mansion' but that 'tacked' onto it was 'a series of more modern buildings in bright brick and straight out of the pattern book of cheery hospitals'.[60] Significantly, Diamond noted, the patient-facing wards were mostly in the newer buildings, and 'it's only in areas like the histopathology department that staff work with the paint falling off the walls'.[61] More recently, particularly in the aftermath of COVID-19, staff areas have gained attention again.[62] As the problem of staff burnout has grown, there is growing attention to the value of providing spaces in hospitals that support staff rest and wellbeing – not just staff work.

Diamond's idea of a 'pattern book of cheery hospitals' has clear echoes in Owen Hatherley's scathing take-down of public architecture. In relation to the buildings of the Private Finance Initiative (PFI) scheme, launched by the Conservative Government in 1992 and expanded by New Labour after 1997, Hatherley described PFI buildings as 'chillingly blank', based on an 'idiom of clean lines, bright colours, red bricks and wipe-clean surfaces'.[63] PFI has been seen by many as a distinctive part of NHS architectural history, and in a King's Fund report from 2000 was criticised for using 'off the shelf' hospital design to cut the costs of private contractors.[64] There are, of course, more recent PFI hospitals where design innovation in architecture and interior design was made possible with the support of NHS Trusts; Southmead hospital's Brunel building, for example, opened in 2014 and drew its inspiration from Norwegian hospital architecture.[65] However, it is broadly true that many PFI hospitals – and PFI buildings in general – had a similar aesthetic. This was not, though, a revolution or a dramatic shift from the trends outlined to this point. The PFI model did not appear out of nowhere, but was the product of many years of evolving thought in hospital design, some of which had previously been part of collaboration between the public and private sectors. When the 'pattern book' was created in the late 1990s, it consolidated decades of movement towards more 'cheery' hospital design, albeit in a way that many critics saw as somewhat soulless.

Architectural shifts and interior design trends were closely interwoven, and by the end of the twentieth century 'warmth' and 'cheer' were more explicitly part of the design of a 'modern' hospital. There is a sense from both Diamond and Hatherley, however, that the reduction of 'cheer' to a 'pattern book' or 'idiom' could have the opposite emotional effect. Bright colours were also used in some NHS Trusts as local branding, for example for hospital charities, making them more a part of visual identity than an emotive signifier. In commercial terms, some bright colour palettes were informed more by hotel and shopping-centre models than healthcare principles. During site visits for this project in 2022–23, I noticed that the most common shade of 'red' across NHS sites is the burgundy Costa Coffee sign. Indeed, in 2008, *The Independent* found that 40 of 170 NHS Trusts had a branded fast food outlet; at the time, 24 were Costa Coffees, and the number has expanded since then.[66] Some of the emotional weight of colour appeared to be lost when it was perceived as a commercial or 'paint by numbers' approach, rather than thoughtful, local design.

Overall, bright colours were widespread by the turn of the century, in a further expansion of the colour palette of modernity. That said, in drawing such conclusions, it is important to remember the issues raised in Chapter 1 about the materiality of paint and colour. Bright colours have been particularly vulnerable to change over time, both as a result of human actions and natural forces such as weathering. Returning to the 'excessive red' of the (now) Dorset County Hospital, a site visit in 2023 revealed the site now to be a range of different shades of red: windows and doors exposed to the weather have faded, while others are brighter red because they have been protected from the elements or replaced. The same is true of some of the interiors, where once vibrant blue floors are now clearly weathered by sunlight to grey in many locations (Figure 5.8).

The hospital of the end of the century was brighter than that of 1948, but many bright colour palettes also faded or changed over

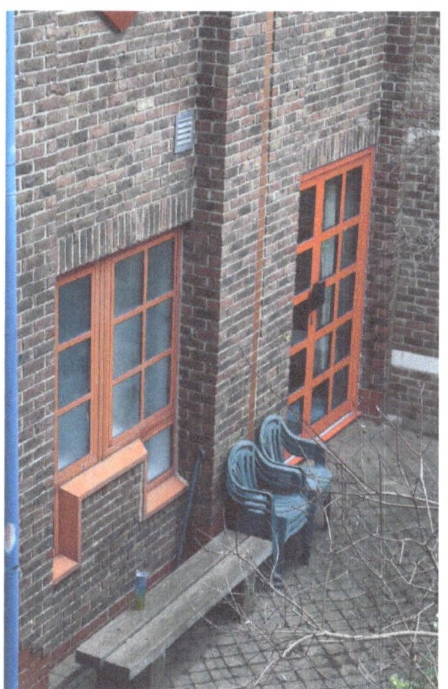

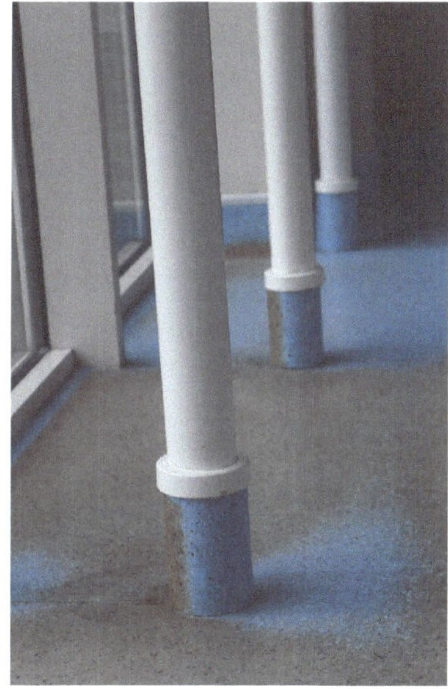

Figure 5.8 Weathering and colour change at Dorset County Hospital, Dorchester (previously West Dorset County Hospital), 2023. © Image: Victoria Bates. Reproduced with kind permission of Dorset County Hospital NHS Foundation Trust.

time. This material history is as important a part of the history of hospital colour as the design history outlined above. Many bright colours were also replaced over time with more neutral ones, but not necessarily as part of a design decision; estates teams needing to repaint walls as part of maintenance sometimes reverted to whites and creams because the paint was available. The brightening up of NHS hospitals might, then, be as much a history of an idea as it is a history of real material change. Brightness represented a new ideal for modern British healthcare, of vibrancy, activity, and efficiency.

Furniture and fittings: splashes of colour

Interior colour schemes in hospitals broadly followed trends outlined in the book to this point: late nineteenth- and early twentieth-century hospitals often used colours such as dark greens and browns, before being replaced by white in the 1930s, and then the early years of the NHS were marked largely by the rise of pastel colour schemes. Focusing on hospital interiors and walls, it would be easy to tell a story in which more vibrant or 'stimulating' colours were largely absent until at least the 1970s. There was some aversion to colours considered 'brash' until the end of the twentieth century, and primary colours were traditionally associated with warnings or with specific groups such as children. However, objects, fixtures, and fittings were often 'bright' much earlier than walls or interiors. They offered splashes and accents of bright colour that were significant in their own right, and should not simply be dismissed as aberrations, or as precedents for later trends.

The case study of red blankets offers an interesting counter-point to the idea that red was largely absent from hospitals until the late twentieth century. Barts Health NHS Trust holds postcard images of wards at the London Hospital, thought to be from the early twentieth century, in which red blankets are a dominant feature (Figure 5.9). In the London Hospital, despite the broad twentieth-century aversion to red in hospitals discussed above, these blankets were viewed very positively. The colour was a significant part of the identity of these blankets: they were known as 'day reds' (shown in the image) or 'night reds' (an older version, kept over the bed

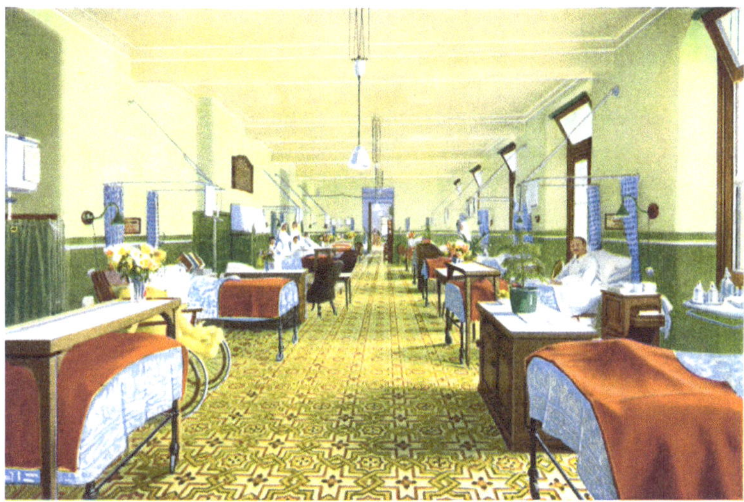

Figure 5.9 Barts Health NHS Trust Archives and Museums, RLHLH/P/2/11/43, London Hospital ward, c. 1900–10.

rail overnight). This terminology appeared to be specific to the London Hospital, and it is unclear how many other hospitals used red blankets or placed such emphasis on their colour. A database search for 'red blankets' and 'hospital' brings up firstly an article on the London Hospital from 1910, reporting a royal visit, in which it is noted that '[t]he garden, which looked delightful in the bright sun, was made still brighter by the blue uniforms of the sisters and the red blankets of the patients, many of whom were on the balconies which run round the quadrangle'.[67] The red blankets of the patients were specifically noted here, as bringing a notable 'brightness' to the hospital site, including when the patients sat under them on hospital balconies to stay warm.

The choice of red is significant in this example, as blankets of any colour would have served the practical function of protecting patients on balconies. As noted in Chapter 1, many hospitals around this time moved away from coloured bedding in the interests of hygiene. Red blankets in hindsight might have represented a more 'homely' or 'humanistic' aesthetic, though the colour also had a strong medical association due to the high profile of symbols such as that of the Red Cross. As with so many colours, the homely and the medicalised were not in tension here. Other sensory and spatial factors were also important in giving meaning to the red blanket, not least the fact that it was a textile object rather than a piece of medical equipment or a geometric, hard object such as a door. A red blanket for wrapping up on a hospital balcony on a cool day was materially and symbolically cosy. In this context, the blanket might have become what Kara Thompson describes (in *Blanket*, a close study of the object) as an 'intimate object [...]. It swaddles and caresses'; in this context the blankets offer a 'caress' to patients who might otherwise feel cold or alone.[68] The blanket could be a familiar and welcoming visual and multi-sensory symbol of care in a specific hospital.

It is, though, important to consider the other side of this picture. In her work on the history of nineteenth-century German hospital beds, Monika Ankele argues that bed treatment for mentally ill people was intended to homogenise patients: '[l]ying in their beds, their blankets pulled up to their chins, every patient's external appearance was similar to that of the next'.[69] The bed, Ankele suggests, 'took on a structuring function within the hospital space', orienting doctors and creating a 'kind of visible classification of patients'.[70] The rows of red blankets in Figure 5.9 could be read through a similar lens. Rather than creating a sense of identity and comfort, such blankets might have been a way of making patients seem homogeneous in their identical beds in long rows. It is difficult to know exactly how such a blanket was experienced or encountered in practice, but there was evidently no straightforward shared cultural meaning of 'red' as 'danger' in this context. Meaning was made by a range of factors, including the object itself, its positioning, the number of blankets in a room, the hospital in which they were used, the weather, and whether they were draped over a body or folded up neatly in lines on beds.

The specificity of hospitals and their local cultures is a crucial part of interpreting the meaning of red and red objects in hospitals, as it is with any colour or coloured object. In this example, the hospital red blanket seems to be a significant part of the visual identify of one particular hospital. Though hospital design was never fully standardised in Britain, hospitals of the early twentieth century arguably had a greater sense of individual visual identity – which extended to objects – because there was no central supply chain from which to draw. Certain colours could become part of the visual lexicon of specific hospitals, as opposed to the later development of a shared NHS colour palette. The meaning of red blankets was therefore site-specific within Britain, though this is not to claim that the London Hospital alone used them. There were also broad trends in what could be conceptualised as shared cultural meanings of red in English hospitals, which did not necessarily translate overseas or carry the same meaning for immigrants and visitors. In 1917, for example, *The Hospital* magazine bemoaned the English habit of sending red blankets to hospitals in Korea: '[p]eople in England commit a grave error of judgment, and, indeed, display a sad want of taste, when sending out a parcel of red blankets. Colours are only worn by juveniles in Korea, a fact which English people never seem to learn'.[71] Red blankets were evidently sufficiently popular in English hospitals at this time for the sending of a 'parcel of red blankets' to Korean hospitals to be noted here as a common problem.

Red is not the only bright colour that existed in early twentieth-century hospitals, and similar case studies could look at other furnishings or fabrics. A close look at red blankets, though, emphasises that bright colours existed in early twentieth-century hospitals and that such colours served specific purposes. Red did not always mean 'danger', when combined with other sensory signifiers of care. In the late 1950s the London Hospital 'reds' were adapted to be 'fixed around patients for medical examinations'.[72] Like curtains, adapted 'reds' were designed to offer comfort and privacy. They were removed from hospital design by this point, and turned into a functional object. The use of older 'reds' may have been the result of budgetary constraints in the 1950s and the wartime 'make do and mend' principle.[73] That said, the continued use of these older red blankets may have been a deliberate choice. As noted, red blankets were part of the visual identity of the London Hospital. As red itself fell out of fashion in material and interior design, the use of familiar 'reds' for patient examinations may have been comforting to long-term patients of that hospital.

A red blanket that was placed over somebody in an emergency had very different symbolism to one that was part of recuperation. In a recent publication *A History of Nursing in the North East and*

Cumbria, one nurse recalled being covered with a red blanket when she was sick as a child. Though the exact date of this memory is unclear, the nurse in question had joined the Royal College of Nursing in 1948, so we can locate it broadly in the early twentieth century. 'My parents were horrified', she notes, 'because I was taken away in the middle of the night in an ambulance, covered in a red blanket, to a remote place in County Durham, and taken into a great old building, to a ward where there were rows and rows of sick children'.[74] The red blanket stands out in this memory as an object of significance, seemingly as a prominent feature of her parents' memories rather than the child's own experience. Being taken away 'in an ambulance, covered in a red blanket' is a striking image, in which the red blanket symbolises alarm, fear, uncertainty, and anxiety.

Red blankets offer just one example of the many ways that vibrant colours – traditionally avoided in paints – were incorporated into hospitals through objects and furnishings. This trend became more widespread and systematic from the mid-century onwards. Harriet Richardson Blakeman notes that 'settees upholstered in yellows and reds' were found in the 'modern' Vale of Leven Hospital outpatients' waiting room in the 1950s.[75] In 1969 John Agate described 'turkey-red bed curtains' adding 'a brilliant splash of optimistic colour' to an old ward; this comment shows the shift towards seeing the stimulating potential of red as something positive, but still as a colour to be used in moderation.[76] In Guy's Tower, in the mid-1970s, the waiting area used 'a soft neutral general background' but with 'visual stimulation and emphasis of individual areas' created through decorative wall panels and 'strongly patterned and coloured furnishing fabrics over simple frames, cheap to buy, easy to move or replace'.[77] In 1971, *Architects' Journal* observed that a new hospital in Eastburn had wards 'lacking in colour except in the bedspread, curtains and decorations' and one in South Cheshire had 'gaily coloured curtains' alongside more colourful carpets.[78]

Doors were also a favoured location for touches of bright colour. Doors often had primary colours in the 'pure' forms, against a background of light or white hallways. The trend for bright coloured doors was in part practical, as doors were easy to change and paint compared with other decorative choices. Introducing bright colours in the form of fixtures and fittings was also increasingly easy over time, as companies started to create products in a wider range of vibrant colours, from entrance matting to railings and doors.[79] Colourful doors also reflected the symbolic and emotional significance of doors in hospitals, as important thresholds and points of potential anxiety. In an article on 'Colour in Hospitals' in 1961, interior architect Elmar Berkovich noted that

> The doors, in so far as they communicate with other rooms, may be given more emphasis by colour to provide a gay note in the colour scheme. It may sound strange, but the outer door of a patient's room plays an important part in the life of a sick person. The doctor, the nurse, the analyst and visitors enter and depart through this door. Hence the colour of this door should be an attractive one to lessen the tension of waiting.[80]

Brightly coloured doors also fitted with a trend to associate vibrant colours with modern, geometric shapes. It is perhaps no surprise to find such a connection between art and architecture; the Rietveld Schröder House built in the 1920s in Utrecht was part of the De Stijl movement with Piet Mondrian, and used blocks of white, yellow, and red.[81] These ideas continued to have influence into the post-war years. Le Corbusier's final building, built in Zurich in the 1960s, similarly used blocks of white along primary colours to dramatic effect.[82] One architect writing on colour in the late 1960s referenced the famous modern artworks of Mondrian from the 1930s: 'Composition in Red, White and Blue', which represented how bright colours – positioned carefully in relation to each other, to whiteness, and to clean lines – could be a balanced, modern aesthetic. The painting is 'an example of a powerful colour stimulus [...] expressed as an abstract rectilinear pattern reminiscent of architectural settings', the author noted, to prevent strong colours from becoming sombre 'without any relieving break between them'.[83] This way of thinking about whiteness was in line with that of Mondrian's abstract peer Wassily Kandinsky, who saw white as equivalent to silence, but emphasised that silence indicated possibility and played a similar role to a break in music; the break was itself full of meaning.[84] Many post-war attempts to brighten up hospital doors did indeed have something of the Mondrian about them. This might be seen as a way to contain or control colour, in line with a point that Lynda Nead raises about colour more generally at this time: 'although colour signified modernity and progress, there was something disturbing about it'.[85] Those who wrote on hospital colour schemes similarly emphasised the need for balance and for careful, contained uses of vibrant colours.

Bright doors were also early 'wayfinding' initiatives. In an article from the 1960s entitled 'Colour in Hospitals', John Agate noted that 'bold colours are rarely successful on a ceiling [...] Doors are a different matter. A variety of brightly coloured doors helps newly arrived or muddled patients to recognise their objectives easily'.[86] Coming more from the medical than the architectural perspective, Agate emphasised that the function of such bright doors was more important than their aesthetics, particularly for older patients or those with limited eyesight, for whom 'strong primary reds, yellows, and blues are ideal'.[87] Bright colours could also serve the specific needs of patients. In some hospitals, bright doors help people with dementia to navigate. With an ageing population, such concerns have become increasingly apparent in hospital design. Some criticise the idea that colours which 'infantilise' are necessary for people living with dementia, and argue that any differentiation in colour palette would achieve the same practical effect, but the use of yellow has been a common practice.[88]

Vibrant fixtures and fittings were often used to remedy some of the perceived limitations of older architecture. In 1982 one medical magazine reported that '[t]here is a porter at St Mary's Hospital for Women and Children in Manchester who delights in directing visitors and patients by telling them: "It's the door with the lion on it"'.[89] The lion doors were in part a navigation device, in line with the trends discussed above; they had value for staff, when giving directions, as well as for patients and visitors in finding their way around. The doors were also part of a wider decorative scheme that went 'a long way to civilising what, in the opinion of one consultant, was a particularly barbaric building which opened in early 1970'.[90] In March 1988, an article entitled 'Bright Ideas for Interiors' noted that 'a lick of paint can achieve as much as a redesign – provided it is chosen well and skilfully done', and advocated changing doorways as a simple way to achieve such change without great time and expense. The article was written by the Director of Works and Estates of Mid-Staffordshire HA, who would be in exactly the kind of role to influence hospital design through repainting rather than full-scale redesign. Instead of a 'dark doorway and down a long institutional hallway', he argued, 'anyone looking down a hallway with doors in each bay painted in a different colour can identify "their" door by its colour, rather than the time it takes to reach it'.[91]

Beds offered another option for low-risk, low-cost experiments with colour. One *Design Guide* on improving hospitals for long-stay residents noted the potential value of painting beds in bright colours in 1973: 'Where an adjustable bed is needed, some models of the King's Fund bed are not too clinical in appearance. Hospital beds can sometimes be reduced in height and their frames painted in bright colours (in non-chip finish)'.[92] Such comments were not just about adding some colour to furniture. They need to be understood in relation to the significance of hospital beds as material sites and symbols of care, a role that grew even more significant from the 1970s as the limited number of beds became a symbol of NHS crisis in the political sphere. Under Enoch Powell's 'Hospital Plan' there had been a deliberate reduction in bed numbers, laying the groundwork for 'community care', which sought to limit hospital long-stay inpatients. In this political and social climate, the hospital bed was symbolically crucial, as it became increasingly rare.[93] The King's Fund bed had been designed in the 1960s for patient comfort and for staff efficiency. It was both a modern and 'humanistic' object, which sought to reduce the uncomfortable, clinical feel of old hospital beds. By painting beds in bright colours, the *Design Guide* built on the principle that they symbolised care and attention rather than institutionalisation. The tone of the *Design Guide* implied that such limited additions of bright colour to selected, meaningful items of hospital furniture and fittings could be a significant change at a local level, perhaps even by ward staff, rather than part of integrated interior design schemes. They made such changes with the needs of patients in mind, though of course there was still a recognition of the practical requirements of the hospital setting with a reference to non-chip paint.

While there were few red or bright orange walls before the late twentieth century, there were many red objects. In addition to the doors, beds, and red blanket discussed here, there were many other colourful objects in hospitals. For example, the next section shows the importance of toys, both provided by hospitals and brought in by families, as part of the colourful chaos of children's play areas. As artist Christopher Tipping noted, in a recent interview,

> For a long time, there was a really big thing about you couldn't use red, for obvious reasons, but actually I think it's nonsense; people bring colour to the hospital in the clothes that they wear, in the cars that they drive, in the landscape that they bring with them and the relatives that come to visit them and all the clinicians that work there. People bring activity and pattern and colour and light and shade and everything to spaces.[94]

While hospitals were primarily decorated in white in the inter-war years, and in muted or pastel colours in the early post-war period, the people moving around them were not necessarily dressed in the same colours. Fabrics, clothing, furnishings, and toys were often much brighter than walls and moved in and out of the modern hospital. To recognise this is an important part of acknowledging that colour schemes were never static, nor did any colour exist in isolation.

Stimulation: play and primary colours

The trends outlined above for the late twentieth century can be seen as the overspill or broadening of some of the principles of children's hospitals, where visual and auditory 'noise' had long been encouraged as markers of play, distraction, and health. This section traces the history of colour in relation to play in design for children, to understand how such principles shaped the rise of bright colour schemes for adults.

Bright colours have long been thought the domain of animals or the young. A recent article on Britain's aversion to colour in *The Guardian* notes that this view was expressed explicitly in important publications, such as Goethe's 1810 *Theory of Colour*, and shared by thinkers, architects, and artists ranging from Aristotle to Le Corbusier.[95] This age-based colour theory explains why children's hospitals had long been brighter and more artistic than their adult counterparts. In a book on the history of hospital tile pictures, John Greene notes that in the late Victorian period it became particularly fashionable to 'brighten the plain tiled walls of children's wards with colourful tile pictures of nursery rhymes, fairy tales and other subjects which would interest and amuse sick children'.[96] At this time, coloured tiles were used widely elsewhere in hospital but often in plain, dark shades such as dark green. Though children's tiles at this time often did not vary dramatically in colour palette, their use of nursery rhyme imagery sought to create the atmospheric characteristics associated with liveliness, play and – to return to Greene's word – 'amusement'. Susan Barclay notes that this trend for hand-painted tiles for children was unique to British hospitals from the late nineteenth century onwards, because of the strength of its ceramic industry at this time.[97] However, some of these tiles were exported, and the use of tiles and mosaics to bring colour into hospitals had a long history across and beyond Europe.[98]

The rise of white 'hygienic' spaces for adults and children alike did not immediately displace colourful tiles for children. Tiles were also viewed as hygienic, and colourful pictures and nursery rhyme tile images were still being installed in many hospitals well into the 1930s. Although Chapter 1 showed that Great Ormond Street embraced the use of all-white tiles, this was an uneven trend. The King's Fund 'model hospital' from 1932 showed that more colourful tiles were still seen as good practice for children at the time.[99] Many of these tile-based images remained fairly traditional and not dramatically different from those of the late nineteenth century, though others did seem to 'modernise'; Phyllis Butler's 'Noah's Ark' panels for children at the Kent and Sussex Hospital, installed in the 1930s, remained traditional in theme but were Art Deco in style.[100] Such tile pictures helped to honour the period's interest in hygiene and children's perceived need for play and stimulation; that said, in wards for infants, they existed as much to be visual signifiers of 'a children's ward' for adults as they did to entertain babies.

Tile pictures were an important example of the way that children's needs were seen as distinct from those of other patients. Coloured tiles fell out of fashion in spaces for children and adults alike, in favour of painted murals or adhesive cartoons and other forms of colourful design viewed as more modern. However, the notion of children's distinct needs continued and indeed strengthened over the course of the century. As Roy Kozlovsky argues, in post-war hospital architecture, children were increasingly seen as an 'exception' whose emotional needs varied dramatically from those of adults.[101] Examples of influential cultural products included a 1952 film called 'A Two Year Old Goes to Hospital' (shown on British television in 1961), a booklet called *Care of Children in Hospital* by the American Academy of Pediatrics that was influenced by this film (1960), the British 'Platt Report' on the 'Welfare of Children in Hospital' (1959), and the 1961 formation of a new patient group Mother Care for Children in Hospital (later renamed the National Association for the Welfare of Children in Hospital).[102] Many of these outputs focused on children's experiences of hospital care and the particularly stressful nature of hospital for children separated from loved ones. In Britain, the Platt Report led to a loosening of restrictions around visiting times, albeit not in a neat or consistent way.

This context fed a renewed vigour around the subject of children in hospitals. Hospital design – including toys, playrooms, interior decorative schemes, and more – offered a way to mitigate some of the issues raised by paediatricians and others. Voluntary organisations, such as Leagues of Friends, often offered to pay for small-scale improvements or to supply toys.[103] The National Association for the Welfare of Children in Hospital even funded a playroom in the grounds of York Hospital.[104] They staffed it themselves as part of supporting visiting times, when they struggled to persuade paediatric staff to allow unrestricted visiting in the late 1960s. Many of the brightest colour schemes for children were in such playrooms. As with recuperating adults, those who designed hospital spaces – including medical practitioners – recognised that only children who felt well enough to play or were in the process of recovery might benefit from stimulating colour schemes. In 1955, for example, two colleagues working in child health wrote that in *The Lancet* that

> much more thought is required about the general design and decoration of children's hospitals [...] The child likes bright colours and attractive pictures, and there is no great difficulty in supplying these [...] Ideally a child who is not too ill should be admitted to a playroom attached to the ward, where the sight of cheerful toys will help him to lose his tension.[105]

This publication indicated that many children's hospitals were still in need of improvement. However, in the mid-1950s they were certainly doing more than many adult-facing spaces in this regard, and much hospital design was implicitly informed by the belief that children and 'bright colours' went hand-in-hand, even if just in the form of toys in playrooms.

The mid-century children's hospital echoed the British city, where the brightest colour was not found in the built environment but in the 'ephemera of everyday life'.[106] Colour was traditionally brought in through toys, while the design could actually be rather plain. Even in the absence of formal interior design or architectural interventions, clinical staff could have an impact on hospital spaces by ordering colourful toys or play materials. This practice echoes some of the 'everyday designing' discussed in Chapter 4 as part of constructing 'homeliness'. One receipt for Great Ormond Street Hospital from August 1958, for example, shows that a matron ordered a range of colourful goods, from rattles to a 'red ball', while other correspondence from the hospital refers to such toys being given as gifts.[107] Records for York District Hospital from across the 1980s and 1990s show the purchase of colourful crafting materials, blocks, and toys in shades ranging from 'scarlet red' to 'lemon yellow'.[108] Though some literature from the US recommended removing red crayons and other colours associated with pain or bruising (blue, black, and purple), there is no evidence of similar concerns in Britain.[109] Colourful objects in playrooms and playgrounds were part of multi-sensory play and engagement with hospital spaces.

Play was a brightly coloured, messy, and unstable process of 'doing' in hospitals.[110] Records of children's hospitals and playrooms depict a rather chaotic scene. One archived letter relating to York District Hospital in 1984, for example, observed the 'clutter and disorder of the playroom' and a health and safety assessment of the same site later observed that 'many cupboards are overflowing [...] many and varied toys out on floor'.[111] Toys were never display objects that were neatly positioned in relation to a chosen interior design or colour scheme; they were material, colourful, visual 'noise' that was constantly being moved, handled, transformed, and encountered in new ways. Great Ormond Street Hospital archives holds the draft of a speech given at some point soon after the publication of the Platt report, to the Annual Meeting of the Association of Mother Care for Children in Hospital, which spoke positively and evocatively about similar disorder:

> In the waiting hall at Great Ormond Street it is almost as easy to be run over by children riding pedal cars and carts as it is in the street! Toys are everywhere, the room is spacious and at the end of an outpatient session the Sister in charge of the Department is happily confronted with a scene that every mother faces after a play session in the drawing room.[112]

Bright colour was just one part of the multi-sensory cacophony that made such a playful atmosphere, and cannot be separated from objects, materials, spaces, and the interactions of children with them. Children also added back into the colour of the atmosphere, not only through their own often bright clothing, but through drawings or their own personal toys. *The Commemorative Book for the Hospital for Sick Children, Great Ormond Street* had a section called 'Impressions from the Children' that stated '[e]verywhere in the Hospital is colour and brightness. Toys and mobiles add to the party atmosphere, but most important of all are the drawings and paintings made by the children and exhibited on ward boards'.[113] Though this promotional book emphasised the 'party atmosphere', historians have shown that play was never 'just play' and that it could be an important way for children to deal with complex emotions or to build relationships.[114] Bright colours were also brought into hospitals not only through new types of playful space, but also through evolving types of playful care; for example, there was more professional and systematic use of hospital clowning for children internationally from the 1980s onwards.[115]

Many hospital playrooms were genuinely difficult to distinguish from schools throughout the late twentieth century. It is no coincidence that school design was such a significant influence on hospital design, including colour schemes, and many children's hospitals included schools for long-stay patients.[116] Much colour in schools and hospitals alike was in primary shades, provided through objects ranging from furniture to toys, creative materials and children's drawings on the walls. These overlaps are worth considering more closely, in relation to the history of school design. Scholars of the history of schools have recently turned away from the idea that school buildings were spaces of discipline and governance. For example, Tom Hulme, in his work on early twentieth-century schools in England and Wales, emphasises 'the emancipatory potential of school environments'.[117] Hulme's work shows that schools and healthcare buildings had long had many overlaps in design principles, even before they were part of a shared welfare state. Early twentieth-century schools shared hospitals' interest in the 'modern' principles of efficiency and hygiene discussed in Chapter 1, with an emphasis on ventilation, light, and air. These buildings were both part of the creation of a certain type of 'citizenship ... not only as a form of cultural identity or political action but also as an everyday concentration on the body to ensure the collective health of the nation'.[118] Over the course of the late twentieth century, the built environments of hospitals and schools alike increasingly facilitated the play and 'individual creativity' that Hulme notes was also a long-term feature of education buildings.

In her work on schools in mid-twentieth-century Britain, Laura Tisdall rightly emphasises a distinction between design ideals and the realities of the schools experienced by most children. She shows that there was growing acceptance of 'child-centred' design in schools, just as there was in hospitals, of which vibrant colour was an important part: in the late 1940s and early 1950s, educational innovators 'promoted brightly painted classrooms with large windows that let in the light'.[119] In practice, in schools and hospitals alike, the ideals of bright, child-centred, playful design did not always align with the practical realities of old infrastructure, budget constraints, and maintenance priorities. That said, the parallels between the two types of space and the growing interest both in brightness and in the idea of 'child-centredness' in both is significant.[120] Children would have experienced school-like hospital spaces as familiar, which may have changed how they responded to them. As Roy Kozlovsky argues, the Platt Report emphasised that 'emotions such as deprivation, fear and despair' felt by children in hospitals were in part the consequence of dislocating children from key familiar environments: 'the intimate environment of the home and the active, playful social life of the school'.[121] Efforts to make hospitals more playful, sometimes deliberately emulating schools, were in part a consequence of such studies. Colours were even sometimes explicitly used for educational purposes in hospitals, outside of hospital schools; when one hospital introduced flooring with a cartoon character holding 'a bunch of eight balloons in bright contrasting colours' in 1980, they reported that it served as an 'educational aid by helping to teach children the colours'.[122] Such work was part of the wider post-war project of a 'welfare-state discourse' in which patients were 'citizens in the making' who needed to be empowered, as part of rethinking and remaking modern healthcare.[123] Strategies such as new colour palettes and repainting offered a relatively easy and budget-friendly route to such goals.

Playgrounds also increasingly integrated artwork and colourful design schemes, and were familiar to many children. In the late 1980s, for example, a 'Children's Play Courtyard' was opened at Basingstoke General Hospital with a mural 'In the Garden of Eden' designed by Sarah Hosking and a 'Noah's Ark for children to play in'.[124] It is also important to remember – to quote two NHS consultants writing on children's playground equipment in 1993 – not only that 'sick children may naturally revert to play if suitable equipment is provided' but also that 'not all children in hospital are ill'.[125] Many spaces for children in hospitals, including some playrooms and playgrounds, were designed to distract young family members visiting sick relatives. As with school-like designs, such playgrounds and play courtyards would have been familiar to children from the wider world outside hospitals. Playgrounds were commonplace in twentieth-century Britain, and had been growing in prevalence since the nineteenth-century expansion of compulsory schooling. Brightly coloured play equipment was widely available for NHS playgrounds, and increasingly so over the course of the post-war years, because it was used so extensively elsewhere.

Trends seen in hospitals – of the rise of play, playgrounds, bright colours, and child-centred design – were part of wider modern British history. They were entwined with the history of schools, parks, leisure, health, and technology. Jon Winder's work on the history of playgrounds argues that they changed in form in around the 1920s and 1930s, with a shift in emphasis from health equipment (to support physical activity such as gymnastics) to more playful swings and slides.[126] The modern playground was child-centred and – rather than purely a mechanism of control or citizenship – increasingly a way 'to combine enjoyment, delight, freedom, and technology, all within an urban garden setting', which also linked to 'other types of amenity landscape'.[127] The playground, then, as a site for enjoyment and delight, was historically contingent, but it certainly had this meaning by the time that NHS hospitals were expanding their playground provision in the post-war years and beyond. Valerie Wright notes that 'in the immediate post-war decades in Britain, an emphasis on the importance of child welfare as an investment in the future coincided with a belief that play was essential to "normal" child development'.[128] In practice, she argues, municipal authorities often had to prioritise housing and schools over play areas, which came 'further down the list, if delivered at all'.[129] However, her work on children living in high-rise flats in post-war Glasgow shows that children were certainly familiar with playgrounds and adapted many different types of space to integrate play into their daily lives.

In architecture and interior design, bright colours often functioned as an invitation for play or interaction. The flooring of Llewelyn-Davies Weeks's 1987 QEQM building at St Mary's Hospital in London, for example, had puzzle pieces that – through a combination of colour, shape, and careful positioning – implicitly encouraged children to hop between them. Similar principles were found in other buildings, including Hull Royal Infirmary, where, in the new children's unit, to quote the Head of Children's Services from 1990,

> little footprints in the flooring indicate the way to the bathroom and toilets [...] there are boards above each bed upon which the youngsters can scribble or stick their own cards, posters and drawings. Incorporated in the playroom floor are giant games of snakes-and-ladders and hopscotch [...] Fun things all help towards therapy.[130]

Images from the Powell & Moya 'Variety Club' building at Great Ormond Street Hospital also show the extensive interior use of colour. Colourful artworks were designed to be interactive and an integrated part of the built environment, including a famous large red bus where children could sit, play, and pretend to drive (Figure 5.10). Other sites included interactive and playful sculptures around this time, again echoing the school playground in many ways. In 1991, for example, Dorset County Hospital installed a 30-foot kinetic artwork that moved with the wind and encouraged playful interaction. It could also be seen from the children's ward. This installation was in the traditional primary colours associated with children, in the form of large crayons (Figure 5.11).

Such works represent an important shift from the tile pictures discussed above. Although viewing has never been a passive or purely visual activity, it is rarely a playful one. There was a subtle shift over the course of the twentieth century in the design of children's

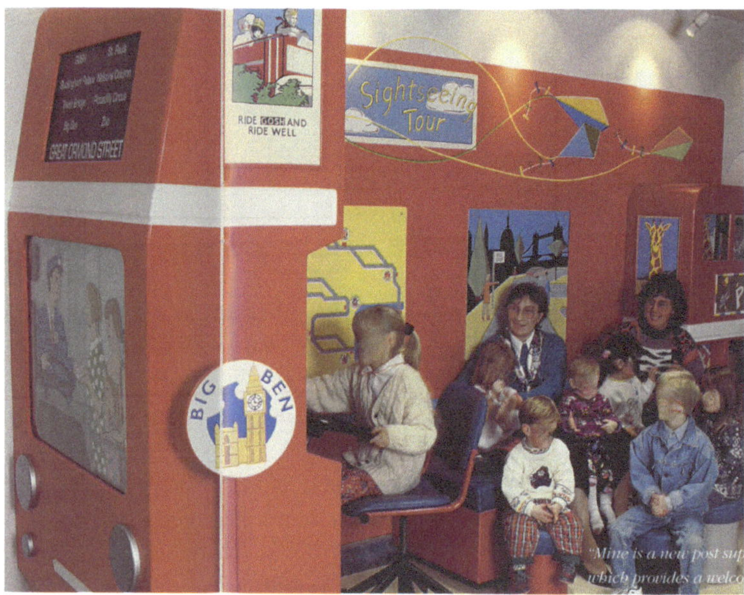

Figure 5.10 Great Ormond Street Archive, B-INT 02702, Great Ormond Street Hospital play bus. © Reproduced with kind permission of Archive Service, Great Ormond Street Hospital for Children NHS Foundation Trust.

hospitals. Children and young people were encouraged – through a combination of colour, shape, and materiality – to interact physically, rather than just emotionally or mentally, with their surroundings. 'Energetic' and 'playful' colour schemes were not simply signifiers of emotional states, in the way that 'cheerful' colour schemes often were. The colours were built into material environments that encouraged interaction, which changed the meaning of stimulation: from something consumed, to something produced through embodiment.

These trends were also evident in international children's hospital design towards the end of the century. *Hospital Development* provided one example of a colourful 'playful and whimsical' design from San Diego in 1993 that was designed in collaboration with staff, visitors, and patients, and which made extensive use of primary colours.[131] In many children's hospitals, it is difficult to distinguish colour schemes from the objects that they tint, as they are so entwined

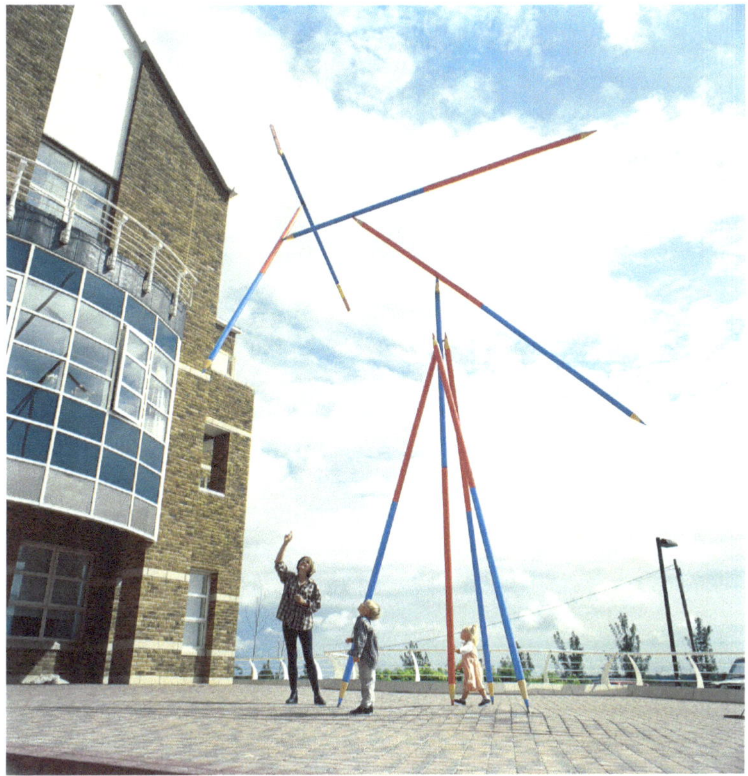

Figure 5.11 'Blue and Red Crayons' by Peter Logan, 1991, Dorset County Hospital, Dorchester (previously West Dorset County Hospital). © Reproduced with kind permission of Dorset County Hospitals (DCH) Arts in Hospital, Dorset County Hospital NHS Foundation Trust. All rights reserved and permission to use this figure must be obtained from the copyright holder.

with the concept of play. In the early 2000s one Oslo hospital paediatric and maternity wing had

> a soft play area, bright colo[u]rs and a fountain. The wing has its own school and a bed for parents in each child's room. Colo[u]rs and furniture in the hospital change constantly, from pinks and blues in the patient rooms to energetic yellows in the physical therapy rooms. Waiting rooms have computers, foosball tables, pianos and television sets.[132]

Such design schemes marked a step away from bright colours and murals in terms of the 'integral' use of colour and child-friendly interiors. The Hospital Sant Joan de Déu Barcelona Children's Hospital, a 1970s building transformed in 2008–18, has a large red slide to connect its floors inside.[133] These trends were happening in parallel and in dialogue with the rise of vibrant colour in more adult-facing spaces in the late twentieth and early twenty-first centuries. They were important in showing the possibilities of colour for stimulating physical and mental recovery, as well as potentially reducing demands on busy staff by keeping patients entertained and supporting whole families.

The idea of a clear difference between spaces for 'children' and 'adults', on which the analysis to this point has been based, is of course simplistic. Children were also not the only people in children's hospitals. A range of adults also inhabited these spaces, from visitors to staff. Some children in hospitals never entered child-facing spaces, but rather were visitors or accompanied family members to other parts of hospitals. Children were also, like adults, a heterogeneous group. One architect recently commented to me that 'there's always been the theory that children like primary colours' but there is evidence that neurodivergent children actually prefer pastels.[134] Children also varied significantly in age. Research in both Britain and Australia has shown that older children can feel alienated by spaces in hospitals that they perceive as 'babyish', often interpreting 'visual cues' such as bright colours and toys as signs that spaces are not for them.[135]

Architects and designers did implicitly show some awareness of this throughout the late twentieth century, in adapting the principles of playful and colourful design for different age groups. In 1974, for example, architect Joyce Bolchover published an article in *Hospital Development* about an adolescent unit at St Mary's Hospital in Manchester where 'very bright colours are used in small areas – a window reveal, balcony walls, day-room wall … The colour scheme does get a reaction – the local newspaper in describing the unit called it "pop"'.[136] In their visit in 1996, the Southern Derbyshire Community Health Council noted 'a graffiti board for the teenagers'.[137] This distinction between children of different ages, or children and adolescents, was evident throughout the late twentieth century, particularly if the site or space allowed for some separation. For example, when a new children's unit was opened at Hull Royal Infirmary in 1990, the Head of Children's Services noted that 'the colour scheme for the older children is lovely and bright, while we've chosen gentler pastels for the babies'.[138] In this sense, grounds emerged on which such principles could be integrated into adult care, as architects and designers started to break down the child/adult binary to show that playfulness could benefit adolescents and young adults.

Towards the end of the century, playfulness started to seep into design for adults. Owen Hatherley, in his comments on the PFI 'idiom', argues that by the end of the twentieth century a great deal of public architecture was designed 'as if furnishing a children's ward'.[139] Hatherley is implicitly critical of this trend. However, for others, the model of a 'children's ward' has marked a helpful way to break free of institutional decorative schemes. There were no adult equivalents to playgrounds or playrooms. However, some of the examples given in the first section of this chapter can be seen as playful, for example in the use of bright colours to encourage laughter and joy. Some patients also used language around play and fun to describe these new, more vivid colour schemes. Giving feedback on the West Dorset County Hospital in the early 1990s, one patient noted that it looked both 'smart' and 'rather Legoland-ish'.[140] In architectural terms, work on US hospital design has argued that modern hospitals have been notoriously 'conservative' with 'cautious' people often making the decisions.[141] However, the playful principles of postmodernism still had some influence. To quote Stephen Verderber and David J. Fine:

> If modern buildings were, according to their critics, severe, conservative, monotonous, minimalist, and restrictive, postmodern buildings could be the opposite: unorthodox in their composition and use of materials, colo[u]rful, ironic, ornamented, and historicist.[142]

There was some evidence of such colourful and unorthodox hospital design in Britain, even if not a full-scale turn to postmodernism.

The history of multi-sensory playful, interactive design shows that brightness was more than just an aesthetic choice. Brightness was part of the making of space and of new ways of encountering and interacting with hospitals. It represented stimulation, positivity, and vibrancy; for those in certain settings, such as children's wards, recovery, or waiting, multi-sensory bright colours invited new and more active ways of being in hospital. The idea of inviting patients to be more active participants in hospital spaces was not simply a decorative choice, but aligned with shifting healthcare principles in the NHS.

Conclusions

Broad design trends, in hospital interiors and exteriors, give the impression of NHS hospitals getting ever brighter over the course of the late twentieth century. Some of the changes were linked to wider shifts in architecture, art, and design. Architects, planners, and citizens in modern Britain, particularly its cities, were embracing more vibrant, non-natural colours in general, and turning towards more playful design. Hospitals were also, in many ways, specific built environments that contained within them a range of different spaces.

Some of the trends outlined here reflected political debates around healthcare, for example for children and the expansion of visitor numbers. Behind these colour changes were shifts in healthcare, health, and illness that allowed brighter colours into hospitals without the fear of 'over-stimulation'. People were spending, in general, much less time in hospitals and moving through them more quickly.[143] The idea that people needed 'restful' colour schemes for lengthy periods of convalescence was no longer relevant. Decorative choices were also part of negotiating what 'patient-centred' care felt and looked like, against a backdrop of the rise of the 'patient-consumer'. Hospitals were increasingly modelled not on 'functional' colour schemes of workplaces and educational institutions as in the post-war period (factories, schools) but increasingly on the more 'decorative' schemes of homes and commercial spaces such as hotels and shopping centres.[144]

This overview story is made more complicated by attention to specific types of colourful object or patient groups. Colours such as red were not avoided to the extent that has often been assumed, and had long been meaningful and important for people in hospitals. The NHS hospital was also not suddenly awash with shades of scarlet. However, splashes of previously avoided 'garish' colours became much more commonplace in hospital design from the 1980s onwards. The idea that hospitals should and could be 'playful' expanded beyond children, to invite a more interactive and active way of existing in the hospital. This change allowed for more vibrant design throughout hospitals, and supported subtle shifts in the healthcare principles that underpinned the NHS. It expanded the colour palette of modernity and changed the meaning of 'brightness' once more, as new vibrant colours continued to exist in dialogue with previous iterations of 'bright' in the form of pastels and whiteness.

Notes

1 Peter Scher, 'Dorset County Hospital, Phase 2', *Hospital Development*, 28 (1997), p. 19.
2 *Ibid.*
3 Iden Wickings, *Improving Hospital Design: A Report on the King's Fund Hospital Design Competition for 1993* (King Edward's Hospital Fund for London, 1994), p. 39; The second phase of the hospital did not repeat this colour palette, in response to 'some criticisms of Phase 1', but the bright colours of Phase 1 remain an important part of NHS hospital history; Scher, 'Dorset County Hospital Phase 2', p. 21.
4 Mark Michael Smith, *Sensing the Past: Seeing, Hearing, Smelling, Tasting, and Touching in History* (University of California Press, 2007), p. 25.
5 Lucy Faire and Denise McHugh, 'Twelve Shades of Grey: Encountering Urban Colour in the Street in British Provincial Towns, c. 1945–1970', *Urban History*, 46 (2019), pp. 288–308; Martin Moore, '"Bright-While-You-Wait"? Waiting Rooms and the National Health Service, c. 1948–58', in Jennifer Crane and Jane Hand (eds), *Posters, Protests, and Prescriptions: Cultural Histories of the National Health Service in Britain* (Manchester University Press, 2022), p. 214.
6 C. P. Biggam, *The Semantics of Colour: A Historical Approach* (Cambridge University Press, 2012), pp. 4–5.
7 For example, in 1934 a hospital in Dublin was described as having 'bright colour schemes of the wards and corridors [which] give an atmosphere of brightness and airiness'; 'Atmosphere of Efficiency. Dublin's Latest Hospital. Elimination of Noise', *The Irish Times*, 17 December 1934, p. 7.

8 Wellcome Library, PP/RMS/A/1, 'Report of Joint Visit by Mr D. J. Petty, Senior Architect, and Dr Shaw, Senior Medical Officer, Ministry of Health to Denmark, Sweden, Finland and Norway, 25th April–28th May 1955'.
9 Jenson and Nicholson, *The Function of Colour in Factories, Schools and Hospitals* (Jenson and Nicholson, c. 1940s/1950s), p. 75 (see Chapter 2, note 11 for details of publication date); see Nuffield Provincial Hospitals Trust, *Studies in the Functions and Design of Hospitals* (Oxford University Press, 1955), p. 113 for an example of this use of accent colours, though at this time they were still considered experimental.
10 Arthur L. Hall, 'Colour in the Hospital', *The Hospital*, June 1951, p. 384.
11 Faire and McHugh, 'Twelve Shades of Grey', abstract.
12 Sarah Street, '"Colour Consciousness": Natalie Kalmus and Technicolor in Britain', *Screen*, 50 (2009), p. 208.
13 Christine Slobogin, '"Something Useful in a National Sense": Percy Hennell's Surgical and Nationalist Colour Photography, 1940–1948', *Visual Culture in Britain* (2023), p. 4. See also Lynda Nead, *The Tiger in the Smoke: Art and Culture in Post-War Britain* (Yale University Press, 2017).
14 Cited in Elle Hunt, 'It's Not Beige, It's Not Grey: It's Greige – And It's Why All Our Houses Look the Same', 25 May 2022, https://www.theguardian.com/lifeandstyle/2022/may/25/greige-color-paint-popular-interior-decorating-design [accessed: 26 February 2024].
15 For example, 'if a nurse in one of the rooms is in an emergency and communicates to one of the nurse stations, a red light appears, accompanied by a high/low 800/680 HZ emergency tone sound'. 'Communications', *Hospital Development*, 11 (1983), p. 32.
16 Joe Moran, 'Crossing the Road in Britain, 1931–1976', *The Historical Journal*, 49 (2006), pp. 477–96.
17 Faber Birren, *New Horizons in Color* (Reinhold Publishing Corporation, 1955), np.
18 London Metropolitan Archives, 'Evaluation of New Guys House', A/KE/I/01/024/059.
19 Brian C. Pierman (ed.), *Color in the Health Care Environment* (Department of Commerce/National Bureau of Standards Special Publication 516, 1978), foreword III.
20 David Howes and Constance Classen, *Ways of Sensing: Understanding the Senses in Society* (Routledge, 2014), p. 41.
21 'Improving with Print', *Hospital Development*, 11 (1983), p. 19.
22 Milton F. Shore (ed.), *'Red is the Color of Hurting': Planning for Children in the Hospital* (National Institute of Mental Health, 1965).

23 For the history of red as a 'dangerous colour' see Michel Pastoureau, *Red: The History of a Color*, trans. Jody Gladding (Princeton University Press, 2017 [2016]), pp. 144–92. For an example of an association between red and danger in Maasai communities, see Josephellah N. Kaburi, *Impact of Applied Colour in Middle Class Interior: A Case Study of Nyayo Highrise Estate in Nairobi* (PhD Dissertation: University of Nairobi, 2007), p. 33.

24 Cited in Amy Yi-Chun Chen, 'Visual Melodies: Design and Evaluation of an Interactive Art Installation for Clinical Environments' (PhD Dissertation: University of Technology, Sydney, 2012), pp. 29–30.

25 This interest was wide-ranging, and can also be seen in the growing interest in views out of windows discussed in Chapter 6.

26 John Agate, 'Colour Can Transform Our Older Hospitals', *Health*, 6 (1969), p. 14.

27 D. W. A. McCreadie, 'A Hospital Colour Scheme', *BMJ* (June 1962), pp. 1687–8.

28 Alistair Fair, '"Modernization of Our Hospital System": The National Health Service, the Hospital Plan, and the 'Harness' Programme, 1962–77', *Twentieth-Century British History*, 29 (2018), pp. 547–75.

29 Susan Black, 'Interior Design Trends', *Hospital Development*, 10 (1982), p. 24.

30 Anna Katrine Hansen, Marie Bitsch Christiansen, Jana Sanyova, and Kim Pilkjær Simonsen, 'Analysis of Poul Gernes' painted folding doors at Herlev Hospital', *Heritage Science*, 6 (2018), p. 1.

31 Tim Edensor, 'What Color is this Place?', *GeoHumanities*, 9 (2023), p. 437.

32 Ulrikka S. Gernes and Peter Michael Nornug, *The Medicine of Colours: Poul Gernes and Copenhagen University Hospital at Herlev* (Borgen, 2003), p. 45.

33 Ronald Weeks, 'Interior Design: Hospitals', *The Architectural Review* (July 1980), p. 46. Though hospital arts have developed a great deal, complaints about the over-use of posters and their contribution to visual noise in hospitals remain commonplace.

34 For more detail on the history of hospital arts, see Chapter 4.

35 'Installations', *Hospital Development*, 8 (1980), p. 15.

36 'Milton Keynes DGH', *Hospital Development*, 12 (1984), p. 28.

37 Ronald Weeks, 'Interior Design: Hospitals', *The Architectural Review*, July 1980, p. 55.

38 Richard Saxon, 'Appraisal', *Architects' Journal*, September 1983, p. 60.

39 'Roundabout: St Mary's Hospital, Paddington', *Hospital Development*, 12 (1984), p. 6.

40 There are differing dates given for Bournemouth Hospital, but the texts lead me to understand that it was completed in 1988 and opened in 1989; 'Design-Build for Poole Clinic', *Hospital Development*, 16 (1988), p. 5.
41 Tony Monk, *HLM50+: Towards a Social Architecture* (Routledge, 2018), p. 81.
42 *Ibid.*; Scher, 'Dorset County Hospital, Phase 2', p. 19.
43 Monk, *HLM50+*, p. 81.
44 *Hospital Development*, 24 (1993), November cover.
45 As Hilary Mantel reflects, '[t]here is a colour of paint that doesn't seem to exist any more, that was a characteristic pigment of my childhood. It is a faded, rain-drenched crimson, like stale and drying blood'. Hilary Mantel, *Giving up the Ghost: A Memoir* (Harper Perennial, 2004 [2003]), p. 25.
46 Susan Barclay, 'When It's Not the Main Game: Art in Hospitals' (PhD Dissertation: University of Western Sydney, 2015), p. 37.
47 Robert Sloane, 'The Healing Arts', *Hospital Development*, 15 (1987), p. 39.
48 Peter Stone, 'Appraisal', *Architects' Journal*, 19 June 1974, pp. 1382–5.
49 Anne Greer, 'Colour Therapy', *Hospital Development*, 30 (1999), p. 19.
50 'Roundabout: St Mary's Hospital, Paddington'.
51 John Davion, 'Ward Conversion for AIDS Patients at The Middlesex Hospital', *Hospital Development*, 15 (1987), p. 13.
52 On the commercialisation model for American hospitals, see David Charles Sloane and Beverlie Conant Sloane, *Medicine Moves to the Mall* (Johns Hopkins University Press, 2003).
53 Greer, 'Colour Therapy', p. 20.
54 *Ibid.*
55 Goldsmiths archive, NNAH/Baron/1/35/a, 'Baron Art in Health Papers: London Hospitals', 1983–99.
56 'From Here to Maternity', *Architects' Journal*, 18 December 2003, https://www.architectsjournal.co.uk/archive/from-here-to-maternity [accessed: 5 March 2024].
57 Hilary Dalke *et al., Lighting and Colour for Hospital Design* (NHS, 2004), p. 19.
58 *Ibid.*, p. 8; Sardar S. Shareef and Guita Farivarsadri, 'The Impact of Colour and Light on Children with Autism in Interior Spaces from an Architectural Point of View', *International Journal of Arts and Technology*, 11 (2019), pp. 153–64.
59 Dalke *et al., Lighting and Colour for Hospital Design*, p. 8.

60 John Diamond, *C: Because Cowards Get Cancer Too…* (Random House, 1998), p. 74.
61 *Ibid.*
62 This issue came up in a number of interviews I did for the 'Sensing Spaces of Healthcare' project. For example, Victoria Shepherdson interviewed by Victoria Bates, 8 December 2022. Victoria Bates, 'Sensing Spaces of Healthcare' interviews, published December 2024, https://doi.org/10.5523/bris.3b8eg2be3ecw52vt38l7nq9kah
63 Owen Hatherley, *A Guide to the New Ruins of Great Britain* (Verso, 2011 [2010]), p. viii.
64 Robert Booth, 'Think Tank Accuses PFI of "Off-the-Shelf" Hospital Design', https://www.architectsjournal.co.uk/archive/think-tank-accuses-pfi-of-off-the-shelf-hospital-design [accessed: 27 February 2024].
65 Vicky Casey interviewed by Victoria Bates, 20 January 2023.
66 'Spending Power: Costa Coffee Colonises NHS', *The Independent*, 30 October 2008, https://www.independent.co.uk/life-style/health-and-families/health-news/spending-power-costa-coffee-colonises-nhs-979802.html [accessed: 27 February 2024].
67 'King George's Visit to the London Hospital', *The Hospital*, 6 August 1910, p. 561.
68 Kara Thompson, *Blanket* (Bloomsbury, 2018), p. xvi.
69 Monika Ankele, 'From a Patient's Point of View', in Rob Boddice and Bettina Hitzer (eds), *Feeling Dis-ease in Modern History: Experiencing Medicine and Illness* (Bloomsbury, 2022), p. 245.
70 *Ibid.*, p. 244.
71 'Life in a Korean Hospital', *The Hospital*, 23 June 1917, p. 230.
72 Barts Health NHS Trust Archives and Museums, RLHINV/1174, 'Adapted Blanket Used for Outpatient Medical Examinations', catalogue entry, 1958.
73 *Ibid.*
74 Royal College of Nursing, *A History of Nursing in the North East and Cumbria: A Report in Celebration of International Nurses' Day* (RCN, 2013), p. 3.
75 Harriet Richardson Blakeman, 'Medicine and Modernity: Fifty Years of NHS Hospital Building in Scotland, 1948–1998' (PhD Dissertation: University of Edinburgh, 2023), p. 51.
76 Wellcome Library, ART/AFH/A/9/9, John Agate, 'Colour in Hospital, *World Medicine*, 20 May 1969, p. 16.
77 London Metropolitan Archives, H09/GY/A/365/025, *Guy's Tower* publication, 1976. Thanks to Agnes Arnold-Forster for drawing my attention to the colour in this source.

78 G. L. Worsley, 'Building Study: Two Hospitals', *Architects' Journal*, November 1971, p. 1071.
79 Such adverts can be found throughout *Hospital Development* magazine across the 1980s and 1990s. See the adverts in the Hospital Interiors special issue of 1988.
80 Wellcome Library, ART/AFH/A/9/9, Elmar Berkovich, 'Colour in Hospitals', *International Lighting Review*, 12 (1961), pp. 121–3.
81 This location was visited by the author in spring 2023; see also John Gage, *Colour in Arts* (Thames & Hudson Ltd, 2006), p. 67. On other examples of such colour use in Modernist architecture see Maria-Cristina Florian, 'The Myth of Pure White Architecture: How Architects of Modernity Used Color', 3 August 2023, https://www.archdaily.com/1004970/the-myth-of-pure-white-architecture-how-architects-of-modernity-used-color [accessed: 14 May 2024].
82 Catherine Dumont d'Ayot, with Tim Benton (eds), *Le Corbusier's Pavilion for Zurich: Model and Prototype of an Ideal Exhibition Space* (Lars Müller Publishers, 2013). This location was also visited by the author in May 2024.
83 H. L. Gloag and M. J. Keyte, 'Rational Aspects of Colouring in Building Interiors', in Alexander C. Hardy (ed.), *Colour in Architecture* (Leonard Hill Books, 1967), p. 34.
84 Heimonen and Kuuva note this, writing on the symbolism of white in hospital corridors in Finland, in Kirsi Heimonen and Sari Kuuva, 'A Corridor That Moves: Corporeal Encounters with Materiality in a Mental Hospital', in Monika Ankele and Benoit Majerus (eds), *Material Cultures of Psychiatry* (Transcript Verlag, 2020), p. 344.
85 Nead, *The Tiger in the Smoke*, p. 146.
86 Wellcome Library, ART/AFH/A/9/9, John Agate, 'Colour in Hospital, *World Medicine*, 20 May 1969, p. 14.
87 Agate, 'Colour in Hospital', p. 13.
88 Anonymous [1001] interviewed by Victoria Bates on 14 July 2023: 'it infantilises everything ... a dementia-friendly room shouldn't look like children should be sitting in there and unfortunately a lot of companies go for that. They have clocked onto the idea that you need contrast so they have gone for bright yellow and red toilet signs'. For an image of yellow doors see Historic England, 'A ward Corridor at St George's Hospital, Tooting', 1988, https://historicengland.org.uk/images-books/photos/item/JLP01/10/34505 [accessed: 28 February 2024].
89 Wellcome Library, ART/AFH/A/9/9, Terence Hogan, 'How a Dismal Children's X-Ray Unit Became a Colourful Jungle', cutting, 18 February 1982, np; on colourful doors in children's hospitals see also 'Hospital

Check-Ups: Two Children's Facilities Put Under Scrutiny, *Architects' Journal*, October 1996, p. 38.

90 Hogan, 'Children's X-Ray Unit'.

91 C. B. Denne, 'Bright Ideas for Interiors', *Hospital Development*, 16 (1988), p. 19.

92 Jean Symons, *CEH Design Guide 1: Improving Existing Hospital Buildings for Long-Stay Residents* (CEH, 1973), p. 22.

93 Agnes Arnold-Forster and Victoria Bates, 'Care and Crisis: Making Beds in the National Health Service', *Journal of British Studies* (2024), pp. 1–27.

94 Christopher Tipping interviewed by Victoria Bates, 25 March 2023.

95 Hunt, 'It's Not Beige, It's Not Grey'.

96 John Greene, *Brightening the Long Days: Hospital Tile Picture* (Tiles and Architectural Ceramics Society, 1987), xiii.

97 Barclay, 'When It's Not the Main Game', p. 118.

98 Uğurgül Tunç kindly shared with me examples of such tiles from her own research, including from thirteenth-century Turkey. She also notes that British tiles made their way overseas. For example, tiles from Wales reached the British Seamen's Hospital in Istanbul completed in 1904. See Uğurgül Tunç, 'Spaces of Healthcare and Hospitals in the Late Ottoman Empire and Early Turkish Republic' (PhD Dissertation: Koç University, 2024).

99 Science Museum Group, 'Model of a Hospital Promoting the King Edward's Hospital Fund, 1932', https://collection.sciencemuseumgroup.org.uk/objects/co122109/model-of-a-hospital-promoting-the-king-edwards-hospital-fund-model [accessed: 7 March 2024].

100 'Kent and Sussex Hospital tiles fail to sell at auction', 17 October 2012, https://www.bbc.co.uk/news/uk-england-kent-19924037 [accessed: 27 February 2024]; 'The Virtual Museum of Poole Pottery', https://www.pooleimages.co.uk/carters-tiles [accessed: 27 February 2024]. Thanks to Robert Proctor for drawing my attention to these.

101 Roy Kozlovsky, 'Programming Emotional Care: The Nuffield Study of the Children's Hospital, 1963', *Childhood in the Past*, 13 (2020), pp. 121–37; on growing post-war attention to children's emotional health see also Teri Chettiar, *The Intimate State: How Emotional Life Became Political in Welfare-State Britain* (Oxford University Press, 2023).

102 Milton F. Shore (ed.), *'Red is the Color of Hurting': Planning for Children in the Hospital* (National Institute of Mental Health, 1965), p. 1; Charlotte Williamson, *Towards the Emancipation of Patients: Patients' Experiences and the Patient Movement* (Bristol University Press, 2010), pp. 80–1.

103 On the wider significance of such organisations see Gareth Millward, '"Its Many Workers and Subscribers Feel That Their Services Can Still Be of Benefit": Hospital Leagues of Friends in the English West Midlands, c. 1948–1998', *Social History of Medicine*, 36 (2023), pp. 433–55.

104 Williamson, *Towards the Emancipation of Patient*, pp. 80–1.

105 R. S. Illingworth and K. S. Holt, 'Children in Hospital: Some Observations on their Reactions with Special Reference to Daily Visiting', *The Lancet*, December 1955, p. 1257.

106 Lucy Faire and Denise McHugh, 'Twelve Shades of Grey: Encountering Urban Colour in the Street in British Provincial Towns, c. 1945–1970', *Urban History*, 46 (2019), p. 288.

107 Archive Service, Great Ormond Street Hospital for Children NHS Foundation Trust, GOS/15/143, 'Gifts of Toys to the Hospital', 1957–68.

108 Borthwick Institute, YDH/1/3/11, 'File of Orders for Equipment and Supplies, 1984–98'.

109 Susan Castelluccio, 'The Relationship of Colour Planning in Designing a Pediatric Oncology Unit to the Symbolic Meaning of Colors as Seen in Patients' Graphic Productions', in Brian C. Pierman (ed.), *Color in the Health Care Environment* (Department of Commerce/National Bureau of Standards Special Publication 516, 1978), pp. 25–6.

110 On 'doing' in histories of play see Stephanie Olsen, 'Learning How to Feel through Play: At the Intersection of the Histories of Play, Childhood and the Emotions', *International Journal of Play*, 5 (2016), pp. 323–8.

111 Borthwick Archives, YDH/1/3/13, Letter regarding Playroom, 1984; Borthwick Archives, YDH 1/3/6, Nursing Support Manager, Playroom Risk Assessment, 1998.

112 Archive Service, Great Ormond Street Hospital for Children NHS Foundation Trust, GOS/15/302, 'Nursing Mothers' Unit', 1959–77. It is not clear from the draft who gave the speech, but presumably someone connected to this Association.

113 *The Commemorative Book for the Hospital for Sick Children, Great Ormond Street* (Manor House Press, 1991), p. 173.

114 Olsen, 'Learning How to Feel through Play'.

115 Anthony Ryan and Grace Neville, '*Le Petit Journal*, Clowns & Children in Hospital in Victorian London', https://hekint.org/2017/01/30/le-petit-journal-clowns-children-in-hospital-in-victorian-london/ [accessed: 25 September 2024]; Peter Spitzer, 'Essay: Hospital Clowns – Modern-Day Court Jesters at Work', *The Lancet*, 368 (2006), S34–S35. This practice was primarily for children, but its potential value for adults has been

increasingly explored recently, see Ludivine Plez, Melissa Holland, Priyanka Kulasegarampillai, Thun-Carl Sieu, and Stefanie Blain-Moraes, '"I Made You a Small Room in My Heart": How Therapeutic Clowns Meet the Needs of Older Adults in Nursing Homes', *International Journal of Qualitative Studies on Health and Well-being*, 18 (2023), 2238989.

116 As noted above, school colour schemes were an explicit influence on Newcastle Regional Hospital Board, *The Use of Colour in Hospitals* (NRHB, 1955); see also 'Play and Education' in 'Children in Hospital', in Department of Health and Social Security and Welsh Office, *The Organisation of the In-Patient's Day*, p. 27.

117 Tom Hulme, '"A Nation Depends on its Children": School Buildings and Citizenship in England and Wales, 1900–1939', *Journal of British Studies*, 54 (2015), p. 408.

118 *Ibid.*, p. 432.

119 Laura Tisdall, '"The School that I'd Like": Children and Teenagers Write about Education in England and Wales, 1945–79', in Sian Pooley and Jonathan Taylor (eds), *Children's Experiences of Welfare in Modern Britain* (University of London Press, 2021), p. 203.

120 *Ibid.*

121 Kozlovsky, 'Programming Emotional Care', p. 123.

122 'Installations: Green Lane Hospital, Ormskirk', *Hospital Development*, 8 (1980), p. 20.

123 *Ibid.*, p. 135.

124 This was given as an example in Wellcome Library, ART/AFH/A/5/2, Peter Senior, 'Art for Health's Sake', *Hospital Development*, 18 (1990), p. 28. There are also records of this playground at Hampshire Record Office, 77A22/1, 'Commission and Purchase of Art and Artefacts for Selected Sites'.

125 Malcolm Miles and John Bennett, 'Product of the Month', *Hospital Development*, 24 (1993), p. 7.

126 Jon Winder, 'Revisiting the Playground: Charles Wicksteed, Play Equipment and Public Spaces for Children in Early Twentieth-Century Britain', *Urban History*, 50 (2023), pp. 134–51.

127 *Ibid.*, p. 145.

128 Valerie Wright, 'Making Their Own Fun: Children's play in high-rise estates in Glasgow in the 1960s and 1970s', in Pooley and Taylor (eds), *Children's Experiences of Welfare*, p. 245.

129 *Ibid.*, pp. 245–6.

130 East Riding Archives, JL/49/1990/Healthview, 'It's Child's Play at Hull', *Healthview [The newspaper for the Health Service in the Yorkshire Region]*, December 1990, p. 9.

131 Jim Brinkley, 'Reaching for the Stars', *Hospital Development*, 24 (1993), pp. 26–9.
132 Lizette Alvarez, 'Where the Healing Touch Starts With the Hospital Design', *New York Times*, 7 September 2004, http://www.nytimes.com/2004/09/07/health/07hosp.html?pagewanted=print&position=&_r=0 [accessed: 27 February 2024].
133 'Transformation Sant Joan de Déu Barcelona Children's Hospital', *EU Mies Award*, https://miesarch.com/work/4917 [accessed: 22 February 2023].
134 Maria Luigia Assirelli interviewed by Victoria Bates, 3 February 2023.
135 Jo Birch, Penny Curtis, and Allison James, 'Sense and Sensibilities: In Search of the Child-Friendly Hospital', *Built Environment*, 33 (2007), p. 412; Rebecca McLaughlan and Julie Willis, 'Atmospheric Inclusiveness: Creating a Coherent and Relatable Sense of Place for a Children's Hospital', *The Journal of Architecture*, 26 (2021), pp. 1197–218.
136 Joyce Bolchover, 'Adolescent Unit: Architects' Approach and Appraisal', *Hospital Development*, 2 (1974), p. 10.
137 Derbyshire Record Office, D6082/182/1, Visit to Children's Hospital.
138 'It's Child's Play at Hull', p. 9.
139 Owen Hatherley, *A Guide to the New Ruins of Great Britain* (Verso, 2011 [2010]), p. viii.
140 Iden Wickings, *Improving Hospital Design: A Report on the King's Fund Hospital Design Competition for 1993* (King Edward's Hospital Fund for London, 1994), p. 35.
141 Stephen Verderber and David J. Fine, *Healthcare Architecture in an Era of Radical Transformation* (Yale University Press, 2000), p. 86; David Charles Sloane and Beverlie Conant Sloane, *Medicine Moves to the Mall* (Johns Hopkins University Press, 2003), p. 94.
142 Verderber and Fine, *Healthcare Architecture*, p. 86. David Charles Sloane and Beverlie Conant Sloane draw on Verderber and Fine's work, noting that critics of existing hospitals were 'borrowing from the work of Robert Venturi, Charles Jenks, and other architectural writers', in *Medicine Moves to the Mall*, p. 94.
143 These trends are outlined in Geoffrey Rivett, *From Cradle to Grave: Fifty Years of the NHS* (King Edward's Hospital Fund for London, 1998).
144 On distinctions between warm/cold and functional/decorative, see discussion of Birren in Chapter 2.

6

Glass: clarity and consumerism

In the 1930s, the modernist architect Le Corbusier wrote a piece for a trade journal entitled 'Glass, the Fundamental Material of Modern Architecture', in which he declared: 'I can state that glass will be a characteristic feature of building in the new machine age because it is the most direct means by which we can find one of the essential conditions for life: sun and light'.[1] He went so far as to call glass an 'architectural revolution' and argued that '[t]he "glass wall" is the conquest of the Modern Age'.[2] Several famous glass buildings had already been built in the nineteenth century, such as the Crystal Palace. Alain Corbin argues that the growing use of windows changed modern ways of seeing, forms of 'visual perception', and 'sensory thresholds' from the nineteenth century onwards.[3] The twentieth century, though, was truly the era of glass and Le Corbusier would soon be proven right. By the end of the century, the use of glass was so extensive that high-profile architects such as Juhani Pallasmaa began to bemoan the trend.[4] Pallasmaa argued that the temporality of buildings was lost in the overuse of materials such as glass, and argued for the value of tactility, darkness, shade, exploration, and glimpses of light, rather than using glass to give too much 'conceptual emphasis'.[5] Glass, then, is a crucial part of the history of architecture, interior design, and experience in hospitals.

Glass was a particularly important material in late twentieth-century hospitals for a range of reasons. Access to the outside and fresh air had long been seen as an important part of curative environments, and more widespread use of (sealed) glass windows facilitated a new kind of 'therapeutic landscape'; there was increased attention to the embodied and emotional processes of looking outside. More extensive use of windows, and interest in the views from windows, emphasised that hospital exteriors were thresholds to be crossed. This differed from walls as boundaries that contained or delineated. It offered people a way imaginatively to exist outside of the hospital's built environment, even as they physically inhabited it. Hospital walls became increasingly transparent at the same time as the boundaries of hospitals became more fluid; people spent more time as outpatients rather than inpatients, and treatments were increasingly moving into the home. The rise of glass in hospitals symbolised the disintegration of the neat boundaries of hospital built environments by the end of the century, as they were increasingly just one part of a system of flowing in and out.

The history of glass, including windows and atriums, brings architecture to the fore of colour history. It shows how hospital buildings and their materials, particularly in the exterior structure of the building, affected the way that colour was experienced and encountered inside them. As one article in *The Architectural Review* noted in 1969, with the rise of glass in buildings 'the colour went from the wall to the window. To the beholder, transmitted coloured light is quite different from reflected […] [t]he type of sky, the seasons and the colour light reflecting surfaces outside the building all affect it'.[6] There is great value in paying attention to transparent materials in histories of colour, and – ultimately – of making glass more visible.

Technology: the rise of glass in the 1980s

Glass was a key feature of modern and modernist architecture. Beatriz Colomina compares the widespread use of glass in the early twentieth century to new forms of medical technology, arguing that 'modern buildings even started to look like medical images' and that early twentieth-century avant-garde architects built structures that looked like X-ray machines.[7] These glass building were, Colomina argues, like 'flowing glass skins revealing inner bones and organs'.[8] This 'X-ray' aesthetic came later to hospitals. However, there are some examples of significant glass use in early twentieth-century healthcare buildings. At first glass was closely entwined with the history of white, hygiene, and lightness. Berthold Lubetkin's Finsbury

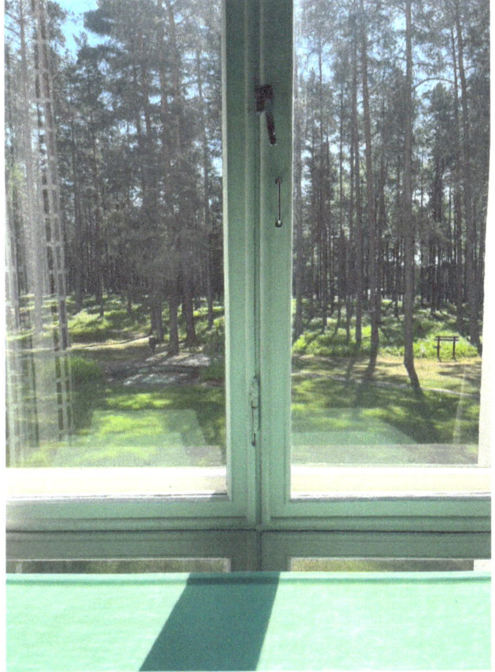

Figure 6.1 View from a Paimio Sanatorium window, 2023. © Image: Victoria Bates.

Health Centre, built over the course of the late 1930s, for example, had a full wall of glass bricks that contributed to its 'cheerful atmosphere' and 'air of efficiency'.[9] Windows had long been thought important for bringing in fresh air and light, and they were used increasingly as part of the structure of buildings. New glass technologies were developed, such as 'Vitaglass' in the 1920s, and the new 'architecture of transparency' arose, with architectural glass products that claimed to maximise healthy ultra-violet rays.[10] Early twentieth-century sanatoria were often built amongst trees, particularly in continental Europe but also in Britain, offering both the therapeutic scent of pine and expansive green views from beds or balconies (Figure 6.1).[11]

With the foundation of the NHS, glass came into its own right as a building material and an increasingly dominant architectural feature. This trend was a consequence both of architectural fashions and of new glass technologies that allowed for larger windows or glass structures. In March 1951, *The Hospital* included a full-page advert from Chance Brothers Limited Glass Works, which declared '[i]t is difficult to picture the ideal hospital or clinic without reference to glass [...] window glass, certainly, and equally interior glass [...] doors, screens, partition walls, light fittings, décor'.[12] The advertised glasses, they declared, 'talk the language of to-day' architecturally, including using particular types of opaque or frosted glass as partitions to 'limit the view without obscuring the light'.[13] Such use of glass became even more the 'language of to-day' over subsequent decades, particularly in large urban and public buildings, as modern architecture in general turned towards glass and transparency. Like white before it, glass was not an absence but an important material addition to hospitals.

In line with broader colour trends in the early post-war years at this time, there was a growing interest in windows and how they could address emotional as well as practical issues in the hospital. An article on 'Glass in the Hospital', published in *The Hospital* in September 1949, noted that the role of glass was primarily to transmit light, for the purposes of creating 'a bright and cheerful atmosphere and a feeling of wellbeing' and supplying the 'best working and seeing conditions' as well as showing up dirt.[14] Glass thus contributed to several of the primary concerns of the modern hospital: hygiene, efficiency, and 'human' emotion. The Nuffield Trust's important 1955 publication on hospital design also recommended that, in smaller wards, more beds could be positioned in parallel with windows to offer both daylight and space efficiency.[15] This recommendation allowed for better use of existing glass, in a context of very limited new hospital building. As Richard Llewelyn Davis – director of the Nuffield Foundation Division for Architectural Studies – noted in 1954, in the old-fashioned ward 'with tall windows between every bed, ample light was available. Indeed, from the patient's point of view, the light was sometimes excessive. When sitting up in bed, he faced a row of bright windows and could not turn away from the light'.[16] By moving beds parallel to the window wall, the patient had more control, and can 'turn away from it if he wishes', though windows and rooms had to be designed carefully to ensure even light distribution in the ward.

Many of these trends had national and international precedents. Brian Abel-Smith locates the 'beginnings of a revolution in hospital architecture' in the 1920s and 1930s, and provides examples of early twentieth-century British hospitals that moved beds parallel to the windows for better access to light and views.[17] The 1949 'Glass in the Hospital' article's reference to a 'cheerful atmosphere' echoed the way that the Finsbury Health Centre conceptualised its use of glass. The 1955 Nuffield publication acknowledged that its ideas about ward layouts were inspired by earlier ward designs from Copenhagen. These trends took hold more firmly under the NHS. Over the course of the 1960s and 1970s, there was increasing attention paid to what glass could do in hospitals. New hospital buildings provided opportunities to be more ambitious about windows. The *West Briton & Royal Cornwall Gazette* reported in 1966 that the Royal Cornwall Hospital, an early new NHS hospital, had a 'hotel air' and that 'in the sixth-storey ward, picture-windows give a fine view over the countryside, with the golf course dominant in the foreground'.[18] Another of the first purpose-built NHS hospitals, the Princess Margaret Hospital in Swindon, was to some extent a test site for glass itself. In 1961 *The Hospital* noted that the Nuffield Trust had funded an evaluation of the first stage of the building, and noted that this building to some extent suffered 'the fate of the pioneer' including temperature problems caused by its extensive use of windows.[19] This indicates the relative novelty of such an approach to hospital building at this time. It further emphasises the importance of recognising that glass changed not only the colour palette of hospitals, offering new exterior views and more weather-based light for interiors, but also had multi-sensory implications, including for warmth.

As the hospital building programme gathered momentum in the 1970s, an increasing number of publications stated not only the need for windows, but explained the rationale for that need. The value of views was described in terms ranging from the 'humanistic' and calming to the stimulating. Some of the hospitals of the 1960s were later discussed and re-evaluated, with those using extensive glasswork being seen as early examples of more 'humanistic design'. Looking back on *50 Years of Health Building* in 1998, for example, Peter Scher noted that Wexham Park hospital (completed 1966) was an example of a pioneering low-rise hospital with 'landscaping and windowed main circulation routes' that 'made a very agreeable human environment'.[20] As Ed DeVane notes, this design approach complemented 'earlier design principles of English modernism set out in texts like Thomas Sharp's 1951 *The Anatomy of the Village*; new buildings should be bold and simple, adaptable to change, and sympathetic to individual places'.[21] A book recommending interior design for the Harness hospital in the mid-1970s noted that 'it is desirable that the location of the dining room within the building should make available landscaped views from the windows or into courtyards, therefore, introducing natural materials' and that the location of the children's ward should 'provide interesting views from the windows to benefit those in bed'.[22] There was a subtle difference in the language here, between soothing 'landscaped' views for adults and implicitly more stimulating, 'interesting' views for children.

People with different physical ailments also needed to be able to engage with windows in specific ways. As the Committee of the Central Health Services Council noted in 1976, '[e]ven an inclined mirror over the bed of an alert bedfast patient will allow him to see the comings and goings of the world outside his window'.[23] There was a shift, then, towards the idea that all patients should be able to see out of windows. There was also greater emphasis on views, rather than light and air alone. As with other interventions, such as hospital artworks that depicted nature, windows were considered to offer both soothing imagery and visual interest. Such ideas gained more widespread attention with the publication of a famous *Science* article by Roger Ulrich in 1984, which indicated that views of nature from a window could improve recovery rates after surgery.[24] Though architectural historian David Theodore has rightly noted that the novelty of Ulrich's work is often over-stated, as windows have long played an important role in hospitals, the publication was highly influential.[25] The 'view through a window' came to be such an important idea in hospital design that it merits consideration on its own, and is discussed further below.

In the 1980s there was also another significant shift in the use of glass in hospitals: the rise of the hospital atrium. This is linked to broader trends in global architecture where, according to Charles Rice, the atrium emerged in the 1960s, reached its 'apotheosis' in the mid-1980s, and 'became the characteristic architectural space of this period'.[26] As an article in *The Architectural Review* noted recently, certain 'typologies – for example the street, the monoblock, the podium with tower or block(s), the campus, the atrium – can be seen in modern hospitals all round the world in various pure and hybrid interpretations'.[27] The atrium had been visible earlier in North America, for example in German-Canadian architect Eb Zeidler's McMaster University Health Sciences Centre in Hamilton in 1972, which had 'important innovations, including an atrium and several landscaped courtyards' that – in the words of one recent article on Zeidler – combined the 'technical and the humanistic'.[28] In the words of Annmarie Adams and David Theodore, writing on hospital atriums in Canada, the atrium drew comparisons with other everyday spaces such as a 'mundane shopping mall'.[29] David and Beverlie Sloane similarly note, in relation to the US, that

> Commercial spaces have long used atriums, in either lobbies or indoor courtyards, as relief from narrow corridors and windowless spaces ... atriums became almost mandatory in luxury hotels built in the 1980s and early 1990s ... [Hospital] designs that resonate of home, hotel, and mall send different messages – of comfort, familiarity, and power sharing between patient and provider.[30]

The atrium could, then, serve a range of functions and emulate several different spaces, with important implications for light, colour, and the 'message' the hospital sent. British atriums similarly evoked non-medical sites, such as shopping centres or airports, and it seems no coincidence that such models were increasingly popular with the rise of the Private Finance Initiative (PFI) hospital at the end of the century.[31] Under PFI, the gap between public and private sectors was much smaller than before. Gesler *et al.* argue that PFI design had a number of goals, including commercial ones,

> while old hospitals are depicted as institutional, uncomfortable, and 'public' – in the negative sense of an absence-of-privacy for patients or staff – new hospitals are compared favourably with privately owned commercial buildings such as hotels, offices, and supermarkets.[32]

The history of glass in hospitals is as much about consumerism and postmodernism, as it is about views from windows. The commonality between hospitals and commercial architecture gained strength in the 1980s, though it was not an entirely new trend. Hospitals had long overlapped with the commercial sphere, even under the NHS. In the post-war period, for example, when there was a turn to pastel shades in hospitals as part of the 'humanisation' agenda, commercial pharmacies such as Boots also turned towards such colour palettes as part of international ideas about 'modern' retail.[33] Commercial and private companies also played important roles in colour research in the mid-twentieth century. Models such as hotels served as a perfect bridge between the post-war model of 'homely' humanistic spaces and more explicitly commercial models of hospital colour in subsequent decades.[34]

The hospital atrium was part of patient-centred design, a trend that was fully formed by the end of the twentieth century. In 1993, *Canadian Architect* hinted at this trend – and how it connected to modernity – in an article on the atrium at Toronto's Hospital for Sick Children, noting that '[t]he hospital remains a well-functioning machine, encased in a user-friendly wrapping'.[35] This idea of the 'user-friendly' wrapping is also an important part of understanding the history of British hospital architecture. Alex Mold notes that the 'patient-consumer' shifted from the 'margins to centre-stage' after Margaret Thatcher's *Patients First* paper (1979), and at a similar time hospitals came increasingly and more self-consciously to emulate 'private' spaces.[36] These two trends were interwoven. To quote *Hospital Development* in 1982, the aim was to make hospitals feel 'like a hotel', and making patients feel 'welcome, at ease and optimistic' became newly aligned with commercial culture.[37] As Sarah Curtis *et al.* argue, responses to recent 'changes in user attitudes' to healthcare such as more 'consumerist' approaches included 'the provision of health-care facilities more resembling commercial outlets such as hotels and shops'.[38] This trend echoed the wider influence of such designs, where the American 'shopping mall' was gradually replacing the British shopping precinct, and the atrium was being imported as a design ideal.[39]

Though not every NHS atrium was inspired by the US and Canada, nor explicitly commercial in its design goals, this context is important. These were not simply superficial changes, and they had particular significance at a time when the negotiation of patients' rights was at the forefront of NHS practice and policy. As Serena Dyer notes in her work on senses and eighteenth-century shopping, senses were a way of 'negotiating' relationships, and shaped how people experienced, moved through, and engaged with retail spaces.[40] The same is true of any space that emulated or echoed those spaces, even if only subtly or subconsciously. By changing materials, colour schemes and other elements of design in emulation of commercial spaces, hospitals might well have changed how they were navigated and the 'negotiation' of relationships between them. The rise of the 'patient as consumer' and consumerist colour palettes were thus interwoven, not necessarily in a neat or linear pattern of cause-and-effect, but as part of ongoing negotiations of what it meant to be a patient in the NHS.

For some commentators, the atrium became a symbol of soulless contemporary hospital architecture. Criticisms of such buildings tend to focus on commercialisation and their 'public–private style'. A *BMJ* book review critiqued such developments in hospital design at some length in 1993:

> We are now dismissing the big block approach to hospitals (and most other services) as mindless and inherently inhumane. But the big block policy was neither mindless nor deliberately inhumane. Unlike today, when there is great uncertainty about the very concept of what a hospital should be, 20 years ago people knew what a hospital could do and consequently what it should look like ... [Now] we see incorporated into hospitals the atriums of the grand airport hotels or the fake vernacular roofscapes of the out of town supermarkets. There is no grand vision emerging in hospital style, just a middling bland decency to make you forget the ministrations of technology and the fears of mortality and make you think of a shopping weekend instead.[41]

Journalist Owen Hatherley also comments on one hospital's 'central atrium at the main Outpatients entrance, where a giant Carillion logo looks over a big branch of Upper Crust, a WHSmith, and a shop which sells a huge range of cuddly toys, amongst other concessions'.[42] There is an obvious politics to such critiques, as well as an aesthetic judgment, as the atrium came to symbolise the rise of private sector influence in the state NHS. Windows and glass became shopfronts, rather than thresholds or symbolic sightlines to recovery.[43] The rise of atriums aligned with other trends, such as the rise of bright colour palettes (of which Hatherley also wrote, with some derision) and a turn towards postmodern hospital design that referenced or evoked non-medical buildings. Not all of these reference points were commercial, but they all connected to the rise of the patient-as-consumer and marked attempts to make the hospital more welcoming.

It is worth distinguishing here between what atriums have come to symbolise – a consumer model of healthcare – and the rationale underpinning their initial introduction. When the Rikshospitalet in Oslo was built, between 1991 and 2001, its large atrium was conceptualised as part of a 'humanistic' design intervention.[44] One of the key architects said 'he and his partners tried to design it with one question in mind: How can this improve the way patients feel and the way employees conduct their jobs?'[45] In an interview with a *New York Times* journalist, he said: 'Let's call it a humanistic hospital: built by humans for humans'.[46] The design of the Oslo hospital, including its use of light, windows, and vibrant colour schemes was apparently so influential that it 'attracted pilgrimages by designers all over the world, including the United States'.[47] Even American atriums should also, then, not be so neatly dismissed as being based on the 'shopping mall'. This was part of a longer tradition of British and American architects alike drawing inspiration from Scandinavian design, which was seen as the forefront of 'holistic' modern architecture.[48] The Oslo atrium most recently influenced the design of Southmead Hospital in Bristol, which also drew on retail and airport environments; the commercial and the humanistic were not seen as incompatible.[49] These types of buildings were not traditionally seen as welcoming places to stay or rest, in the same way as hotels, but they offered useful and familiar templates for flow, movement, wayfinding, and navigation. The Southmead and Oslo atriums can be seen in Figures 6.2 and 6.3.

By the end of the twentieth century, the use of glass in hospital architecture was in full force. This trend changed the colour palette of hospitals dramatically, including changing the quality of light that entered buildings and altering views out of them. As Barbara Erwine notes, light itself can be seen as an architectural 'material' because 'the quality and shape of light in a place sets its character'.[50] More extensive natural light would have changed the colours within hospitals and connected those colours more closely to daylight, weather, and seasons. There was also increasing interest in the opportunities that glass offered for looking outside, as a therapeutic tool. With the widespread use of glass, hospitals also emulated other building types such as airports and shopping centres.

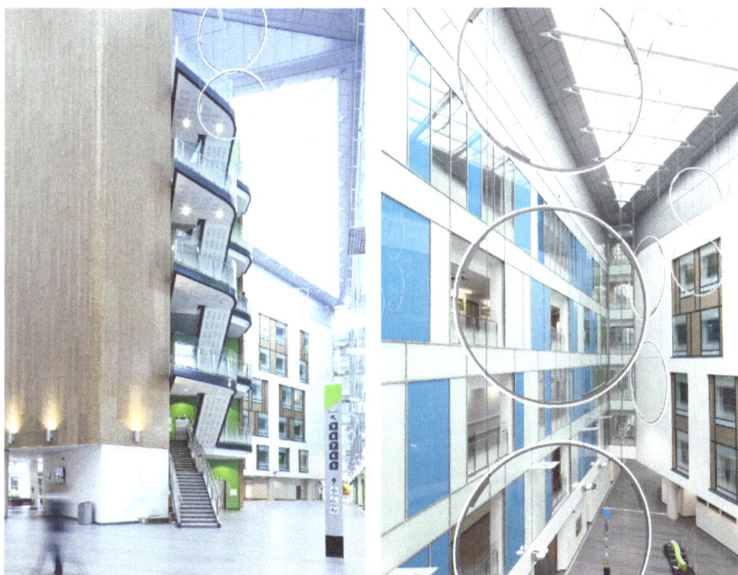

Figure 6.2 Southmead Hospital atrium. © Images: Building Design Partnership (BDP). Reproduced with kind permission of BDP. All rights reserved and permission to use this figure must be obtained from the copyright holder.

Overall, glass expanded, rather than replaced or dramatically altered, ideas about modern hospital architecture and design. The atrium, for example, was an extension of many other trends, including more 'humanistic' design, the introduction of nature (and natural colours) into hospitals, and the desire to make hospitals more 'vibrant' and playful for those who sought stimulation. They were additionally and newly, rather than *only*, consumerist in influence and expression. Just as layers of paint accumulated and held the multiple, expanding meanings of the 'modern' hospital, glass reflected the concerns of the time.

Thresholds: the window

Glass had multiple roles in hospitals, with increasing emphasis on the ability to see outside. In the wake of Roger Ulrich's influential

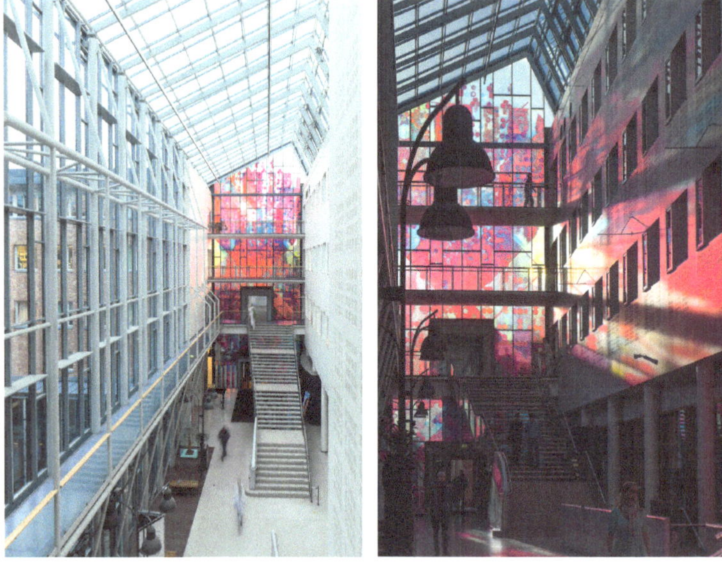

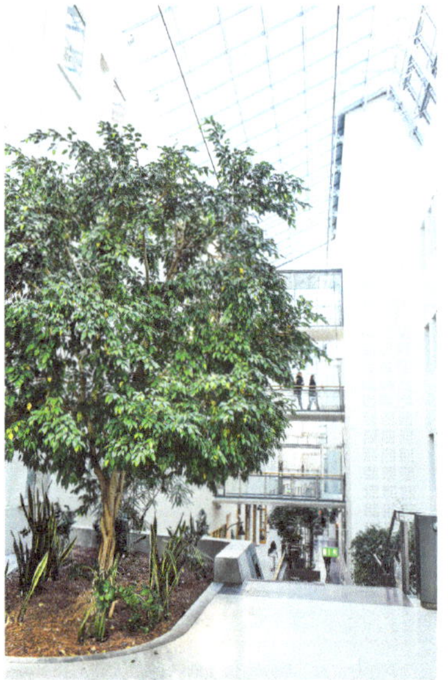

Figure 6.3 Atrium at Rikshospitalet in Oslo. © Glass images: Øystein Horgmo, University of Oslo; Tree image: Kristin Ellefsen, University of Oslo. Reproduced with kind permission of the Medical Photography and Illustration Service, University of Oslo.

publication, which argued that views of nature hastened recovery from surgery, from the 1980s onwards there was a dominant cultural model for glass in hospitals: the 'view through a window'. Ulrich was disproportionately influential because he offered 'evidence-based' research that apparently 'proved' the value of windows in quantitative terms.[51] There were undoubtedly limits to this research, including the simple binary offered between views of nature and a brick wall, but his continued international influence and legacy remains significant. One of the most important parts of Ulrich's work was its emphasis on recovery, rather than just on the aesthetic value of windows. It also emphasised the healthy nature of windows in terms of *views* rather than the more traditional models of air, ventilation, and other sensory stimuli. Indeed, considering that windows were increasingly sealed in modern hospital buildings for purposes of 'environmental control', the emphasis on views from windows and their therapeutic role was important.[52] This section turns to the question of what it meant to look 'through' windows, including how landscapes and exteriors affected the experience of colour in hospitals. As with the other modernist architectural favourite, the 'white wall', consideration of windows as material objects also shows the limits of conceptualising them as 'transparent'.

It is not difficult to find examples of historic hospitals, including pre-modern buildings, for which engagement with nature was an architectural feature. However, it would be a mistake to take this as evidence that 'therapeutic landscapes' are trans-historical.[53] Shan Jiang notes that hospital courtyards were often functional, while many gardens were ornamental or viewed only from the outside: 'the people–nature relationship' in many early hospitals, she argues, 'was incidental' because many plans were adapted from other types of buildings such as palaces or churches.[54] Nightingale wards had windows as a key feature of design but with an emphasis on cross-ventilation. Most beds in these wards had windows behind and opposite them, but more for the purposes of light and air than scenery, and they were often too far away to offer views. Florence Nightingale did advocate the value of seeing the 'bright colours of flowers' from a window, though light and air were given much greater emphasis in her published work.[55] Specific types of healthcare building, such as the sanatorium, had included balconies for patients with some interest in the therapeutic potential of views (see Figure

6.1 for the view from Paimio Sanatorium). Again, though, the emphasis tended to be on light and fresh air, and the physiological benefits such as the power of sunlight to kill bacteria.[56] These were all important ways in which people engaged with nature, and understood the benefits of doing so, in hospital design. However, they differed from the late twentieth-century concept of the 'view from a window' as part of the therapeutic process.

Ulrich's work connected to, and accelerated, growing international emphasis on the visual stimulus that windows offered. What Jiang describes as 'the current revival of hospital greenspaces' came with 'the rejection of modernism and the exploration of patient-centred environmental design' in the late twentieth century.[57] This interest was particularly visible in regions with large institutions such as North America, Australia, and Europe, where there was a fear that connections to nature might be lost.[58] This linked to many of the trends discussed in previous chapters, such as concerns about the 'dehumanisation' of hospitals and increasing interest in the role of stimulation as part of recovery. Ulrich's work tapped into many prevailing trends in thought about hospital architecture and design, packaging them into an 'evidence-based' model that could be used to make economic arguments for more 'humanistic' architecture. David Theodore notes that, by the late 1960s, the hospital had declined as a 'healing machine', because 'health could now be delivered as a systematic effect of the operation of the whole hospital, and not as a therapeutic effect of the architecture on the individual patient'.[59] The hospital window in the 1980s, however, offers an example of the return of the idea of healing architecture and the power of 'therapeutic landscapes' on individuals.

The hospital window was increasingly seen as a symbol of potential recovery. Its emotional aspects can only be understood in relation to the experience of confinement: wanting to access the world outside but being unable to do so.[60] As Duncan Patterson notes in his history of the window in art and architecture, 'one side is cast as hopeful and filled with possibility relative to the other'.[61] Writing in 1990 about St Mary's Hospital on the Isle of Wight, Richard Burton noted that '[v]ery ill patients want little stimulation, but later, as the patient gets stronger, he or she will be able to sit in the conservatories at the end of each ward, which look down on the garden with its lake and island'.[62] Windows were therefore carefully positioned in some hospitals to correspond to the recovery process; while patients in spaces such as ICU did not need 'views', they offered stimulation – and sometimes options for ambulation, as in the Isle of Wight example – for those moving towards leaving the hospital. The window, in this model, offered hope of a world outside to which patients could return.

Colour was an important part of the view from a window. As Sarah Bell, Clare Hickman, and Frank Houghton argue, encounters with so-called 'therapeutic landscapes' are often 'framed in terms of colour – be they green, blue, white or yellow spaces'.[63] Garden designers showed close attention to colour. *Architects' Journal* reported that, in Suffolk Hospital in 1980, for example, a hospital roof garden was planned with

> broad bands of foliar colour, i.e. light green, dark green, yellow, white, and purple which were to run across the roof with the lightest colours tending to be towards the top. It was then intended that different areas of the planting would flower or fruit in a random sequence so that there would be some area of particular attention throughout the year.[64]

Some contemporaries referred to engagement with landscapes and courtyards as 'passive' when consumed through windows, compared with physical immersion.[65] This could be a particular problem for courtyards that were physically inaccessible to staff and patients.[66] Others focused on more active forms of looking and imagination. One architect in 1980 even claimed that residents of a home for blind people still

> insisted upon describing to each visitor the environment around them in minute detail – all of course based on what they had learned from nurses and visitors, whether it be pictures on their wall, flowers in window boxes or views from the windows.[67]

In this school of thought, the visual interest offered by windows could also offer rich material for description and imagination, even in the absence of the ability to see. In this framework, engagement with windows was an active process.

In general, there was a growing belief at this time that looking itself could be an engaged embodied act. Bell, Hickman, and Houghton also argue that there is value in 'going beyond such palettic framings to engage with the processes and temporalities of intimate, visceral place sensing'.[68] Some contemporary architects and landscapers did think more expansively about hospital windows, as a mode of engagement with the living natural world, rather than as the passive consumption of 'green' or 'blue' landscapes. In the late 1980s, for example, Pat Hartridge won an Institute of Social Inventions' Ecology Award for her ideas about facilitating hospital wildlife and supported the development of hospital gardens, with an emphasis on liveliness and interaction. She referred implicitly to Ulrich in her writing, advancing his ideas to emphasise what nature could offer beyond 'landscape':

> A scientific study in America has shown that those patients with access to a window whilst in hospital need fewer drugs than those in a windowless environment. How much saving in drugs would there be if there was also something interesting to see outside that window.[69]

For Hartridge, presenting a view shared by many others working on hospital gardens and courtyards at this time, nature was not just 'a view' but something alive and engaging. She wrote, for example, that 'I hope that those patients who were keen naturalists before their hospitalisation might be able to record sightings of various species from their ward windows' and reflected on her own experience of hospitalisation, during which a robin 'perched outside the window of my room in the isolation unit'.[70] She advocated planting shrubs that would specifically encourage or appeal to wildlife, offering not just 'green spaces' but the ever-shifting colours of birds, butterflies, bees, and more. These flows, changes, and movements were crucial for distinguishing the process of looking out of a window from the process of engaging with more static artwork.

The discussion to this point has focused largely on ideals and design principles. In practice, many hospital sites were old, with windowless rooms and corridors. These were often tackled with artwork, light panels, or more recently digital screens that emulate windows' changeable views of the outside.[71] Even where windows did exist, their views were highly variable between hospitals, depending on factors ranging from geography to garden design.[72] Some hospitals were able to offer the gardens and lakes of the Isle of Wight site, or even views of the sea, but others were new, out-of-town sites with little greenery. The rise of car use meant that newer hospitals often prioritised car parks over gardens, whether on urban or rural sites, meaning that the 'view from a window' was often a courtyard rather than a sweeping landscape.[73] Changing land use meant that, just when hospitals embraced the importance of window views, such views were increasingly limited. The views of 'blue' and 'green' spaces were also largely conceptual; even where water was present, it was rarely 'blue', and trees could range from red to brown, depending on the season.[74]

Contemporary sources that show people's experiences of hospital windows 'on the ground' were mixed, in old and new buildings alike. Patient feedback from the King's Fund evaluation of New Guy's House in 1962 noted '[m]y only complaint, looking down from the dining room window, the shocking insanitary buildings ajacent [sic] to the Hospital'.[75] There was also a neglect of the views that staff encountered in their work and the role of windows in the workplace, beyond the need for light, at least in comparison with the extensive attention paid to patients' views and the role of windows in recovery. In relation to a residential training school in Bristol, adapted in 1950, for example, one report noted that the window faced a wall.[76] These problems were not limited to the post-war years. As influential hospital architect Howard Goodman noted, as part of the Arts for Health conference 'A Vision of Caring Environments' in 1989:

> We might consider the view from the patient's window. He might be lucky and have a room with a view of rolling countryside and no-one would, or probably could, improve on that. But the chances are that what he sees is an adjoining building or the general tat and squalor which seems to surround so many hospitals.[77]

Windows could introduce 'grey' or 'brick' to the hospital colour palette as much as they could introduce 'green' or nature. Outside areas also often needed maintenance to preserve its visual appeal. One arts strategy paper, for example, for the new hospital in Hastings in the late 1980s, noted that the hospital's 'extensive southfacing windows […] look out into and over a large courtyard and the coast beyond […] This design strength is also a potential weakness, for if the courtyards are not properly treated they will be unattractive and depress the viewer'.[78] Sometimes window areas with far-reaching views of 'green space' have also not been sufficiently protected. Under the pressures of spaces and resources in the NHS, for example, a glazed balcony area can end up being used for storage.

Instead of leaving undesirable views as transparent lenses on the outside world, many hospitals adapted windows and added artwork. To understand glass as simply transparent is to misunderstand its role in hospital spaces, and hospital colour schemes. Glass has never been an absence or a neutral in colour terms. At St Mary's on the Isle of Wight, for example, stencils of natural imagery were added to windows to distract from less pleasant views without limiting light. In an oral history interview, Guy Eades – now retired as the director of Healing Arts, the arts and health programme for the Isle of Wight NHS Trust – noted that these transfers were part of an integrated art programme using local artists, and that they were intended to create 'privacy', but also that they were to block unpleasant external views:

> it kind of informed the design of St Mary's that every ward, bed arrangement, should have a view out … natural light during the day is so much better than artificial light. And again, if there are windows and you can see out, I mean I prefer that. What you look out onto is another matter. I mean if you look out onto a busy market or whatever and you're in a city or a street then it's fascinating. If you look out onto a brick wall opposite, it can be very depressing … although you've got a window it's obviously what it looks out onto. So that's why we ended up doing lots of window transfers because often someone would just put a portacabin outside the thing and then the view was lost. So we tried to replace it with a window transfer so that it mitigated that negative impact.[79]

It is significant that for Eades the emphasis is on visual interest rather than nature. Though the Isle of Wight site offered natural views, he notes that a window in a city could also offer 'fascinating' views for people; the problem, in his opinion, is when any such view is absent, blocked, or lost. Eades raises the important point that hospitals are constantly evolving, and it was not uncommon for interesting views to be replaced by new structures. Others suggested that 'if there are windows that look out into dead areas… stained glass is a wonderful way of letting in the light and blocking out the view which may be depressing'.[80] This quote is from a 1989 hospital art strategy, again indicating that windows could be forms of artwork, and how features such as stained glass moved from specific spaces (such as hospital chapels) to more widespread use in architecture. Coloured glass, curtains, window ledges, stencils, and other artistic or interior design choices could provide colourful distraction when the world outside failed to do so.

The materiality of windows is also important in a number of ways. Hospital windows were as reflective as they were transparent, with significant implications for light and colour. As Juhani Pallasmaa notes, 'the increasing use of reflective glass in architecture reinforces the dreamlike sense of unreality and alienation'.[81] Pallasmaa argues that the reflective quality of windows makes it difficult to 'see or imagine life behind these walls' of glass.[82] As noted above, many NHS hospital beds were in parallel with windows rather than facing them, because of the problems of reflection and glare created by glass. Hospitals often tried to reduce glare in the day, and the coldness of windows at night, with curtains, drapes, or blinds. Even if windows did offer views outside, at the right angle or in low light they were often dirty and needed regular cleaning to fulfil their 'transparent' purpose. One Cornish hospital visitors' report from 1951 stated that '[t]he hospital windows are not clean and Matron tells us that it is many months since any window cleaning has been done'.[83] Similar comments were made on a hospital visit in Derbyshire over three decades later, emphasising that hospital sites could also be dirty and noisy because of building work: 'We drew attention to the very dirty windows on Ward 8'.[84] In some wards, window cleaning contracts were suspended for 'financial reasons'.[85] This did not go unnoticed by patients or visitors: in a response to a 1997 Mass Observation directive on the NHS, for example, one person noted:

> I was a bit suprised [sic] when I visited my daughter at one of the most famous London maternity hospitals to see really dirty windows and sills … It is so sad to see the effects of lack of money.[86]

The challenge of cleaning windows was made increasingly difficult by the tendency to build high-rise hospitals in the early years of the Hospital Plan. Window cleaning sometimes was a battle with local elements, such as the geography of the land making cleaning difficult, or high levels of dirt from traffic pollution or seagull droppings. Such dirty windows affected how views outside, and light inside, were experienced by patients and staff. While they did not constitute

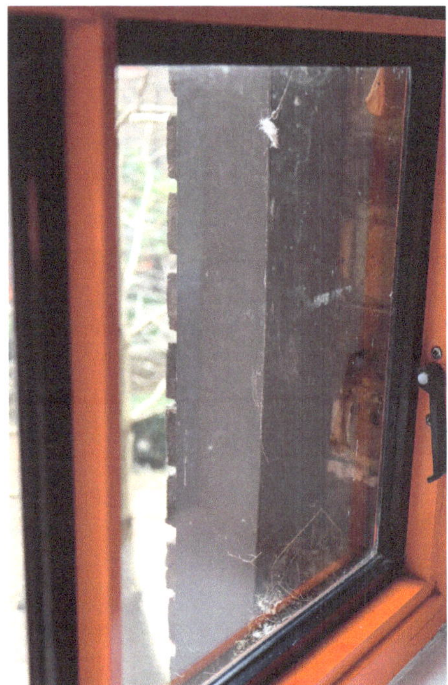

Figure 6.4 A bird's nest on a window sill at Dorset County Hospital, Dorchester (previously West Dorset County Hospital). © Image: Victoria Bates. Reproduced with kind permission of Dorset County Hospital NHS Foundation Trust. All rights reserved and permission to use this figure must be obtained from the copyright holder.

a colour palette in themselves, nor did they offer a transparent view out onto the exterior world, but a mediated, sometimes hazy, threshold between the hospital and the world 'out there'. This is not to assume that dirty or visible glass was always a negative feature of hospitals. Alvar Aalto even apparently preferred the softer quality of light that filtered through unclean windows and illuminated the colours within.[87] Some windows also created new environments for wildlife and offered views not of the designed or managed nature of a courtyard, but of the more unruly natural world in the form of webs or nests (see Figure 6.4).

Though most contemporaries focused on the transparent qualities of windows, some emphasised that they could also be used strategically to create privacy. Cicely Saunders spoke of the range of qualities that windows at St Christopher's hospice offered:

> Man is a social being and he needs to see life going on [...] to see the world from his window, however ill he is [...] But I do not wish only to emphasize activity. Space is also planned for a change of scene for the patients, for silence and also for privacy. Beds can be pushed right up into the bay windows with their splendid view.[88]

Though hospices had their own specific architectural features and goals, the balance between transparency and privacy was also important in hospital design and for a range of different patient groups.[89] Windows could offer a view of other people or protection from them, depending on the needs of a patient, though they were often dependent on staff to facilitate these views. As in the hospice described by Saunders, hospital windows offered the opportunity to create barriers or booths, through deliberately opaque glass, or shapes such as a 'carrel or bay window' for 'children who are shy or upset'.[90] In practice, most windows were carefully controlled to create the illusion of transparency: contemporaries writing on hospital design noted examples where glass was designed to facilitate 'a panoramic view of green, wooded countryside from all windows. But they cannot see staff or visitors', although staff could still monitor and 'keep an eye on the ward' from their side.[91] Windows could, then, also create a sense of privacy through careful design that created the illusion that people were only looking out, not being looked at. Some hospitals introduced coloured glass doors, again seeking to balance privacy and transparency. Coloured glass doors offered permeable thresholds that were welcoming *and* suggested the ability to leave.[92] Coloured security screens were also used because they offered a material presence that 'blended in' with the interior design scheme.[93]

Windows, overall, played an increasingly important part in hospital design over the lifespan of the NHS. They were significant partly because of their visual and symbolic permeability, and partly because of their role as material structures or physical thresholds; they were never merely an absence or a 'gap' in a building. A view 'through' a window has always, in practice, also been a view 'of' a window. As a material intervention into the hospital, windows are best understood as part of design – including colour schemes – rather than 'authentic' or unobstructed lenses onto the outside world. Windows reflected, amplified, and existed in relation to interior colour schemes.

Reflections: window to the soul

Healthy spaces and places within hospitals have never simply been built. They have always been made in relation to a patient's embodied and affective feelings about illness and recovery. This is true for all colours, but perhaps particularly so for glass because of its role as a symbolic threshold and barrier. There are rich records from the 1980s onwards that show how people have engaged with glass in hospitals, ranging from oral histories, Mass Observation, surveys, and the flourishing genre of illness memoir. Each of these is a narrative form, rather than a direct lens into 'experience', but they still have value.[94] They aid an understanding of the personal and relational nature of people's encounters with the 'therapeutic landscape' and its windows, as later remembered and understood.

As a relatively young genre, illness memoirs can be of value to contemporary history. They offer rich and detailed accounts of people's experiences of healthcare services, which often includes hospitals. Windows regularly feature in accounts of hospitals in these texts, often as symbols or metaphors, and sometimes in accounts of boredom or the 'everyday' in hospitals. The latter is more common when people spent extensive or repeated periods of time in hospitals. In musician Ben Watt's *Patient* from 1996, for example, he writes at great length about watching the view from a London hospital window in 1992:

> My hospital bed was by the window – old French windows that opened on to a small balcony with a black iron railing [...] The room overlooked a garden – the public garden I'd walked round on that first Sunday – an umbrella of tall and leafy trees, council flower-beds and a tarmac path. During the day it served as a short cut for most people. Few stopped off to sit on the benches, only drinkers and solitary people. On sunny lunch-times the grassy lawns attracted builders and secretaries [...] At night the garden was different. The pub on the far side looked neo-thirties, and after hours the awning lights were left on, casting a soft orangey light over the streets. Cars

> would glide by. Garage doors would open and close at 3 a.m. Figures on the pavements. Leaf shadows dancing on the blind. It made my life seem cinematic and even more extraordinary than it already was.[95]

This account must be understood in relation to his illness: Watt was in intensive care, slowly recovering from surgery due to a rare auto-immune condition. At this point he was still in significant pain and not sleeping well, hence experiencing the view from the window at many different times of day and night, but alert enough to appreciate distraction. This extract offers rich and evocative detail of life outside a hospital window, and its relationship to the viewer, rarely found in interviews or other insights into memory. It shows how the view from the window changed the atmospheric conditions – and the colour palette – of the hospital room over day and night: from green space, to soft orange light, and black/white shadows. As Watt's windows opened – not typical of a hospital in the 1990s – he could also experience what Tim Ingold describes as the 'taskscape' and temporalities of activity.[96]

Of particular importance, in relation to colour, is the way that Watt describes light. Again, Ingold places great emphasis on light as a 'phenomenon of experience'.[97] Light and weather are crucial to understanding the role of windows in shaping hospital atmospheres; as Shanti Sumartojo, Tim Edensor, and Sarah Pink note, 'light often exceeds material boundaries [...] bouncing off surfaces and angles in unexpected ways [...] light also carries and communicates atmospheric impressions because it resists perfect control'.[98] This lack of control is also emphasised in *Patient*, in which light and colour change over the course of a day and are not stable; they would also, by extension, change with the weather, the seasons, and more. Sumartojo, Edensor, and Pink note that designers often try to work with light and colour, for example through coloured glass or 'tuned' spaces in which light is designed to enhance or interact with colour schemes in interiors, but emphasise that '[a]tmospheres [...] cannot be perfectly designed, simply because they are taken up in individual experience by people with their own imaginations, histories and subjectivities'.[99] Watt's account shows how his own 'imaginations, histories and subjectivities' are part of shaping his encounters with the window and the world outside. He focuses very much on activity and distraction, and on the window as 'cinematic' rather than as equivalent to a picture or landscape. This way of thinking about the window is shaped by his feelings of living an 'extraordinary' life, and of his memories of the space. Even the view of a park from a window, then, is never neutral. This memoir shows how extremely personal and relational the experience of viewing colour and life through windows can be. Reducing 'views of nature' to 'therapeutic landscapes' misses some of the richness of these more embodied, emotional, relational, and more unstable encounters with hospital windows.[100]

Similar conclusions can be drawn from traditional historical sources, such as oral history archives and Mass Observation records. Recollections shared on postcards for a 'Sensory Memory Bank' as part of the 'Sensing Spaces of Healthcare' project show the personal nature of encounters with windows (and their colour schemes). One contributor wrote:

> I remember [...] When I woke from the general anaesthetic that I had when my second son was born I opened my eyes to see the silvery wallpaper in front of me swirling around in the most psychedelic fashion – most unnerving! Then I looked out the window to see a green hillside with small shrubs that were definitely moving up and down the hill! This went on for quite a while and I told my visitors that they couldn't leave me till everything stopped moving around![101]

Such personal encounters between windows, colours, and individual people are not accounted for in any of the design or 'therapeutic landscapes' literature in which windows looking at green spaces are assumed to be healing. Colour is, here, a significant part of the person's memory, but not in any of the ways discussed in literature on hospital windows.

Other contributors to the 'Sensory Memory Bank' project emphasised that windows could be barriers, rather than symbols of hope. A former staff member, who worked in an 'asylum' that became a psychiatric unit, also commented on the potential frustrations of windows for people detained in hospital:

> One of the more subtle cruelties of the hospital was how it used perspective to really make you feel imprisoned. Apart from the obvious locked wards and imposing buildings, it gave the occupant (staff or resident) beautiful grounds to look at. Ancient trees, field gardens, flowers, so on [...] residents would look upon these grounds behind secure windows and only leave once Section 17 was arranged.[102]

This comment emphasises that windows overlooking green space and flowers could only offer hope if people were free to leave. Another contribution to this 'Memory Bank' from a visitor to an old-fashioned 'Nightingale' style ward in the 1980s noted a strong memory of 'small windows up high making it feel depressingly like a prison'.[103] The inability to see out of these windows, combined with other features of the space, created a strong emotional and atmospheric memory for this person. The window was formed in relation to their feelings about visiting someone, and a sense of being trapped, even though they were able to leave the hospital themselves. Both of these responses are also important reminders about the range of people using hospitals at any given time, and that windows could be encountered in different ways by staff, patients, and visitors.

In the light of the 'therapeutic landscapes' literature that was flourishing at this time, it is perhaps surprising that oral histories and Mass Observation records are not filled with descriptions of views of gardens, birds, or courtyards. Negative memories – of windowless rooms, or being stuck behind glass – appear to have been stronger.[104] There are, though, some notable exceptions to this trend. For the 'Voices of Our NHS' project one interviewee (Sandra), who worked in NHS finance, recalled having her appendix out as a child in 1969:

> I was in hospital for two weeks ... it was a very unpleasant experience ... I really didn't like it at all. The one overriding memory I have of that is that there were no real windows I could see out of in the ward apart from a skylight at the top ... I didn't have access to a clock ... but I knew when the sky went this very dark blue colour my dad was coming to visit me, and I love that colour now ... aquamarine. I used to look for the colour.[105]

This is an extremely important memory in relation to windows and colour. As a child, Sandra formed an important relationship with a specific shade of blue because it represented a positive part of an otherwise very difficult hospital journey. For her, it was not a view from the window that was important, but the way that the window gave access to time – which, for a seven-year-old, was important information. It is unlikely that anybody else in the same ward at the same time was engaging with the skylight, and the blue sky visible through the skylight, in this way. It is also significant that Sandra's hospital experience went on to form her relationship with that colour; she did not appreciate aquamarine through the hospital skylight because she liked it, but liked it *as a result* of her hospital experiences. The window could, then, be a formative experience in people's life stories and memories, if it played an important role in a childhood stay. The role of windows in marking time was also important for some others, in their oral history interviews, for example the view from windows – including some 'eye-opening' nocturnal activities in post-war cities – featured in accounts of working night shifts.[106] There is a significant difference, then, between a young child telling the time through the darkening blue of a skylight, and working staff at night observing the bright lights and activity of a nearby hotel.

Courtyards and gardens did occasionally appear in Mass Observation records, including two directives on attitudes to the NHS from 1997 and 2008. Even stories that support the 'therapeutic landscape' literature, though, show the personal and emotional nature of people's encounters with windows and colour. One 1997 respondent, for example, emphasised the importance of the colour green and light in their positive hospital experience: '[w]hen one is confined within the bounds of an institution these things are so important, so is being able to see GREEN outside. "My" hospitals were constructed to allow light in and views of the outside green world'.[107] For this individual, the window and its greenery was bound up with the positive smiles and words of staff, as part of a positive experience of care. Other records of hospital memories show, similarly, how windows became meaningful to people in relation to specific experiences. In a booklet compiling memories of Withington Hospital, for example, a contributor described the shock of her first labour. She recalled pain and discomfort after the birth, but also her appreciation of the hospital windows: 'At quiet times I loved to cradle my son, crooning whilst gazing on the outside world and the beautiful May flowers and sunsets. I still glance up at that window whenever I pass, and smile at those memories'.[108] The window, with its flowers and sunsets, gained meaning for this woman because of the association with her son and shared 'quiet times' in the hospital; the flowers, sunsets, and window did not, in this account at least, carry innate meaning in themselves.

For other Mass Observation respondents, the view from windows was not experienced as intended. One person, writing in 2008, noted that they were admitted to a psychiatric unit in 2005 and that it 'was basically run by care assistants' with poor treatment options:

> The ward was very dark [...] and all the windows looked inward onto a central courtyard not out to the countryside around. There was no way of getting exercise and the food was appalling. As a fellow patient said to me 'this is not an environment which is going to do anything to make depressives feel better'. This was a modern, purpose-built unit![109]

This kind of account challenges some of the 'progress' narratives found in design literature about improvements in hospital design and landscaping. For this individual, echoing some of the specific comments above about long-stay psychiatric patients, the view of a courtyard served not as beautiful 'green space' but as a reminder of what they could *not* access (a rolling countryside out of view, exercise, and implicitly freedom). Windows, and the views from them, always existed in relation to a viewer.

Illness narratives and individual memories are important reminders that social and cultural factors have always interacted with individual bodies, emotions, experiences, and more. A return to the concept of 'atmospheres', discussed previously in relation to 'homeliness', may be useful here. In an article on affect, atmosphere, and secure psychiatric units, Steven Brown *et al.* note that atmosphere must be grounded in 'socio-historical settings' but that

> There is a danger that in describing the 'quasi thing-like' character of feelings 'poured into place' atmospheres can seem to be 'just there' awaiting the person who experiences them. Yet clearly the way in which we engage with an atmosphere is crucial to what it is we feel.[110]

They argue for the value of thinking about 'modes of engagement' with atmospheres, including in healthcare settings.[111] This careful balance, which recognises the co-existence of 'a' culturally informed shared sense of atmosphere and various individual atmospheres, is useful for historians of design, architecture, space, and place.[112] It is a more relational approach, which helps us to shift away from histories in which either buildings or people are the centre, and offers a more entangled way of thinking about hospitals.

Conclusions

The story of glass at the end of the twentieth century offers many points of comparison with whiteness. Glass is often discussed as a transparent material, partly explaining its connection with modernist architecture. It is often overlooked in histories of hospital design perhaps precisely because of the assumption that its primary role is transparency and lightness. As Stephen Eskilson argues in *The Age of Glass*, '[c]orporate atria, hospitals, museums, schools, malls, airports: nowadays structural glass facades may be literally transparent but they are also largely invisible in the public's imagination'.[113] Like white walls, glass has too often been treated as neutral or absent in colour terms, when it was anything but. Glass itself was an important material addition to the hospital, whether dirty, clear, or reflective.

Glass has a long – and ongoing – role in introducing colour (in stained glass), in providing privacy (in frosted glass), and in reflecting back a building's interior. The assumption that glass is purely a visual phenomenon is also flawed, as glass has always affected other sensory qualities of space such as temperature. In relation to the history of colour, even transparent glass is an important and often neglected part of the story. The changing positioning of beds in relation to hospital windows, for example, has meant that more patients can look out of them; whether the view is of trees or a car park, this is an important part of the colour palette that they inhabit. The growing use of glass is actually perhaps the most important shift in modern architecture for the history of colour. Light (both natural and electric) and weather have also always affected the way that colours look, change over time, and are experienced. In hospitals with more glass, all of the decorative trends outlined to this point would have been experienced differently.

The history of glass in hospitals is the story of a shift in ways of seeing and experiencing colour. The expansion of glass walls, windows, and atriums – along with other shifts such as new bed positions and an increasing number of single rooms – meant that people saw colour through, in, and on glass more than ever before. Windows were increasingly sealed, but they were also more widespread, meaning that they were particularly important as part of the history of light in hospitals. As sounds and air from outside were cut off, by the end of the century light poured in, moved, fell on new (often bright) colour schemes, and changed the hospital colour palette more than ever before. More widespread use of glass changed other aspects of the atmosphere of hospitals, for example by creating more of a commercial feel, again in dialogue with new colour schemes and other architectural features. The prevalence of windows in people's memories of hospitals also shows that they were highly meaningful. They could operate as thresholds, barriers, or powerful embodied encounters with the world outside the hospital. Overall, then, the history of glass is one of the most important – and most overlooked – stories in the history of hospital design and experience.

Notes

1 Le Corbusier, trans. Paul Stirton, annot. Tim Benton, 'Glass, the Fundamental Material of Modern Architecture', *West 86th: A Journal of Decorative Arts, Design History, and Material Culture*, 19 (2012 [1935]), p. 292. Though unbuilt, Le Corbusier also experimented with the importance of skylights in hospital design in the infamous 'New Venice Hospital' in the 1960s; Mariabruna Fabrizi, 'The Building is the City: Le Corbusier's Unbuilt Hospital in Venice', *Socks*, https://socks-studio.com/2014/05/18/the-building-is-the-city-le-corbusiers-unbuilt-hospital-in-venice/ [accessed: 28 February 2024].
2 Le Corbusier, 'Glass', p. 294.
3 Alain Corbin, 'Urban Sensations: The Shifting Sensescape of the City', in Constance Classen (ed.), *A Cultural History of the Senses in the Age of Empire* (Bloomsbury, 2014), p. 48.
4 Juhani Pallasmaa, *The Eyes of the Skin: Architecture and the Senses* (John Wiley & Sons, 2005 [1996]).
5 Zoë Blackler, 'Juhani Pallasmaa in Praise of Shadows at the Cooper Union in New York', *The Architectural Review*, https://www.architectural-review.com/essays/new-york-usa-juhani-pallasmaa-in-praise-of-shadows-at-the-cooper-union-in-new-york [accessed: 28 February 2024].
6 'Windows and Environment', *The Architectural Review*, 1 December 1969, pp. 11–12.
7 Beatriz Colomina, *X-Ray Architecture* (Lars Müller Publishers, 2019), p. 136.
8 *Ibid.*, p. 137.

9 These quotes are taken from an exhibition board, see RIBApix, RIBA35370, 'Exhibition Display Panels', https://www.ribapix.com/Exhibition-display-panels-explaining-features-of-the-design-of-Finsbury-Health-Centre-Pine-Street-Finsbury-London-Cheerful-atmosphere_RIBA35370# [accessed: 28 February 2024]; see also John Allan, '1938: Finsbury Health Centre, London', *C20th Society*, https://c20society.org.uk/100-buildings/1938-finsbury-health-centre-london [accessed: 28 February 2024].
10 John Sadar, 'The Healthful Ambience of Vitaglass: Light, Glass and the Curative Environment', *arq: Architectural Research Quarterly*, 12 (2008), pp. 269–81.
11 See Clare Hickman, 'Pine Fresh: The Cultural and Medical Context of Pine Scent in Relation to Health – From the Forest to the Home', *Medical Humanities*, 48 (2022), pp. 104–13.
12 Chance Brothers Limited Glass Works Advert, *The Hospital*, March 1951, p. xiii.
13 *Ibid.*
14 'Glass in the Hospital', *The Hospital*, September 1949, p. 569.
15 Nuffield Provincial Hospitals Trust, *Studies in the Functions and Design of Hospitals* (Oxford University Press, 1955), pp. 20–1.
16 R. Llewelyn Davis, *The Scottish Design Congress* (The Council of Industrial Design Scottish Committee, 1954), p. 6.
17 Brian Abel-Smith, *The Hospitals, 1800–1948: A Study in Social Administration in England and Wales* (Heinemann, 1964), p. 402.
18 RIBA Archive, AHP/25/4, Adams, Holden + Pearson, Cuttings concerning the Royal Cornwall Hospital at Treliske near Truro.
19 'Commissioning a Hospital', *The Hospital*, March 1961, p. 1.
20 Peter Scher, 'The Low-Rise Era', *50 Years of Health Building: A Supplement to HD* (1998), pp. 22–3; on landscaping and Wexham Park see also Edward Patrick DeVane, 'Building the NHS: Planning, Publics and Britain's New State Healthcare Facilities, 1945–74' (PhD Dissertation: University of Warwick, 2022), pp. 79–81.
21 DeVane, 'Building the NHS', p. 80.
22 The National Archives, MH166/1136, Harness Interiors produced by the interior designers from the Regional Health Authorities and the Department of Health & Social Security, part of the papers of the 'Technical Design Group', 1973–75, pp. 19, 24.
23 Department of Health and Social Security and Welsh Office, *The Organisation of the In-Patient's Day: Report of a Committee of the Central Health Services Council* (HMSO, 1976), p. 68.
24 Roger Ulrich, 'View Through a Window May Influence Recovery', *Science*, 224 (1984), pp. 420–1.

25 David Theodore, 'Better Design, Better Hospitals', *CMAJ*, 188 (2016), pp. 902–3.
26 Charles Rice, *Interior Urbanism: Architecture, John Portman and Downtown America* (Bloomsbury, 2016), pp. 2–3.
27 Sunand Prasad, 'Typology Quarterly: Hospitals', *The Architectural Review*, 27 April 2012, http://www.architectural-review.com/essays/typology-quarterly-hospitals/8629443.article [accessed: 28 February 2024].
28 Alex Bozikovic, 'In Eb Zeidler's World, Architecture is "Everything"', *The Globe and Mail*, 23 November 2013, http://www.theglobeandmail.com/life/home-and-garden/architecture/in-eb-zeidlers-world-architecture-is-everything/article15554908/ [accessed: 28 February 2024].
29 Annmarie Adams and David Theodore, 'The Architecture of Children's Hospitals in Toronto and Montreal, 1875–2010', in Cheryl Krasnick Warsh and Veronica Strong-Boag (eds), *Children's Health Issues in Historical Perspective* (Wildred Laureier University Press, 2005), p. 466.
30 David Charles Sloane and Beverlie Conant Sloane, *Medicine Moves to the Mall* (Johns Hopkins University Press, 2003), p. 107.
31 The perceived link between the spatial patterns of hospitals and airports had a long history, and is famously evoked in Philip Larkin's poem 'The Building' (1972). At this time, other kinds of healthcare structures were also even more directly linked to commercial buildings, for example see Ed DeVane on West Midlands welfare centres that used 'adapted premises such as shops and cinemas'; DeVane, 'Building the NHS, p. 134.
32 Wil Gesler, Morag Bell, Sarah Curtis, Phil Hubbard, and Susan Francis, 'Therapy by Design: Evaluating the UK Hospital Building Program', *Health & Place*, 10 (2004), p. 123.
33 For example, Boots noted the use of pastel colours in their visits to American commercial pharmacies in the 1950s; Walgreens Boots Alliance Heritage, WBA/BT/12/17/1, 'International Wholesale Visit Reports' (1958–59). Thanks to Jack Moss for drawing my attention to this source, which he found as part of his University of Nottingham PhD research on the history of Boots.
34 Sloane and Sloane, *Medicine Moves to the Mall*, pp. 94–5.
35 Mary Lou Lobsinger, 'Animation for Sick Kids', *Canadian Architect*, 1 April 1993, p. 16.
36 Alex Mold, 'Making the Patient-Consumer in Margaret Thatcher's Britain', *The Historical Journal*, 54 (2011), pp. 509–28.
37 Susan Black, 'Interior Design Trends', *Hospital Development*, 10 (1982), p. 24.

38 Sarah Curtis *et al.*, 'Therapeutic Landscapes in Hospital Design: A Qualitative Assessment by Staff and Service Users of the Design of a New Mental Health Inpatient Unit', *Environment and Planning C: Government and Policy*, 25 (2007), p. 595.
39 On the spread of the American shopping mall to the UK see Sam Wetherell, *Foundations: How the Built Environment Made Twentieth-Century Britain* (Princeton University Press, 2020), p. 49; on the rise of the atrium in late twentieth-century US hospitals see Annmarie Adams, David Theodore, Ellie Goldenberg, Coralee McLaren, and Patricia McKeever, 'Kids in the Atrium: Comparing Architectural Intentions and Children's Experiences in a Pediatric Hospital Lobby', *Social Science & Medicine*, 70 (2010), pp. 658–67.
40 Serena Dyer, 'Shopping and the Senses: Retail, Browsing and Consumption in 18th-Century England', *History Compass*, 12 (2014), p. 698.
41 P. Dormer, 'Review: Improving Hospital Design', *BMJ*, 29 October 1993, p. 309.
42 Owen Hatherley, *A Guide to the New Ruins of Great Britain* (Verso, 2011 [2010]), p. viii.
43 This trend also had deeper roots. For example, 'the shops will have displays of goods in their windows', in The National Archives, MH 166/1136, Harness Interiors produced by the interior designers from the Regional Health Authorities and the Department of Health & Social Security, part of the papers of the 'Technical Design Group', 1973–75, p. 9.
44 Ratio, 'Rikshospitalet', https://www.ratioark.no/en/projects/rikshospitalet-oslo [accessed: 20 March 2024].
45 Lizette Alvarez, 'Where the Healing Touch Starts With the Hospital Design', *New York Times*, 7 September 2004, http://www.nytimes.com/2004/09/07/health/07hosp.html?pagewanted=print&position=&_r=0 [accessed: 28 February 2024].
46 *Ibid.*
47 *Ibid.*
48 This interest was explicit in a number of ways. For example, the international influence of Scandinavian design is discussed in Nuffield Provincial Hospitals Trust, *Studies in the Functions and Design of Hospitals* (Oxford University Press, 1955); N. H. B. Duncalfe, 'A Scandinavian Tour of Hospitals', *The Hospital*, July 1962, p. 446; Wellcome Library, PP/RMS/A/1, 'Report of joint visit by Mr D. J. Petty, senior architect, and Dr Shaw, senior medical officer, Ministry of Health to Denmark, Sweden, Finland and Norway, 25th April–28th May 1955'.

49 Vicky Casey interviewed by Victoria Bates, 20 January 2023. Casey also compares atriums to cathedrals. See also Ruth Richardson, 'Building Healing Environments: An Historic Perspective', in Deborah Kirklin and Ruth Richardson (eds), *The Healing Environment: Without and Within* (Royal College of Physicians, 2003), p. 25.
50 Barbara Erwine, *Creating Sensory Spaces: The Architecture of the Invisible* (Routledge, 2017), p. 43.
51 On 28 February 2024 Google Scholar showed that this article had been cited 8,337 times. Though no single citation tracker is authoritative, this can be taken as broadly indicative of the influence of this scholarship.
52 The 'environmental control' quote relates to American history, but is equally applicable in the UK. See Jeanne Kisacky, 'When Fresh Air Went Out of Fashion at Hospitals: How the Hospital Went From Luxury Resort to Windowless Box', *Smithsonian Magazine*, 14 June 2017, https://www.smithsonianmag.com/history/when-fresh-air-went-out-fashion-hospitals-180963710/ [accessed: 28 February 2024].
53 As Clare Hickman notes, many of the trends of the late twentieth-century hospital landscape design would have been 'familiar' to those in the late nineteenth century, but their contexts, meanings, and technologies were distinct. See Clare Hickman, *Therapeutic Landscapes: A History of English Hospital Gardens since 1800* (Manchester University Press, 2013), p. 216.
54 Shan Jiang, *Nature through a Hospital Window: The Therapeutic Benefits of Landscape in Architectural Design* (Routledge, 2022), eBook np.
55 Though Nightingale did mention one large ward window with 'beautiful views' and did speak of the value of seeing out, she placed emphasis more on three functions: '1. Light; 2. Ventilation; 3. To enable patients to read in bed'; Florence Nightingale, *Notes on Hospitals* (Longman, Green, Longman, Roberts and Green, 1863 [1858]), p. 63; 'bright colours of flowers' cited in Clare Cooper Marcus and Marni Barnes, *Gardens In Healthcare Facilities* (The Center for Health Design, 1995), p. 8.
56 Richard A. Hobday, 'Sunlight Therapy and Solar Architecture', *Medical History*, 41 (1997), pp. 455–72.
57 Jiang, *Nature through a Hospital Window*.
58 The term 'international' is used broadly here to reflect the fact that Ulrich's work was undertaken in the US and was read, cited, and used in many countries. It also reflects the fact that many of the trends discussed in this chapter were not specific to the UK. Similar stories

can be told about many countries, for example, on Australia and the way it has embraced so-called 'biophilic' design see Kate Copeland (ed.), *Australian Healthcare Design 2000–2015: A Critical Review of the Design and Build of Healthcare Infrastructure in Australia* (International Academy for Design and Health, 2013), p. 54. The Australian example also offers a reminder that many cultures and countries were already closely connected to 'nature'. The design of many Indigenous healthcare buildings, for example, was embedded in ideas about connecting to place and land, and architects in Australia and New Zealand have turned to local communities to learn from them. See Julian Soper, 'Designing Culturally Inclusive Health Facilities', *Arup*, https://www.arup.com/perspectives/designing-culturally-inclusive-health-facilities [accessed: 1 March 2024]. Glass was only seen as necessary to reconnect to nature, then, in places and communities where that connection had apparently been lost through big institutional structures.

59 David Theodore, 'The Decline of the Hospital as a Healing Machine', in Sarah Schrank and Didem Ekici (eds), *Healing Spaces, Modern Architecture, and the Body* (Routledge, 2017), p. 195.

60 Albeit in the context of Victorian and Edwardian public schools, Jane Hamlett argues that '[e]nclosure or confinement in space is also fundamental to emotional life'; cited in Rob Boddice, *The History of Emotions* (Manchester University Press, 2018), p. 172.

61 Duncan P. R. Patterson, '"There's Glass between Us": A Critical Examination of "the Window" in Art and Architecture from Ancient Greece to the Present Day', *FORUM Journal*, 10 (2011), p. 3.

62 Richard Burton, 'St Mary's Hospital, Isle of Wight: A Suitable Background for Caring', *BMJ* (December 1990), pp. 1423–5.

63 Sarah L. Bell, Clare Hickman, and Frank Houghton, 'From Therapeutic Landscape to Therapeutic "Sensescape" Experiences with Nature? A Scoping Review', *Wellbeing, Space and Society*, 4 (2023), pp. 1–11; see also Sarah L. Bell, Ronan Foley, Frank Houghton, Avril Maddrell, and Allison M. Williams, 'From Therapeutic Landscapes to Healthy Spaces, Places and Practices: A Scoping Review', *Social Science & Medicine*, 196 (2018), pp. 123–30.

64 In this case there was an issue with the supplier that limited this colour scheme in practice, but the principle remains important and potentially indicative of practices elsewhere; Stephen Scrivens, 'Suffolk Hospital: Roof Gardens', *Architects' Journal*, 16 April 1980, p. 782.

65 P. R. Thoday, *Hospital Courtyard Design* (DHSS, nd), p. 9. Though there is no date given for this publication, its references run up to

1974 and it has a British Library stamp from 1981, so must have been published between these dates.

66 Hickman, *Therapeutic Landscapes*, p. 221.

67 Ronald Weeks, 'Interior Design: Hospitals', *The Architectural Review*, 1 July 1980, p. 46.

68 Bell, Hickman, and Houghton, 'From Therapeutic Landscape to Therapeutic "Sensescape"; see also Bell *et al.*, 'From Therapeutic Landscapes to Healthy Spaces, Places and Practices'.

69 Wellcome, ART/AFH/A/12/3, Pat Hartridge, 'Garden of Healing'. This article isn't dated but it talks about projects from the 1980s as if they are recent, up to 1987. The influence of these ideas is indicated by the fact it was collected as part of the 'Landscape and Healthcare' collection of AFH. See also Pat Hartridge, 'Hospital Wildlife Gardens', *Professional Horticulture*, 3 (1989), pp. 51–5.

70 Hartridge, 'Garden of Healing'.

71 Wellcome Library, ART/AFH/A/5/2/, 'Computer-Driven Scenes Give Patients Room with a Healing View', 9 April 1990; Wellcome Library, ART/AFH/A/5/2/, 'A Sickroom with a View: A New Artificial Window Brightens Patients' Days', *Newsweek*, 26 March 1990, p. 61. Wellcome Library, ART/AFH/A/5/2, 'Behind Closed Doors', *Hospital Development*, 24 (1993), p. 35. These examples are all from a UK arts for health collection of cuttings and articles, though many of their early examples of digital windows were from the US.

72 There is a rich history of hospital gardens, which – while it is not the focus of this book – shows some of the differences in what landscapes hospital windows might have offered; see in particular Hickman, *Therapeutic Landscapes*. Hickman has also contributed to the Hospital Senses Collective work on wildlife and its relationship to hospital windows, including for example how birds have historically been able to enter open ones. See Hospital Senses Collective, 'Birds', *Thresholds*, https://hospitalsenses.co.uk/birds/ [accessed: 28 February 2024] and Clare Hickman, '"Sick Hands, Thin and White, Were Always Slipping Offerings Across my Windowsill, Offerings for the Little Birdlings": Multispecies Encounters Within and Around the Rural Modernist Medical Institution', *Modernist Cultures*, 19 (2024), pp. 8–32.

73 Hickman, *Therapeutic Landscapes*, pp. 206, 217.

74 For example, Hannah Pitt, 'Muddying the Waters: What Urban Waterways Reveal about Bluespaces and Wellbeing', *Geoforum*, 92 (2018), pp. 161–70.

75 London Metropolitan Archives, 'Evaluation of New Guys House', A/KE/I/01/024/060.

76 The National Archives, DT 33/1328, 'Southmead General Hospital', 1946–70.
77 Wellcome Library, ART/AFH/A/1/1, Howard Goodman, 'A User Friendly, Quality, Healthy Environment', 1989, p. 12.
78 Wellcome Library, ART/AFH/A/8/1, South East Thames Regional Health Authority, 'The New Hastings Hospital', c. 1987.
79 Guy Eades interviewed by Victoria Bates, 13 March 2023. On creating privacy through window art, see also Christopher Tipping interviewed by Victoria Bates, 25 March 2023.
80 Wellcome Library, ART/AFH/A/8/1, 'Recommendations for Inclusion of Artworks for Medway DGH: Mental Illness and Geriatric Block', 1989.
81 Pallasmaa, *The Eyes of the Skin*, p. 34.
82 *Ibid.*
83 Kresen Kernow, AHA/372, 'Minutes, Liskeard Hospitals' House Committee', 1948–54.
84 Derbyshire Record Office, D6082/18/2/3, Southern Derbyshire Community Health Council visit to Derbyshire Royal Infirmary.
85 *Ibid.*
86 Mass Observation Archive (University of Sussex), Replies to Spring 1997 directive [M2290].
87 I was told this on a tour of Paimio Sanatorium, and it has been repeated anecdotally online, though I cannot trace the original source; for example Minna Jones, 'Household Tip by Alvar Aalto', 14 November 2012, http://www.minnajones.com/2012/11/household-tip-by-alvar-aalto.html [accessed: 28 February 2024].
88 King's College London Archives, K/PP149 3/1/8, Address by Dr C. Saunders, at St. Christopher's Annual General Meeting, 22 July 1966, p. 3.
89 On hospice design and the specifics of their architecture, see Ken Worpole, *Modern Hospice Design: The Architecture of Palliative Care* (Routledge, 2009).
90 The National Archive, ED 173/63, *Meeting the Educational Needs of Children in Hospital: Design Note 38* (Department of Education and Science, 1984), p. 5. Department of Health and Social Security Welsh Office, *Hospital Accommodation for Children: Health Building Note 23* (HMSO, 1984).
91 RIBA Archive, Adams, Holden + Pearson Press Cuttings, Elizabeth Prosser, 'Sister Patricia Finds her Paradise', AHP/25/4.
92 Bill Murray, 'Changing the Face of Patient Care', *Hospital Development*, 16 (1988), p. 25.
93 'Products: Security Screen', *Hospital Development*, 24 (1993), p. 25.

94 On genre see Angela Woods, 'The Limits of Narrative: Provocations for the Medical Humanities', *Medical Humanities*, 37 (2011), pp. 73–8.
95 Ben Watt, *Patient: The True Story of a Rare Illness* (Viking, 1996), pp. 50–1.
96 Tim Ingold, *The Perception of the Environment: Essays on Livelihood, Dwelling and Skill* (Routledge, 2000), p. 199.
97 Tim Ingold, 'The Eye of the Storm: Visual Perception and the Weather', *Visual Studies*, 20 (2005), p. 99.
98 Shanti Sumartojo, Tim Edensor, and Sarah Pink, 'Atmospheres in Urban Light', *Ambiances* [Online], 2019, https://doi.org/10.4000/ambiances.2586 [accessed: 8 September 2023].
99 Sumartojo *et al.*, 'Atmospheres in Urban Light'.
100 It falls outside the timeframe of this book, but I have also written on the significance of windows in the graphic memoir *Probably Nothing* by Matilda Tristram (2014); see Victoria Bates, 'Sensing Space and Making Place: The Hospital and Therapeutic Landscapes in Two Cancer Narratives', *Medical Humanities*, 45 (2019), pp. 10–20.
101 'Sensing Spaces of Healthcare: NHS Sensory Memory Bank', Memory 7 https://hospitalsenses.blogs.bristol.ac.uk [accessed: 9 February 2024]. This research was conducted by the author.
102 'Sensing Spaces of Healthcare: NHS Sensory Memory Bank', Memory 66 https://hospitalsenses.blogs.bristol.ac.uk [accessed: 9 February 2024]. This research was conducted by the author.
103 'Sensing Spaces of Healthcare: NHS Sensory Memory Bank', Memory 15 https://hospitalsenses.blogs.bristol.ac.uk [accessed: 9 February 2024]. This research was conducted by the author.
104 For example, Mass Observation Archive (University of Sussex), Replies to Spring 1997 directive [B1440 and P1637].
105 British Library Sounds, C1887/204, Sandra Adcock interviewed by Naomi Weaver, July 2019, Voices of Our National Health Service © University of Manchester.
106 British Library Sounds, C1887/141, Alice Woods interviewed by Gwen Crossley, March 2019, Voices of Our National Health Service, © University of Manchester.
107 Mass Observation Archive (University of Sussex), Replies to Spring 1997 directive [W1893]. Capitalisation in original.
108 Roger Sim and Helen Kitchen, *More than a Place of Healing: An Anthology of Memories, Memorabilia and Anecdotes of Withington Hospital* (Hospital Arts, 1999), p. 62.
109 Mass Observation Archive (University of Sussex), Replies to Spring 2008 directive [P3213].

110 Steven D. Brown, Ava Kanyeredzi, Laura McGrath, Paula Reavey, and Ian Tucker, 'Affect Theory and the Concept of Atmosphere', *Distinktion: Journal of Social Theory*, 20 (2019), pp. 11, 13.
111 *Ibid.*, p. 13.
112 *Concerning Astonishing Atmospheres: Aisthesis, Aura and Atmospheric Portfolio* (Mimesis International, 2018), p. 42.
113 Stephen Eskilson, *The Age of Glass: A Cultural History of Glass in Modern and Contemporary Architecture* (Bloomsbury, 2018), p. 154.

Conclusions: white to bright

Hospitals are not drab subjects. Though hospitals lost much of their colour in the early twentieth century, they were more colourful than ever by its end. Shifts in hospital colour schemes broadly aligned with societal, cultural, and political changes. The all-white hospital of the early twentieth century, for example, symbolised hygiene and efficiency; the turn towards pastel, homely, and 'humanistic' hospitals represented a growing interest in patients' emotions and experiences, which aligned with the rise of the welfare state and post-war social democracy; and, finally, bright colours and glass link to histories of consumerism and neo-liberalism. There are also several other important stories in modern history with which this narrative connects. Changing colour palettes met the shifting medical needs of staff, patients, and visitors, from the rising number of maternity service users, to the decline in long-stay patients, the increase in visiting hours, and the ageing population. Hospital colour schemes also responded to wider trends in international and national architecture and interior design.

In many ways, the 'big' story outlined here is one of modernity or modernisation. Hospitals were part of modern Britain, including building the welfare state and building cities. In the post-war period, some even saw hospital design and city planning as 'analogous'.[1] Hospitals and their colour schemes were key to the construction of 'modernity' and its meanings, both within and beyond healthcare. Irrespective of the colour and time period, the idea that that colour was 'bright' and 'modern' was commonplace: white, pastels, artworks, patterns, vibrant shades, and glass alike were all discussed in these terms. The language stayed consistent but each new colour palette, or coloured material, represented a shift in the meaning of modernity.

The modern hospital environment – including its colour schemes – was intertwined with questions about what it meant to provide good medicine and care, particularly after the introduction of the NHS. The conundrum of the modern hospital, specifically with the rise of the large District General Hospital, was well expressed in *Architects' Journal* in 1963:

> The size and complexity of building necessary to accommodate a large general hospital presents aesthetic and technical problems which are not easy to reconcile. How to achieve a scale which is reasonably intimate rather than oppressively imposing? An environment which is disciplined but not authoritarian, clinically efficient yet also comfortable? Above all how to establish an atmosphere which, while paying due respect to the mystique associated with the medical profession, nevertheless enables the patient to feel at home.[2]

A more recent commentator, writing in *The Architectural Review* on the hospital as 'building type' in 2002, made similar comments about the challenges of reconciling 'technology and humanity'.[3] The hospital was the 'perfect Modern building', it noted, and a 'technical building par excellence ... a great machine, reassuring in its efficiency, yet it could also be a labyrinth in which the patient felt lost'.[4] Hospitals – including their architecture and design – became a symbol of the many requirements of modern healthcare, and the challenge of balancing them.

Many people in the late twentieth century found themselves generally troubled by how modernity was shaping up, and conversations about colour (or the lack thereof) became a shorthand for such concerns. There were broad critiques of 'Enlightenment notions of progress' in the 1960s and 1970s, and these were often expressed through attacks on architecture.[5] The white modern, and modernist, hospital was similarly under attack at this time and perhaps more than any other building represented these 'notions of progress'. Concerns about modernity were often heightened, or expressed, in relation to hospitals as symbols of an increasingly high-technology healthcare system that seemed to prioritise efficiency and hygiene over humanity. As a range of contemporary commentators sought to redefine 'modern' healthcare, colour came to represent some of these principles: efficiency and hygiene, humanistic and homely, and eventually also patient-centred and even consumerist. On a more practical level, it also offered the flexibility that architects increasingly embraced and associated with modernity.[6]

The past also had a role in constructing modernity, and colour schemes were an important part of this process. Older colour schemes were often dismissed as 'forbidding', 'gloomy', 'dehumanising', or 'old-fashioned', partly to construct new ones as 'modern' and 'humanistic'.[7] Such views were in tension with the rhetorical romanticisation of Victorian hospitals, for example with repeated references to Florence Nightingale and the way she embraced 'brilliancy of colour', alongside critiques of modernist, functionalist architecture and design.[8] Yet, critiques of the past were grounded in rhetoric as much as reality. Many hospitals still had, and complained about, the large Nightingale wards and long corridors of Victorian buildings. Criticisms of the old-fashioned dark greens of Victorian hospitals sat alongside positive discussions of the fresh light, air, colour, and flowers found in Nightingale wards. Complaints about the sterility and dehumanisation of all-white hospitals failed to note that there was often quite extensive and careful use of colour in modernist hospitals.

The story of colour and 'modernisation' is not about progress; it is about the building up of new layers of meaning. Continuity and change often sat side by side in material terms as well as cultural ones, and change over time was not linear. Just as paint in hospitals was layered, creating different strata that can tell us different things about how the space and function of the hospital was viewed, we need to see modernity as multi-layered. This conceptual framework offers a new way to understand the multiplicities of modernity, which transcends ideas of transformation, tension, or co-existence. It also facilitates new ways of understanding change over time, by putting material history – rather than political or social history – at the centre of historical narratives.

Colour also tells a story about everyday life and its relationships with the 'modern'. Many colour schemes were entirely practical and followed no obvious order or timeline, revealing the disjointed and localised nature of modern British hospitals. Some hospital colour schemes were chosen by professional interior decorators, others by estates teams; some were chosen for aesthetic qualities, others for economy and practicality. Some local decision-makers pushed back against architects' decisions or recommendations, while in other locations painting was done on a more ad hoc basis. Many of these local negotiations over colour schemes were important, and shaped principles such as patient-centred design, showing that such ideas were not just 'top down' or driven by a centralised, coherent NHS.

A history of colour is always, in part, a history of experience. Colour was a material, emotional, and multi-sensory phenomenon. Studying hospital history through these lenses further disrupts politics-based periodisation, and has an unstable chronology. Hospital colour was experienced and encountered in different ways according to physiology and colour perception, cultural contexts, and social factors such as demography, including gender, age, and race, and geography. Tim Edensor argues for 'more extensive geographical research, including ethnographic explorations into the meanings and feelings attributed by local residents to the colo[u]rs they live amidst' and this plea could easily be extended to historical research.[9] Going beyond social and cultural histories, a relational approach to histories of hospital colour shows that colours could be experienced (or remembered) in a wide range of ways by different people, or even by the same person on a different day. Colour was itself an unstable and important actor, changing through human intervention (from damage to maintenance) and non-human intervention (such as weather, and weathering). Colour moved in and out of hospitals, through objects, in a way that did not always neatly align with decorative schemes.

There is great value in understanding the history of colour as a messy ongoing process, rather than a neat history of ideologically informed decisions. This approach to the history of colour conceptualises it as part of the history of everyday life, a framework that makes sense of change over time by showing how the 'apparently universalizing processes of modernity are shot through with historical survivals and local differences'.[10] A colour-based chronology, with its literal and figurative layers, offers a new timeline for the architecture, design, and mundane life of the modern British hospital. It guides historians away from the idea of novelty, particularly in relation to the idea of the NHS as a turning point, and shows subtle shifts in hospitals over the course of the twentieth century.

Many of the trends discussed in this book are still influential, and a multi-layered model of colour and modernity continues to exist. This point is well illustrated by the outcomes of a series of workshops at

Great Ormond Street Hospital in London and Southmead Hospital in Bristol in 2022, run by Rebecka Fleetwood-Smith as part the 'Sensing Spaces of Healthcare' project, in which colour emerged as a key theme. The research involved talking to people about their sensory experiences and their 'dream hospitals', using a range of creative methods including mapping, collage, and clay. Reflecting on a collage, one staff member said 'I remembered how important colour is in the hospital environment. You know, I can remember being at hospital as a kid, and it's quite sterile'.[11] Another made a similar point, that 'some people say, oh, it is just a colour on the wall, [but] it actually does play a part' in supporting people having a difficult time.[12] In terms of the colours chosen, from a selection offered as part of the activity, there was a range of responses (see Figure 7.1). Many staff members emphasised 'natural' and neutral shades, including 'warm colours and different shades of these colours, organic shapes and gentle textures' and colours that represent 'the

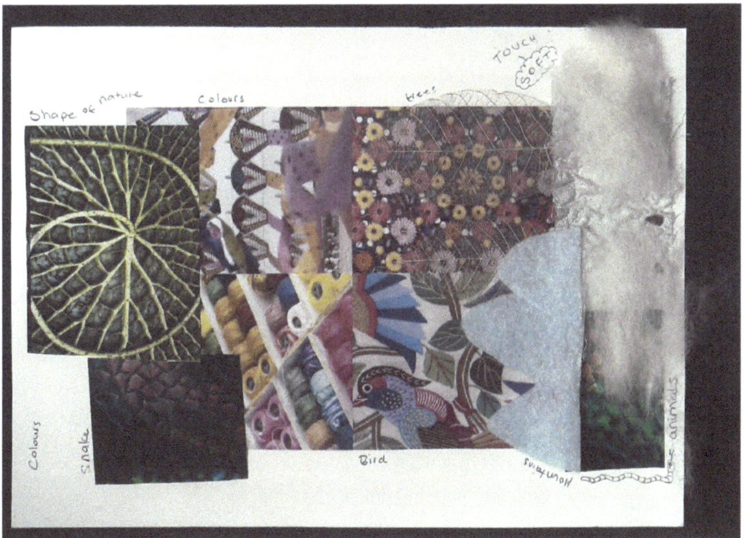

Figure 7.1 Participant collages from the 'Sensing Spaces of Healthcare' project. Clockwise from top left: A1004, A2003, and A1013.

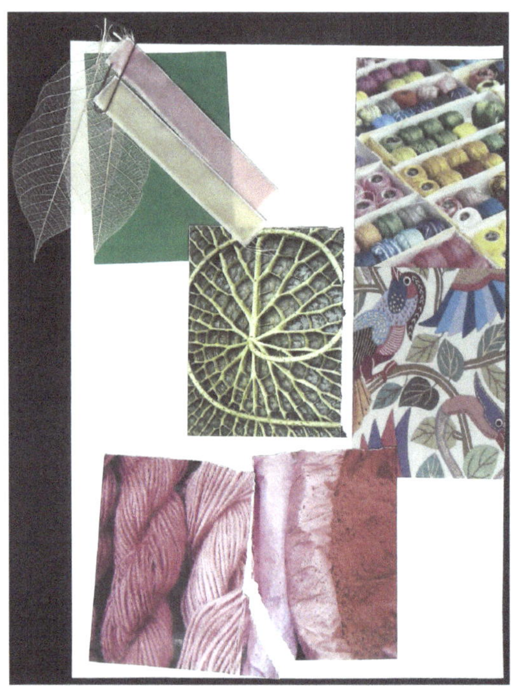

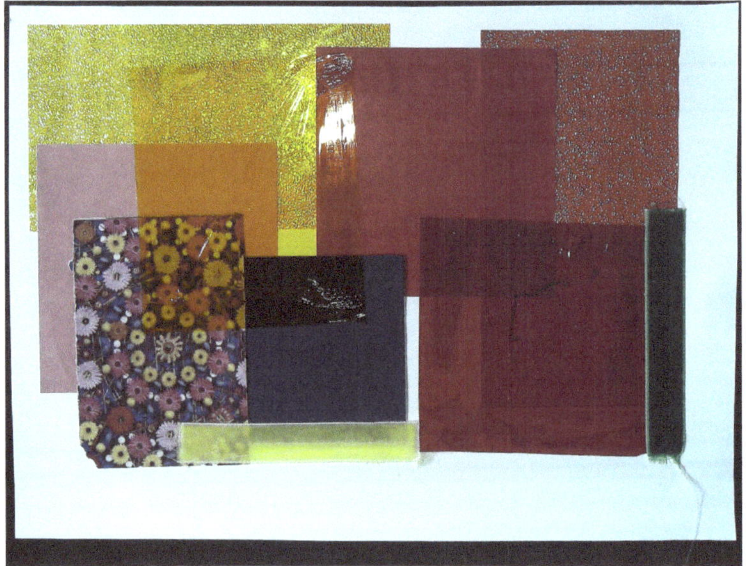

Figure 7.1 Continued

environment and colour and shapes that exist in nature'.[13] One maternity service user went for a different colour scheme, noting that 'initially after considering the words "calm", "relaxing", and "homely" I started to gather pale/neutral/pastel colours, but it did not feel friendly or inviting, rather bland and impersonal. I found looking at brighter colours and patterns felt friendlier, less clinical and [more] inviting'.[14]

The variety of responses reinforces the personal nature of colour and colour preferences, and shows some of the different cultural scripts that have built up around colour over time and which continue to co-exist. The intertwining of ideas about nature and soft, pastel colour palettes has roots in the story of 'humanisation'. As one participant noted, pastels and natural shades are the colour palettes of words such as 'homely' and 'relaxing', which remain design goals in many hospitals. The brighter colour palette offers an expansion of what colour can be in hospitals, emphasising the potential to go beyond 'homely' and towards concepts such as 'friendly' and 'inviting'. The interest in vibrant schemes, including colours such as red, is a relatively recent one but it has not displaced pastels and natural colour palettes.

Overall, rather than thinking about linear stories, with twists and turns, the history of colour offers a way to think about change over time as a series of layers and palimpsests. Each layer exists in dialogue with the other, rather than replacing what came before, and each of these layers is itself textured and complex. Colour is a rich and vivid subject of enquiry. It is time to stop treating colour as a backdrop, and instead bring it to the foreground of our narratives.

Notes

1 Guy Ortolano, *Thatcher's Progress: From Social Democracy to Market Liberalism through an English New Town* (Cambridge University Press, 2019), p. 93.
2 'Building Study: Hospital', *Architects' Journal*, 25 December 1963, p. 1366.
3 'Comment: The Hospital as Building Type', *The Architectural Review*, 1 March 2002, p. 43.
4 *Ibid.*

5 Owen Hopkins, *Architectural Styles: A Visual Guide* (Laurence King Publishing, 2014), p. 194.
6 Colours could not only be easily changed or replaced, to suit the changing needs of a building, but by the early twenty-first century architects were using colours that were themselves 'versatile' and able to 'transform'. See Juan Serra, 'The Versatility of Color in Contemporary Architecture', *Color Research & Application*, 38 (2013), pp. 344–55.
7 Susan Black, 'Interior Design Trends', *Hospital Development*, 10 (1982), p. 24.
8 Such references are present from the post-war years to the twenty-first century. For example, see Nightingale quoted on colour in Nuffield Provincial Hospitals Trust, *Studies in the Functions and Design of Hospitals* (Oxford University Press, 1955), p. 109; John Wells-Thorpe, 'Healing by Design: Feeling Better?', in Deborah Kirklin and Ruth Richardson (eds), *The Healing Environment: Without and Within* (Royal College of Physicians, 2003), p. 12; Fiona McWilliam, 'Care in the Community', *Architects' Journal*, 28 October 2004, p. 5; The King's Fund, *Celebrating Achievement: Enhancing the Healing Environment Programme 2003–2005* (TSO, 2006), p. 2.
9 Edensor, 'What Color is this Place?', *GeoHumanities*, 9 (2023), p. 442.
10 Joe Moran, 'History, Memory and the Everyday', *Rethinking History*, 8 (2004), p. 55.
11 A2002 interviewed by Rebecka Fleetwood-Smith, 2022.
12 A1001 interviewed by Rebecka Fleetwood-Smith, 2022.
13 A2003 interviewed by Rebecka Fleetwood-Smith, 2022, and A1004 interviewed by Rebecka Fleetwood-Smith, 2022.
14 A1013 interviewed by Rebecka Fleetwood-Smith, 2022.

Index

Please note that page references in italics refer the reader to photographs, tables or other images. Movements and schools of thought, along with exterior, more permanent aspects of hospital buildings such as the size, number and shape of windows, appear under 'architectural ideas and features'; interior, more easily altered furnishings, colour schemes and design decisions can be found under 'hospital buildings'. All hospitals can be found under 'hospitals and institutions', with those located outside Britain identified in parenthesis. While it is best practice to allow no more than eight page numbers or ranges for each heading (excluding those that denote images), exceptions have been made here for the sake of completeness, most noticeably in relation to some of journals, periodicals and newspapers mentioned.

EU authorised representative for GPSR:
Easy Access System Europe, Mustamäe tee 50,
10621 Tallinn, Estonia
gpsr.requests@easproject.com

www.ingramcontent.com/pod-product-compliance
Ingram Content Group UK Ltd.
Pitfield, Milton Keynes, MK11 3LW, UK
UKHW062008040626
6253IPUK00010B/56

* 9 7 8 1 5 2 6 1 6 8 5 1 1 *